Handbook of Nursing Case Management

Health Care Delivery in a World of Managed Care

Dominick L. Flarey, PhD, MBA, RN,CS, CNAA, NP-C
Health Care Management
 Consultant
Higman Health Care, Inc.
St. Petersburg, Florida

Suzanne Smith Blancett, EdD, RN, FAAN
Editor-in-Chief
Journal of Nursing Administration and *Nurse Educator*
Philadelphia, Pennsylvania

AN ASPEN PUBLICATION®
Aspen Publishers, Inc.
Gaithersburg, Maryland
1996

Library of Congress Cataloging-in-Publication Data

Handbook of nursing case management : health care delivery in a world
of managed care / [edited by] Dominick L. Flarey, Suzanne Smith
Blancett.
p. cm.
Companion v. to: Case studies in nursing case management.
Includes bibliographical references and index.
ISBN 0-8342-0790-7
1. Nursing care plans—Handbooks, manuals, etc. 2. Nursing-
-Effect of managed care on—Handbooks, manuals, etc. 3. Hospitals-
-Case management services—Handbooks, manuals, etc. I. Flarey,
Dominick L. II. Blancett, Suzanne Smith. III. Case studies in
nursing case management.
[DNLM: 1. Nursing Process—organization & administration.
2. Managed Care Programs. 3. Economics, Nursing. WY 100 H2359 1996]
RT49.H36 1996
362.1'73'068—dc20
DNLM/DLC
for Library of Congress
95-50683
CIP

Orders: (800) 638-8437
Customer Service: (800) 234-1660

About Aspen Publishers • For more than 35 years, Aspen has been a leading professional publisher in
a variety of disciplines. Aspen's vast information resources are available in both print and electronic
formats. We are committed to providing the highest quality information available in the most appropriate format for our customers. Visit Aspen's Internet site for more information resources, directories,
articles, and a searchable version of Aspen's full catalog, including the most recent publications:
http://www.aspenpub.com
Aspen Publishers, Inc. • The hallmark of quality in publishing
Member of the worldwide Wolters Kluwer group.

Editorial Resources: Ruth Bloom

Library of Congress Catalog Card Number: 95-50683
ISBN: 0-8342-0790-7

Printed in the United States of America

2 3 4 5

Table of Contents

Contributors xi
Foreword xv
Preface xvii

**1—Case Management: Delivering Care in the Age of
Managed Care** **1**
Dominick L. Flarey and Suzanne Smith Blancett

    Managed Care and Case Management 2
    Case Management 4
    Characteristics of Case Management Systems 6
    On the Horizon 13
    Conclusion 14
    Appendix 1-A. Critical Path Maps 16

**2—The Early Years: The Evolution of Nursing
Case Management** **23**
Karen Zander

    Nursing as the Industry Catalyst 24
    From Case Management Plans to CareMap®
       Medical Record 27
    Skipping Steps, Losing Theory Base as Application
       Expands 35
    Outcome-Based Critical Paths as Core 35
    Nursing Case Management: A Classic 38
    Conclusion 41

3—New Challenges and Opportunities in Integrated Health Care Systems **46**
Joanne Ritter-Teitel

Driving Forces behind Integrated Health Care Systems   47
Definitions   49
Dimensions   50
Surrogate Terms   54
Attributes of Integrated Health Care Systems   55
Forerunner Hospital Systems   59
Model Systems   60
Organizational Outcomes   61
Challenges and Opportunities for Nurse Executives   63
Conclusion   65

4—Developing a Successful Hospital Case Management System **68**
David Bach, Carolyn Hope Smeltzer, and Allen J. Baler

History   68
Requirements for Effective Hospital Case Management   69
Creating an Effective Case Management Program   75
Conclusion   78

5—Developing and Implementing Critical Paths in Case Management **80**
Magdalena A. Mateo, Cheryl L. Newton, and Karen K. Kanatas

Definition and Uses of Critical Paths   80
Developing Critical Paths   82
Implementation of Critical Paths   85
Issues in the Use of Critical Paths   86
Evaluation   88
Conclusion   88
Appendix 5-A. Sample Critical Pathways   91

6—Documentation To Achieve Patient Outcomes through Critical Pathways **100**
Pamela E. Windle and Susan Houston

Case Management/Outcomes Management   100
Benefits   103

Desirable Patient Outcomes 104
Critical Pathways 104
Collaboration. 109
Conclusion 110
Appendix 6-A. Critical Pathways and Examples of
  Reporting Tools 112

7—Outcomes Assessment through Protocols **136**
Nancy Shendell-Falik and Katherine B. Soriano

Protocol Overview 137
Protocol Development and Implementation 138
Variance Analysis 141
Outcomes 142
Conclusion 145
Appendix 7-A. Examples of Protocols and Documentation
  Records 148

8—Improving Quality through Nursing Case Management . . . **170**
*Ann Scott Blouin, Jodi A. Lewis, Nancy A. Malone, and
  Katherine E. Metz*

Quality of Care: Growing Interest in a Changing
  Environment 170
Quality Defined 171
Care Giver versus Patient Perceptions of Quality 173
The Cost/Quality Relationship 174
The Role of Case Management 175
Evidence in the Literature. 177
The Role of Leadership. 179
Conclusion 181

**9—Evaluating the Effectiveness of Case
  Management Plans** **184**
Hussein A. Tahan and Toni G. Cesta

Variance Analysis 185
Expected Outcomes of Care. 187
Outcomes Management 188
Conclusion 191

10—Variance Analysis **194**
Barbara Barth Frink and Larry Strassner

Strategic Initiatives of the Organization: Managed Care 195
Variance Analysis 200
Information Management of Critical Path Data 206
Conclusion 220

**11—Improving Accreditation Results through
Case Management** **224**
Diane B. Williams

The Joint Commission on Accreditation of Healthcare
    Organizations 226
The National Committee for Quality Assurance 233
Conclusion 238

12—Strategies for Operationalizing Case Management **239**
Magdalena A. Mateo, Cheryl L. Newton, and Barbara H. Warner

Laying the Groundwork 239
Implementation Process 244
Evaluation of Outcomes 248
Issues and Strategies Related to the Case Manager Role 250
Conclusion 251

13—Training and Education Needs of Case Managers **254**
Hussein A. Tahan

Length of the Curriculum 255
Defining a Knowledge Base for the Curriculum 255
Delineating the Goals and Objectives of the Curriculum 256
Curriculum Outline 257
Preceptorship Program 265
Performance Evaluation of Case Managers 266
Conclusion 270

**14—Roles of the Professional Registered Nurse in
Case Management and Program Direction** **272**
*Donna McNeese-Smith, Gail Anderson, Cheryl Misseldine,
    and Gabriele Meneghini*

Roles of the Case Manager 273
Roles of the Case Management Director 284

Education of the RN Case Manager   291
Graduate Programs for Case Manager Preparation   292
Certification/Case Management Associations   292
Conclusion   293

15—Alternate Case Management Models   295
Karen A. Clark

Private Case Management   296
Social/Community-Based Case Management   298
Primary Care Case Management   301
Vendor/Gatekeeper Model of Case Management   301
Conclusion   302

**16—Relationship Building in Developing the Continuum of
Care Concepts 305**
Rhonda M. Anderson

Relationship Building   308
Consumer Relationships   308
Team Relationships   309
Payer Relationships   310
Continuum of Care Provider Relationships   310

17—Physician/Nurse Collaboration in Case Management   315
*Rella A. Adams, Pam M. Warner, Eric G. Six,
and Ben M. McKibbens*

Collaboration: A Concept Analysis   316
Model of Clinical Collaboration   316
Physician/Nurse Liaison Committee   318
From Managed Care to Case Management   319
Collaboration in Case Management   320
Development of Restorative Care Paths   323
Conclusion   328
Appendix 17-A. Stroke Protocol   329

18—Managed Care and the World of Capitated Payment   336
Leanne M. Hunstock

Evolution of Managed Care and the Capitated
Payment System   336
Evolution of Integration   338

Stages of Market Evolution 339
Success Factors in the World of Capitated Payment 342
Using Case Managment Effectively To Manage
   Clinical Resources. 343
Model for Integration, Capitation, and
   Successful Outcomes 345
Conclusion 346

19—Working with Managed Care Networks:
Strategies for Success. 348
Marilyn D. Harris and Sharon A. Lynch

Managed Care versus Case Management 348
Advantages and Disadvantages of Contracting with
   Managed Care Companies. 350
Role of the Home Care Clinical Case Manager versus
   Payer Case Manager 351
Strategies for Cultivating a Successful Relationship 352
Quality Assessment/Performance Improvement
   (QA/PI) Issues 355
Conclusion 360

20—Cost Savings and Financial Analysis of Case Management
Models 362
Sandra Pelfrey and Mary Lou Wesley

Standards 363
First Critical Pathway 366
Patient Care Project Team 367
Creating the First Critical Pathway 367
Evaluating Critical Pathway Results 369
Variance Analysis 372
Potential Variance Analysis Models 373
Data Retrieval 375
Maximizing Reimbursement. 376
Conclusion 378

21—Data Management through Information Systems 379
Catherine Noone and Cathy A.R. McKillip

Increased Need for Access to Information 379
System Readiness. 380
Consumer Impact 382

Benefits of Data Management through Information
    Systems   383
Impact on Nursing Management   384
Steps in Planning and Implementing an Information
    System   385
Conclusion   386

**22—Case Management As a Service Economy Job Design:
    Toward a Theoretical Model** **388**
Mary Crabtree Tonges

Job Design for a Service Economy   389
Job Design Theory and Research   393
Theoretical Extensions: Situational Constructs   406
Theoretical Extensions: Dispositional Differences   410
Theoretical Model: Antecedent Conditions Related to
    Nurses' Satisfaction and Performance   413
Research Opportunities and Needs   417

23—Legal Liabilities in Case Managment **424**
Deborah J. Nichols

Professional Responsibility   426
Standards of Practice   427
Patient Confidentiality   429
Malpractice/Negligence   431
Benefit Decision Making versus Case Management   432
Negligent Referral   436
Abandonment and Patient Discharge   437
Vicarious Liability   438
Interference with Physican-Patient Relationship   439
Incompetence, Malpractice, Misconduct, and Reporting   439
Contracting   440
Conclusion   440

24—Ethical Issues in Case Management **443**
Winifred J. Ellenchild Pinch

Advocacy   444
Justice   446
Functioning at the Interface of Advocacy and Justice   448
Ethical Issues   450

Ethical Decision Making   456
Conclusion   457

Epilogue—Case Management: The Shape of Things
       To Come **461**
Suzanne Smith Blancett and Dominick L. Flarey

Continuity of Care   461
Patient Issues   462
Reimbursement Systems   463
Evolving Goals   463
Evolving Roles   464
Conclusion   465

Appendix A—Discussion Topics for Each Chapter **466**

Index **475**

Contributors

Rella A. Adams, PhD, RN, CNAA
Senior Vice President, Nursing
Valley Baptist Medical Center
Harlingen, Texas

Gail Anderson, MN, RN, CPHQ
Director, Case Management
Glendale Adventist Medical Center
Glendale, California

Rhonda M. Anderson, MPA, RN, CNAA, FAAN
Executive Vice President
Hartford Hospital
Hartford, Connecticut

David Bach, MD
Senior Associate
APM, Inc.
New York, New York

Allen J. Baler, BA
Research Associate
APM, Inc.
New York, New York

Suzanne Smith Blancett, EdD, RN, FAAN
Editor-in-Chief
Journal of Nursing Administration
Philadelphia, Pennsylvania
Editor-in-Chief
Nurse Educator
Philadelphia, Pennsylvania

Ann Scott Blouin, PhD, RN
Senior Manager
Ernst & Young, LLP
Chicago, Illinois

Toni G. Cesta, PhD, RN
Director of Case Management and
    Case Management Consultant
Long Island College Hospital
Brooklyn, New York

Karen A. Clark, MS, RN
Clinical Nurse Specialist, Intensive
    Care
Sarasota Memorial Hospital
Sarasota, Florida

Dominick L. Flarey, PhD, MBA, RN,CS, CNAA, NP-C
President
Health Care Seminars, Inc.
Niles, Ohio
Vice President and Administrator
Primary Health Care Group, Inc.
Niles, Ohio

Barbara Barth Frink, PhD, RN, FAAN
Director of Nursing Systems and Research
The Johns Hopkins Hospital
Baltimore, Maryland

Marilyn D. Harris, MSN, RN, CNAA, FAAN
Executive Director
Visiting Nurse Association of Eastern Montgomery County/
A Department of Abington Memorial Hospital
Willow Grove, Pennsylvania

Susan Houston, PhD, RN
Director, Outcomes Measurement and Research
St. Luke's Episcopal Hospital
Houston, Texas

Leanne M. Hunstock, MBA, MEd, RN, CS, CNAA
Patient Care Executive Consultant
APM, Inc.
San Francisco, California

Karen K. Kanatas, BSN, RN
Staff Nurse III
Department of Critical Care Nursing
The Ohio State University Medical Center
Columbus, Ohio

Jodi A. Lewis, MS, MBA, RN
Senior Consultant
Ernst & Young LLP
Milwaukee, Wisconsin

Sharon A. Lynch, MSN, RN
Clinical Supervisor
Visiting Nurse Association of Eastern Montgomery County/
A Department of Abington Memorial Hospital
Willow Grove, Pennsylvania

Nancy A. Malone, MBA, MPH, RN
Manager
Ernst & Young LLP
Chicago, Illinois

Magdalena A. Mateo, PhD, RN, FAAN
Research Associate
Department of Physical Medicine and Rehabilitation
The Ohio State University Medical Center
Clinical Assistant Professor
College of Nursing
The Ohio State University
Columbus, Ohio

Ben M. McKibbens, MHA, FACHE
President and Chief Executive Officer
Valley Baptist Medical Center
Harlingen, Texas

Cathy A.R. McKillip, MPA, BA
Operations Manager
In-Home Health Services
An Affiliate of Newton Memorial Hospital
Sparta, New Jersey

Donna McNeese-Smith, EdD, RN
Assistant Professor and Coordinator
Nursing Administration Graduate
  Program
UCLA School of Nursing
Los Angeles, California

Gabriele Meneghini, MN, RN
Case Manager
Community Health Plan
Los Angeles Department of Health
  Services
Long Beach, California

Katherine E. Metz, MBA, RN
Manager
Ernst & Young LLP
Chicago, Illinois

Cheryl Misseldine, BSN, RN
Lead Case Manager
USC University Hospital
Los Angeles, California

**Cheryl L. Newton, MSN, RN,
  CCRN, CNRN**
Director, Continuous Quality
  Improvement/Education
American Transitional Hospital
Columbus, Ohio

Deborah J. Nichols, JD, MBA, RN
Oklahoma City, Oklahoma

**Catherine Noone, MS, BSN, RN,
  CNA**
Administrator
In-Home Health Services
An Affiliate of Newton Memorial
  Hospital
Sparta, New Jersey

Sandra Pelfrey, MBA, CPA
Associate Professor, Accounting
School of Business Administration
Oakland University
Rochester, Michigan

**Winifred J. Ellenchild Pinch, EdD,
  RN**
Professor
School of Nursing and Center for
  Health Policy and Ethics
Creighton University
Omaha, Nebraska

Joanne Ritter-Teitel, MA, RN
Doctoral Candidate
School of Nursing
Center for Health Services and
  Policy Research
University of Pennsylvania
Philadelphia, Pennsylvania

Nancy Shendell-Falik, MA, RN
Assistant Vice President, Nursing
Robert Wood Johnson University
  Hospital
New Brunswick, New Jersey

Eric G. Six, MD, FACS, ABQAURP
Medical Director
Staff Neurosurgeon
Valley Baptist Medical Center
Harlingen, Texas

**Carolyn Hope Smeltzer, EdD,
  MSN, RN, FAAN, FACHE**
Principal
APM Management Consultants
Chicago, Illinois

Katherine B. Soriano, MS, RNC
Head Nurse
Pediatric and Adolescent Units
Robert Wood Johnson University
  Hospital
New Brunswick, New Jersey

Larry Strassner, MS, RN, CNA
Director of Critical Paths
The Johns Hopkins Hospital
Baltimore, Maryland

Hussein A. Tahan, MS, RN, CNA
Clinical Nurse Manager
Cardiac Care Center
Mount Sinai Medical Center
New York, New York

**Mary Crabtree Tonges, MBA,
  MSN, RN**
Consultant
The Center for Case Management,
  Inc.
South Natick, Massachusetts
Doctoral Candidate, Organization
  and Policy Studies
Baruch College
New York, New York

Barbara H. Warner, MS, RN
Director, Department of Psychiatric/
  Rehabilitation Nursing
The Ohio State University Medical
  Center
Columbus, Ohio

Pam M. Warner, RN, CPHQ
Administrative Director
Valley Baptist Medical Center
Harlingen, Texas

Mary Lou Wesley, MSN, RN
Visiting Faculty Consultant
School of Nursing
St. Joseph Memorial Hospital
Rochester, Michigan

Diane B. Williams, MSHA, BSN
Consultant
T.P. Williams and Associates, Inc.
Portland, Oregon

**Pamela E. Windle, MS, RN, CNA,
  CPAN, CAPA**
Nurse Manager
Day Surgery/Post Anesthesia Care
  Unit
SLMT Ambulatory Preop and
  Recovery Room
St. Luke's Episcopal Hospital
Houston, Texas

Karen Zander, MS, RN, CS
Principal and Co-owner
The Center for Case Management,
  Inc.
South Natick, Massachusetts

Foreword

Ten years ago, a graduate student asked me how she should respond to a professor who questioned the student's plan to write a paper about case management. The professor believed case management had "nothing to do with nursing." Ah . . . where to start?

As this book illustrates, case management by any definition is "a natural" for nursing. Some may even say that provider-controlled, clinical case management *is* nursing because it demands a total and effective integration of every skill a nurse has used in working with many people to meet patients' needs.

In addition, case management is a natural for the current state and predicted future of the health care industry. At its most immediate level, case managers facilitate the services of all disciplines so that they are delivered in a timely fashion and at the lowest cost to produce the desired results (*e.g.*, the use of a pulse oximeter rather than an arterial blood gas analysis). Case managers strive to keep a patient's length of stay within reimbursable limits. They also expedite smooth transfers and discharge planning wherever possible, thereby not only helping the patient but also securing the financial well-being of the agency and physicians in a managed care reimbursement system.

As managed care evolves into capitated contracts, case management models that cover "at-risk" populations living in the community will become increasingly needed to control resources. Although these case management services will not be cheap, they will prevent more expensive interventions because the case managers will assist clients in maintaining their highest level of wellness.

By definition, case management is a strategy used to create a complete loop or network of services for a predefined population of patients. Case management is a model designed specifically to cut across formal hierarchies and departments to produce a matrix of services at or near the direct care level. Case management differs from traditional management because a case manager oversees processes rather than people.

As you will read, case managers are evaluated on their success in achieving measurable clinical and financial outcomes. They may use clinical pathways as tools to assist the management of processes. Negotiation skills, however, are what they use the most as they strive to identify, expedite, and evaluate care. Because they work in and between complex organizations brimming with experts of every imaginable variety, their authority base must be constantly earned rather than given.

As you will deduce, case managers cannot conduct their enormous responsibilities alone. The most successful case managers are seen as expediters, greasing the wheel of health care bureaucracies and payer formulas to conduct as smooth, effective, and efficient an episode (course) of care for a person as possible. They are not police of clinical path compliance, physician practice, or the status quo. Their job is often to make something out of nothing—structure out of confusion and cooperation out of diverse agendas and personalities.

In ten years, the simple notion that an entire episode of care for patients, moving across units and time, could be better managed than traditional plans, physician orders, and assignment patterns could offer has hit a responsive nerve. Nurses have begun the reorganization required to provide the infamous seamless system for disease and/or wellness management.

Enjoy reading how nurses are using clinical paths, unit-based care coordination, and agency or community-based case management as powerful methods to help their patients, organizations, and themselves adapt and even conquer new rules, regulations, and financial realities. From the lessons learned here, you too can create a caring and care-giving nursing infrastructure that will become the heart of the managed care world.

Karen Zander, MS, RN, CS
Principal
The Center for Case Management
South Natick, Massachusetts

Preface

Since the early 1980s, our health care delivery system has been undergoing radical changes, and the journey is far from over. What is impressive is that with each major transition in health care reform, the professions of nursing and other health care disciplines have emerged more powerful, more professional, and more important to the delivery of quality, cost-effective care. As front line providers of care, nurses had the most to lose and everything to gain. It is at this time that nursing is reaping the rewards of its efforts.

As we look back over the past ten years of change, we have witnessed many health care agendas, fads, and "quick fixes" come and go. Many were discarded because they simply did not do what the theorists promised. We experienced the same phenomenon in the redesign of delivery systems and models of care. Newer models and systems were being designed so rapidly that it was impossible to keep pace with what was happening in our profession.

Only one model of care delivery has withstood the test of time—case management. The model is not new; it was implemented by Karen Zander and her colleagues as early as the mid-1980s. What is amazing is that the answer to the delivery of cost-effective quality care has been staring us in the face for so many years and we failed to realize it until recently. It required an intense, chaotic, and painstaking journey to bring us to the point of this realization today. Our journey is very similar to that of Dorothy in the wonderful story, *The Wizard of Oz.* Although Dorothy always possessed the power to return to Kansas, she had to learn this for herself by journeying through the Land of Oz.

So, too, our journey for the best delivery system of care has come to an end. Case management is here to stay. However, we are now embarking on a new journey. We must develop the case management system of care continually to meet the demands of the ever-changing environment in which we live and practice. We see this new journey as the beginning of another milestone for nursing and other health care disciplines. One can only imagine what will come to pass in the next century because of our efforts to continue the evolution of case management.

Because we are now entering another new era in health care, we thought it essential to produce a comprehensive work on case management. We believed that there was a great need for a foundational reference and resource that highlights the evolution of case management to the present time. With this book, we hoped to provide a solid foundation that will be used to develop further the world of case management in the years to come as this dynamic system for managing care delivery continues to evolve.

We use the phrase *world of case management* because that is what it is. As we began this book project and really explored case management, we discovered so much essential material that needed to be made available. As a result, this project is published in two volumes, which are companions to each other. This volume presents theories, methodologies, and concepts related to case management as a delivery system of care. The companion volume, *Case Studies in Nursing Case Management: Health Care Delivery in a World of Managed Care,* presents the operationalization of the material presented in this book. The case studies provide the real-life experience complement to this material.

One of our goals for this project was to develop a comprehensive work that would be a classic in the foundation for the future transformation of case management. To achieve this goal, we brought together the finest people in the field today to share their knowledge and expertise. Each of them worked very hard to bring this project to completion. We extend our sincere thanks to them for their dedication and commitment. We believe they are the current and future experts in the world of case management.

As this project came to a close, we realized the overwhelming contribution that nursing has made and is continuing to make to our nation's health care delivery system. We hope that readers of this book and its companion will experience this same intense sense of nursing accomplishment and pride. We also hope that these books will provide you with the knowledge and skills necessary to continue the development of case management as nursing's model of care.

For a project such as this to come to fruition required the intense support of many behind-the-scenes people. The support and encouragement we received was overwhelming. We especially thank the staff at Aspen Publishers who worked hard to make our lives a little less hectic over the past year. Our thanks and love to our families who encouraged us daily to pursue our goals.

And a sincere thanks to our friends and colleagues who so earnestly support the continued development of nursing. This book is dedicated to all case managers—past, present, and future. It is their hard work and efforts that drive the delivery of quality health care in our nation everyday.

Dominick L. Flarey, PhD, MBA, RN,CS, CNAA, NP-C
Suzanne Smith Blancett, EdD, RN, FAAN

■ 1 ■

Case Management: Delivering Care in the Age of Managed Care

Dominick L. Flarey, PhD, MBA, RN,CS, CNAA, NP-C
Suzanne Smith Blancett, EdD, RN, FAAN

> Although no one model has proven to be a panacea for health care institutions, health care delivery models projected to be the most successful in the future are those that incorporate clinical and economical case management into operational redesign.
> —W. Crawley, *Health Care Supervisor*

The dramatic change in our system of health care delivery has been realized. But it is useless to speak of change—health care *is transformed.* Our challenge today is to make the change work through innovative delivery systems offering high-quality care at an affordable price. Over the past decade, we have witnessed care delivery systems come and go. We have redesigned, restructured, downsized, up-sized, right-sized, and created new entities that we cannot manage. Throughout this period of reform, only one delivery system withstood the test of time—case management. The popularity of case management grows daily. Everyone is either implementing it or investigating its potential. Could it be that case management is the delivery system that will meet health care reform objectives well into the next century? We believe the answer is an emphatic *yes!*

This chapter provides an introductory look into the concept of case management as the most definitive delivery system in health care. It paves the way for the sequential presentation of the major concepts and issues related to case management in the following chapters. This chapter also provides the foundational elements for fully understanding the operationalization of case management presented in the companion volume, *Case Studies in Nursing Case Management: Health Care Delivery in a World of Managed Care.*[1]

MANAGED CARE AND CASE MANAGEMENT

We now live in a world of managed care. At least 56 million people in the United States receive health care today in a health maintenance organization (HMO).[2] The number of preferred provider organizations, point-of-service plans, and physician networks is increasing at a rapid rate. The real drivers of health care reform are our nation's employers. It was their demands to cut health care costs and reduce spending that led to the need to manage care formally.[3]

In response to employer demands, the aim of most health care reform bills has been the encouragement of people to join managed care networks. It is no secret that managed care is the structure that drives costs and spending down. Managed care has been conceptualized in many ways. It is basically an organized brokerage of health care services for specific groups of the population with an emphasis on quality of care and controlled costs. One study showed that if the entire U.S. population in 1990 had been receiving care via an HMO, we would have spent 12.2 percent less on health care.[3]

Such study outcomes create compelling reasons for encouraging more people to join managed care plans and networks. As managed care models increase, case management will be the preferred delivery system to meet reform's challenges. Bartling[2] identified seven major trends that will shape managed care. These trends will be instrumental in shaping case management systems in the near future. The seven trends are:

1. *Capitation:* This evolving system of reimbursement and managed care provides for a more coordinated, more efficient team-based approach to care delivery. The major focus is on the efficient and effective management of resources. With capitation, providers receive a fixed amount of reimbursement per enrollee. Providers receive this fixed amount regardless of services provided. It is through case management that quality care will be delivered under a capitated system.

2. *Information systems:* These systems will flourish; the delivery of care will be data base intensive and driven. These systems will ensure appropriate management and integration of all care delivery. This is happening to meet the need to move more quickly and efficiently when dealing with complex, multisystem information. Information systems will fully support the operations of case management models.

3. *Physician control:* These providers must and will provide the degree of leadership necessary to be successful in the world of managed care. They must and will play major roles in the development and implementation of case management models and systems. Although nurses are

the driving force behind case management systems, physician support and leadership are needed to ensure commitment to the model.

4. *Medicare/Medicaid increases:* To save money, states are requiring that greater percentages of their Medicaid recipients be in managed care plans or networks. The same is true for the federal government and Medicare recipients. Because each group presents its own unique health care needs, case management systems will be modified and redesigned to address this trend.

5. *Carve-outs:* Managed care organizations will escalate their practice of subcontracting for various health care services. Nurse case managers practicing in case management models will be in great demand as subcontractors of health care delivery. This trend will foster the rapid development of entrepreneurial nurse case managers and move the nursing profession to the forefront of point-of-service care.

6. *Insurance company ownership:* These entities will own their own networks. They will use case management systems and nurse case managers to drive the efficient and cost-effective delivery of care. Nurse case managers will play significant roles in insurance-owned groups.

7. *Increased decentralization:* Managed care organizations will seek out relationships and models that move them closer to patients. Case management is the ideal model to realize this goal.

We are already seeing these trends emerge in what is now known as integrated delivery systems. These systems operate in response to managed care initiatives.

> A fully integrated delivery system is one that unites a financing group with all providers—from hospitals, clinics, and physicians to home care and long-term care facilities to pharmacies. The system is built on a foundation of primary care, and all facets of it operate under capitation, so everyone involved shares risk.[4(p.8)]

We are fast approaching the time when integrated delivery systems will be the predominant infrastructure of our health care system. This infrastructure will be supported and driven by case management models and systems. A recent survey of health care leaders from across the country revealed that 71 percent of their organizations belong to or are in the process of organizing an integrated delivery system. In the same sample, 81 percent said that their health care organization would not operate as a stand-alone in five years.[4]

CASE MANAGEMENT

It is beyond the scope of this particular chapter to define in detail the concept of case management. The entire book and its companion[1] serve that overall objective. Instead, basic elements inherent to any and all case management models are presented.

To begin to understand case management, examination of a few universal definitions that have shaped its development is necessary. Zander[5] tells us that the origination of case management in the mid-1980s was for the purpose of lending structure to health care delivery where it was sorely lacking. The model developed by Zander and her colleagues was the first initiation of case management in acute care settings, a needed response to the initiation of a prospective payment system. Since this inception, case management as a system of care delivery has evolved significantly. Today, two reputable definitions of case management are available. The first is supported by the American Nurses Association (ANA):

> Case management has at its heart a systematic approach to care. The American Nurses Association defines the goals of case management as providing quality health care along a continuum, decreasing fragmentation of care across many settings, enhancing the client's quality of life, and cost containment. The framework for nursing case management includes five components: assessing, planning, implementing, evaluating, and interacting.[6]

This description by the ANA focuses heavily on the nursing process as the foundation for nursing case management. It includes the important element and added dimension of collaboration into the case management definition. Through case management, nursing is in the vanguard of encouraging collaboration when delivering health care services. Recently, other professional associations have focused on the concept of collaboration in care delivery, which nursing has owned for some time. "Collaboration is the cornerstone of the Agenda for Change set forth by the Joint Commission on Accreditation of Healthcare Organizations and the basis for continuous, systematic, and organization-wide improvement in performance standards and patient care outcomes."[7] The Joint Commission's position on collaboration likewise provides support for the use of case management as the delivery system of health care today. The National Case Management Task Force definition of case management also focuses on the collaborative nature of this system of care delivery:

> Case management is a collaborative process which assesses, plans, implements, coordinates, monitors, and evaluates the options and services to meet an individual's health needs, using communication and available resources to promote quality, cost-effective outcomes.[8(p.9)]

The goals of case management flow from the working definitions. Many goals have been defined for case management. The following are the major goals for any case management model today.

1. *Quality of care:*[9–11] Case management has its roots in a strong focus on the quality of health care delivery. Services must be therapeutic and beneficial to the population being managed. Quality outcomes must be identified and interventions planned to meet them. Outcomes must demonstrate that care delivery through case management has had a therapeutic effect on the client's condition, problems, and needs.

2. *Length of stay:*[10,11] Inherent in the concept of case management as a cost-control mechanism is a focus on reducing the inpatient length of stay. The system is designed to move patients rapidly through the care process while maintaining quality of care. Timeliness of the process becomes paramount. This is also achieved by reengineering systems and processes to support the efficiency of the case management model. Studies show that the best-run hospitals have reduced their length of stay to one-half the national average.[3] Thus, length of stay is correlated to systems' efficiency.

3. *Resource utilization:*[10] Case management reduces and controls resource utilization. This is achieved by protocols that guide care delivery based on research and the evaluation of patient outcomes. Protocols define a plan of care that is careful to avoid inappropriate resource utilization. This is a hallmark goal of case management.

4. *Continuity:*[9] Case management provides continuity of care during each episode of delivery. Models are designed to provide clients with a full range of services by familiar professionals. Continuity evokes client ownership and collaboration of services received. Case management also focuses on the entire episode of illness.[10] This concept of continuity also merges nicely with the collaborative approach inherent in case management systems.

5. *Cost control:*[9] A most important goal in this era of capitation, case management achieves reduction of costs and decreased spending through the interface of the previously stated goals. In this way, cost control becomes the primary outcome of the system.

Defining the goals of case management is important as they in turn become the definite measure for evaluating case management systems. When developing and designing any case management system, it is imperative that these major goals be defined and supported by everyone. The operationalized goals provide a road map for the construction of a case management system and lead to the development of its major objective: the coordination of care and services for patients and families requiring extensive interventions.[10] Other goals of case management include staff satisfaction, job satisfaction, patient/family satisfaction, learning, wellness, and prevention.

CHARACTERISTICS OF CASE MANAGEMENT SYSTEMS

Case management as a system of care delivery has proved itself over time. Positive outcomes using many variations of case management models are well documented.[12–22] This book and its companion[1] present the latest documentation of outcomes and successes through case management. Throughout the evolution of case management model design, there have been consistent elements and characteristics, which continue today in model development. These characteristics are important to define and clarify as they are the building blocks of most case management models. The presentation of consistent characteristics provides us with the framework necessary to design a case management system today. The ten major characteristics of most case management models are as follows.

1. *Nurse driven:* Case management development and use in health care settings was largely the result of a nursing effort. Nurses have always been the managers of care. The complexity of a case management system of care requires the knowledge and skills of professional registered nurses. They are the only professionals involved in the entire episode of care. As such, case management will always be a system managed by nurses. Although technical nursing personnel assist in the delivery of health care services, professional registered nurses, through the nursing process, drive the entire care process and maintain responsibility for achieving quality outcomes. Professional nurses are also well prepared to function as advocates for patients.

2. *Family focused:* In a case management system, the importance of the family or significant others to the patient's recovery becomes a major focus of the overall plan. Case management is designed to include family in all aspects of care and during the episode of illness. Socialization theory provides us with the framework to design case management models so that family participation is included. People do not get sick in isolation, and so healing cannot take place in isolation. Case management systems recognize the position of the patient within his or her family system and use that reality to the maximum benefit of the patient. Case management is designed to bring the patient closer to the family unit during episodes of illness and to draw on their support to assist in recovery. Case management models incorporate family teach-

ing. An in-depth understanding of the illness process and the patient's needs allows the family to provide the needed support, and often resources, that the patient needs to recover from illness or disease. Case management as a vehicle of care delivery also focuses on care of the family during a member's illness. Health care professionals view the patient and family as a unit in need of services.

3. *Protocols:* Medical, nursing, and treatment protocols are one of the evolutionary hallmarks of a case management system. Although many terms have been used to define them, their objectives and goals are all similar. To appreciate fully their integral role in case management, it is necessary to clarify the concepts through a sound definition:

> Clinical guidelines are the distillation of the best collective thinking from literature, practicing physicians and academic experts on how to treat a particular medical situation. Guidelines (also called practice parameters and protocols) are targeted to physician intervention, while critical pathways and CareMaps® pertain to the patient care activities of entire multidisciplinary teams.[23(p.70)]

Exhibit 1-1 presents the current consensus on the definitions for the various types of protocols used in case management systems. It is essential when designing case management systems that we use a uniform nomenclature for protocols. As case management becomes the dominant delivery model, confusion over protocol terms must be eliminated. Exhibit 1-A-1 (in Appendix 1-A) presents a sample critical path focusing on medical and nursing interventions for a patient with congestive heart failure. Exhibit 1-A-2, a sample of a CareMap® for congestive heart failure, focuses on patient and family outcomes. Exhibit 1-A-3 presents a revised CareMap® for congestive heart failure in which the concepts of a critical path are incorporated into one comprehensive protocol. This type of comprehensive protocol is preferred as it supports the collaborative and multidisciplinary nature of case management systems.

Both the critical path and the CareMap® are essential protocols for managing the entire process and episode of patient care. Each protocol complements and is synergistic with others in moving the patient along the entire continuum of care.

The importance of protocols and guidelines in case management systems cannot be stressed enough. They are, in actuality, the multidisciplinary teams' written map to achieving the goals of case management as previously discussed. In concert with these defined goals, the benefits of using protocols and guidelines are:[23]

Exhibit 1-1 Nomenclature for Case Management Guidelines and Protocols

CLINICAL PRACTICE GUIDELINES: The National Academy of Sciences' Institute of Medicine, Washington, D.C., adopted this term to refer to standards developed to assist practitioner and patient decisions about appropriate care in specific clinical circumstances.*

PRACTICE PARAMETERS: The American Medical Association refers to them as educational tools that enable physicians to obtain the advice of recognized clinical experts, stay abreast of the latest clinical research, and assess the clinical significance of often conflicting research findings.*

CLINICAL PATHWAYS/CRITICAL PATHS: These are clinical management tools that organize, sequence, and time the major interventions of nursing staff, physicians, and other departments for a particular case type, subset, or condition.**

CAREMAPS®: These are more elaborate critical pathways that show the relationship of sets of interventions to sets of intermediate outcomes along a time line. They merge standards of care with standards of practice in a cause-and-effect relationship across time.**

Data from: *Clinical Paths: Tools for Outcomes Management, American Hospital Publishing, Inc., 1994.
**Center for Case Management, Inc., 1994.
Source: Reprinted from *Hospitals & Health Networks,* Vol. 68, No. 20, by permission, October 20, 1994, Copyright 1994, American Hospital Publishing, Inc.

- They provide increased efficiency in the delivery of health care.
- They improve decision making by health care professionals, as well as assist in improved decision making by patients and families.
- They reduce costly variations in practice, both medicine and nursing.
- They eliminate inappropriate procedures.
- They rationalize approaches to care.

Because of the intense benefit of protocols to the delivery of health care, in 1989 the federal government, through the Department of Health and Human Services, funded the Agency for Health Care Policy and Research[23] to develop expert, comprehensive protocols for uniform care delivery. These protocols are available from the department and should be reviewed and incorporated into the design for use in case management models.

To date, most protocols have been developed around acute care problems, especially related to high-cost diagnosis-related groups (DRGs). Such an initiative was appropriate at the time as hospital costs traditionally make up 40 percent of all medical spending.[3] Today, however, protocols are being developed and implemented in all types of case management settings, including physicians' offices. This is occurring as the experienced benefit of protocols goes far beyond cost savings.

Once protocols are in place, the health care team must continually evaluate their effectiveness in practice. Revisions must be ongoing and based on evaluations as well as current published literature. Protocols must be considered tools that are always evolving in the case management system. When developing and/or revising protocols, three crucial questions must be answered:

> a. What is the work required to get patients with certain case types to desired outcomes?
> b. What is the best way to produce these outcomes?
> c. Who is accountable for the results?[24]

Answering these questions helps ensure the development of sound protocols that will assist in achieving the goals of the case management system.

4. *Outcome driven:* To be effective, all case management systems must be outcome driven. They must be designed to move the patient through the process of care delivery toward the attainment of defined outcomes. Outcomes must be clearly defined and measurable. They must also be communicated to the entire health care team, as well as to the patient and family. An outcome-driven model will assist in the continued development and revisions of protocols and guidelines. Guidelines can then be defined to lead the patient to the achievement of outcomes.

Outcomes for the entire case management system must also be defined and agreed on by all disciplines involved. This is essential to the maintenance of the system. These outcomes are also useful in the overall evolutionary process of the case management system and guide needed revisions in the system. Exhibit 1-2 presents generic outcomes for most case management models.

5. *Multidisciplinary:* Case management requires case managers and other health professionals to function as multidisciplinary and multiservice integrators.[25] Case management is changing the role of the professional nurse. We have witnessed the implementation of reorganization roles and responsibilities of nurses who are case managers.[11] The role of the nurse case manager continues to evolve. Its core feature is the multidisciplinary direction it has taken. Today, nurse case managers provide leadership for a multispecialty, multidisciplinary staff of professionals and assistants. As the nature of case management is to provide compre-

Exhibit 1-2 Outcomes for a Case Management Model

Cost Effectiveness
The case management model is a cost-effective vehicle for the delivery of health care services. Costs are controlled, spending is reduced, and quality care is provided in a capitated reimbursement system.

Improvement in Health Status
Patients leave the case management system in a healthier state than that in which they entered, or the patient leaves the system with the knowledge, resources, and support needed to care for him- or herself with a chronic disease process.

Social Responsiveness
The entire community becomes involved in the care of the client receiving services through case management. Community resources are used and maximized for the benefit of the patient and family. Community agencies participate in the overall care of the patient.

Patient Knowledge
Patients and families leave the case management system with a good working knowledge of the disease process and health care needs and the strategies and interventions needed to maintain health and prevent relapse.

Collaboration
The case management system facilitates total collaboration in the care of populations. All disciplines are intricately involved in the delivery of services, and each discipline supports the others in the quest for the delivery of quality, cost-effective care.

Psychological Equilibrium
Patients, families, and care givers experience a sense of psychological well-being after experiencing health care delivery through case management. There is acceptance of the disease state and the plan of care.

Responsibility
Patients emerge from the case management system with a good sense of responsibility for their overall health and life style. Patients accept and participate in fiscal responsibilities of their care.

Prevention
Patients have a greater sense of the need for preventive health care practices and begin to incorporate prevention into their daily living. This prevention practice results in healthier people and communities.

Provider Knowledge
Everyone involved with the case management system becomes more knowledgeable of the system's potential and effectiveness. Research of goals and outcomes provides the knowledge needed to redesign the system toward greater efficiency and effectiveness.

Death with Dignity
Patients in the case management system with life-threatening, incurable diseases receive full, multidisciplinary support and experience death with dignity.

hensive, full continuum services to populations, the case manager role has become multidisciplinary.

The case management model itself is designed to be multidisciplinary. All professionals come together for the common good of the patient. This multidisciplinary approach is another hallmark feature of case management systems and has been instrumental in breaking down the barriers to and fragmentation of health care delivery. The actual process of care delivery is defined and designed in a multidisciplinary format with a multidisciplinary approach using written protocols. All care givers are equally important to the patient and the case management system.

6. *Multiservice:* Case management systems provide for a wide array of health care services. One service line is not responsible for the entire delivery of care. Multiple services, rather, come together to provide a comprehensive system of care. Services frequently used in case management models include social services, community services, extended and skilled care services, psychological services, and nutrition services.

A system that does not integrate all available service lines into the case management model is not really a case management system. When services integrate, care delivered is of a greater quality, the episode of care is more rapid, and the outcomes are superior. As such, a case management system should integrate all services into one model.

7. *Brokerage of services:* In line with the multiservice dimension, a case management system provides for brokering services. This role of broker is played by the professional registered nurse. In a case management system, the professional nurse case manager assumes a primary responsibility for ensuring that clients are referred to all available services in the system. He or she advocates for the patient and family for the necessary services.

Brokerage of services is another element and dimension of case management that has rapidly moved professional registered nurses to the forefront of health care delivery in this country. Here nurses have been able to operationalize the concepts of patient advocacy to the fullest. This dimension has empowered professional nurses and allowed them to take the lead in managing and implementing a superior delivery system of care. The role of broker is being designed more and more into the redesign of professional nursing roles. This trend will continue well into the future.

8. *Specialized:* Case management systems have been and will be specialized. They are specialized in the sense that they have come into their own right; they are an art and a science unto themselves. We can witness this

specialization of the case management delivery system by the abounding literature on case management models and outcomes, the creation of a specialty association for case managers, and the more recent process of certification for case managers.

Role development has also molded case management as a specialty. Many organizations have their own internal case management training, education, and development programs. Credentialing for case managers in institutions is fast becoming a norm. Another important feature of the growth of case management as a specialty is the recent emergence of collegiate courses in case management. As the debate continues over educational preparation for nurse case managers, we believe that in the near future, case management will require graduate education to fulfill the most important roles in case management systems. The trend toward specialization in case management will continue to evolve well into the next century.

9. *Continuum of care:* Case management systems do not look at patients or episodes of illness as isolated objects or events. Rather, case management acknowledges that people evolve along a continuum that requires life-long health care services. In line with this philosophy, we are witnessing more disease prevention and wellness counseling incorporated into overall case management systems. We also have an emerging trend of managing critical life points and are focusing on the types of needs that populations have for services.

Case management has been the driving element in the development of integrated delivery systems that offer a full continuum of care. We believe that the continuum of care concept that emerged during the recent push for health care reform originated from concepts inherent in existing case management models. The definitive difference being that an integrated delivery system is actually a very large model of case management. The two concepts mirror each other.

10. *Research based:* The development and design of case management systems are based in research. The structure of a case management model facilitates the incorporation of ongoing research. It is designed so that its elements and its outcomes can be adequately evaluated. This ongoing evaluation leads to the professional responsibility of recreating the system continually to greater levels of perfection. Because case management is a research-based system, it enjoys more fully the status of a professional model of care.

ON THE HORIZON

Case management continues to evolve as a model of care delivery.[10] With health care reform in full motion, case management models will proliferate, and we will witness their continual redesign. Despite such redesign, however, the fundamental characteristics of case management will remain unchanged.

Two major trends occurring in health care are increasingly driving the redesign of case management systems. The first is the growing trend toward disease prevention and wellness; the second is the trend for using more fully advanced practice nurses in health care delivery. Both are worth considering.

The trend toward wellness and disease prevention is very strong. This trend was highly visible in health care reform agendas, and rightfully so. A recent publication purports that preventable illnesses account for approximately 70 percent of all medical treatment in this country.[3] If we prevent disease through comprehensive wellness programs, overspending in health care might be virtually nonexistent. A major U.S. corporation recently released some data that support this premise. This corporation discovered that behavioral risks among its employees, such as smoking and obesity, cost the company $71 million per year in lost work and medical expenses.[3]

This growing trend for wellness will soon reshape case management. We will witness the emergence of health-focused case management models. Protocols will be developed to case manage populations throughout the life span, with a focus on maintaining wellness and health life styles. Nurse case managers are well educated and prepared to take the lead role in facilitating this transition.

The appropriate utilization of advanced practice nurses will escalate significantly over the next few years. There are two compelling reasons for this growing trend: (1) their quality and cost-effectiveness have been documented time and again, and (2) the public accepts and welcomes them. The following supports this premise:

> A recent national public survey found that fully 66 percent of responders would either strongly favor or somewhat favor receiving much of their routine care from a well-trained nurse rather than from a doctor.[26(p.23)]

As health care reform continues to unfold, we will witness advanced practice nurses playing major roles in our health care system. They will become more intensely involved in case management systems, and many will assume advanced case manager roles.

CONCLUSION

After a decade of rethinking, restructuring, and redesigning our health care delivery system, we have finally come to the place where we have developed the best delivery system of our time. Case management is the delivery system of the present and of the future. Yes, it too will change, as all things do, but its basic concept, premises, and characteristics will stand the test of time for many years to come.

Because of case management and its painstaking development by the nursing profession, nursing has moved to the forefront of health care delivery in this country, and we must be proud of that accomplishment. This book is a tribute to the nursing profession and its significant role in health care delivery through case management.

REFERENCES

1. Blancett SS, Flarey DL. *Case Studies in Nursing Case Management: Health Care Delivery in a World of Managed Care.* Gaithersburg, Md: Aspen Publishers, Inc.; 1996.
2. Bartling A. Trends in managed care. *Healthcare Executive.* 1995;10(2):7–11.
3. Faltermayer E. Why health care costs can keep slowing. *Fortune.* 1994;129:75–82.
4. Bartling A. Integrated delivery systems: fact or fiction. *Healthcare Executive.* 1995;10(3):7–11.
5. Zander K. CareMap systems and case management: creating waves of restructured care. In: Blancett S, Flarey D, eds. *Reengineering Nursing and Health Care: The Handbook for Organizational Transformation.* Gaithersburg, Md: Aspen Publishers, Inc.; 1995:203–222.
6. Hemphill S, Biester D. Case management in a reformed health care system. *J Pediatr Nurs.* 1994;9:124–125.
7. Vautier A, Carey S. A collaborative case management program: The Crawford Long Hospital of Emory University model. *Nurs Adm Q.* 1994;18:1–9.
8. Mullahy C. *The Case Manager's Handbook.* Gaithersburg, Md: Aspen Publishers, Inc.; 1995.
9. Crawley W. Case management: managing the nurse case manager. *Health Care Supervisor.* 1994;12(2):84–89.
10. Hill M. CareMap and case management systems: evolving models designed to enhance direct patient care. In: Flarey D, ed. *Redesigning Nursing Care Delivery: Transforming Our Future.* Philadelphia, Pa: J.B. Lippincott; 1995:173–185.
11. Edelstein E, Cesta T. Nursing case management: an innovative model of care for hospitalized patients with diabetes. *Diabetes Educ.* 1993;19:517–521.
12. Allred C, Arford P, Michel Y, Carter V, Veitch J. A cost-effective analysis of acute care case management outcomes. *Nurs Econ.* 1995;13:129–136.
13. Johnson K, Proffitt N. A decentralized model for case management. *Nurs Econ.* 1995;13:142–151.
14. Wimpsett J. Nursing case management: outcomes in a rural environment. *Nurs Manage.* 1994;25(11):41–43.

15. Cohen E, Cesta T. *Nursing Case Management: From Concept to Evaluation.* St. Louis: C.V. Mosby; 1993.

16. Erkel E. The impact of case management in preventative services. *J Nurs Adm.* 1993;23(1): 27–28.

17. Cesta T. The link between continous quality improvement and case management. *J Nurs Adm.* 1993;23(6):55–61.

18. Mahn V. Clinical nurse case management: a service line approach. *Nurs Manage.* 1993;24(9):48–50.

19. Esher R, Bentz P, Sorensen M, Von Orsow T. Patient-centered pneumonia care: a case management success story. *Am J Nurs.* 1994;94(11):34–38.

20. Hampton D. Implementing a managed care framework through caremaps. *J Nurs Adm.* 1993;23(5):21–27.

21. Fox S, Ehreth J, Issel LM. A cost evaluation of a hospital-based perinatal case management program. *Nurs Econ.* 1994;12:215–220.

22. Quick B. Integrating case management and utilization management. *Nurs Manage.* 1994;25(11):52–56.

23. Bergman R. Getting the goods on guidelines. *Hosp Health Networks.* 1994;68:70–74.

24. Zander K, McGill R. Critical and anticipated recovery paths: only the beginning. *Nurs Manage.* 1994;25(8):34–40.

25. Allred C, Arford P, Michel Y, Veitch J, Dring R, Carter V. Case management: the relationship between structure and environment. *Nurs Econ.* 1995;13:32–41.

26. Buerhaus P. Managed competition and critical issues facing nurses. *Nurs Health Care.* 1994;15(1):22–26.

Appendix 1-A
Critical Path Maps

Exhibit 1-A-1 Critical Path Focused on Interventions

COLUMNS: ER—Day 3
DRG:
Prescribed LOS: 6 days

Congestive Heart Failure CareMap®
CAREGIVER INTERVENTIONS CRITICAL PATH
SECTION 1

CareMap® is a registered trademark of The Center for Case Management, Inc., 6 Pleasant Street, So. Natick, MA 01760, tel. 508-651-2600

ADDRESSOGRAPH

Date				DAY 1 ER 1–4 Hours	N	D	E	DAY 1 Floor Telemetry or CCU 6–24 Hours	N	D	E	DAY 2 Floor	N	D	E	DAY 3 Floor	N	D	E
Interventions																			
Assessments				Vital signs q 15 mins Nursing assessments focus on lung sounds, edema, color, skin integrity, jugular vein distention Cardiac monitor Arterial line if needed Swan Ganz Daily weight Intake and output				VS q 15 minutes Repeat nursing assessments Cardiac monitor Arterial line Swan Ganz Weight I & O				VS q 4 h Repeat nursing assessments D/C cardiac monitor at 24 hr D/C arterial and Swan Ganz Weight I & O				VS q 6 h Repeat nursing assessments Weight I & O			
Consults																			
Specimens/Tests				Consider TSH studies Chest x-ray EKG CPK q 8h × 3 ABG if pulse OX:___ Lytes, Na + +, K, Cl, CO2, GLU, BUN, Creatinine Digoxin: (range)___				B/G				Evaluate for ECHO Lytes, BUN, Creat							
Treatments				O2 or intubate IV or Heparin Lock				O2 IV or Heparin Lock				IV or Heparin Lock				D/C pulse Ox if stable D/C IV or Hep lock			

Exhibit 1-A-2 CareMap® Focused on Outcomes

COLUMNS: ER—Day 3

DRG:

Prescribed LOS: 6 days

Congestive Heart Failure CareMap®
Standard of Care
PATIENT/FAMILY OUTCOMES
SECTION 1

CareMap® is a registered trademark of The Center for Case Management, Inc., 6 Pleasant Street, So. Natick, MA 01760, tel. 508-651-2600

ADDRESSOGRAPH

Problem/Focus	DAY 1 ER 1–4 Hours	N	D	E	DAY 1 Floor Telemetry or CCU 6–24 Hours	N	D	E	DAY 2 Floor	N	D	E	DAY 3 Floor	N	D	E
Date																
1. Alteration in gas exchange/perfusion and fluid balance due to decreased cardiac volume	Reduced pain from admission or pain free Uses pain scale O2 Set improved over admission baseline on O2 therapy				Respirations equal to or less than on admission				O2 Set = 90 Respiration 20–22 Vital Signs Stable Crackles at lung bases Mild SOB with activity				Does not require O2 VSS Crackles at base Resp 20–22 Mild SOB with activity			
2. Potential for shock	No S/S of shock				No S/S of shock				No S/S of shock				No S/S of shock Normal lab values			
3. Potential for consequences of immobility and decreased activity: skin breakdown, DVT	No redness at pressure points No falls				No redness at pressure points No falls				Tolerates chair, washing, eating and toileting				Has bowel movement Up in room and bathroom with assist			
4. Alteration in nutritional intake due to nausea and vomiting, labored breathing					No c/o nausea No vomiting Taking liquids as offered				Eating solids Takes in 50% of each meal				Taking 50% of each meal			

Source: Reproduced by special permission of The Center for Case Management, South Natick, Mass. All rights reserved, and reproduced with permission of JB Lippincott Co., Philadelphia, Pa. Reprinted from: Hill M. CareMap and Case Management Systems: Evolving Models To Enhance Direct Patient Care, in Flarey DL., *Redesigning Nursing Care Delivery: Transforming Our Future.* Philadelphia, Pa: JB Lippincott Co., 1995.

Exhibit 1-A-3 Congestive Heart Failure CareMap®

Location / Problem	Day 1 — ER 1–4 hours	Day 1 — Floor Telemetry or CCU 6–24 hours	Day 2 — Floor	Day 3 — Floor	Day 4 — Floor	Day 5 — Floor	Day 6 — Floor
			Benchmark Quality Criteria				
Alteration in gas exchange/profusion and fluid balance due to decreased cardiac output, excess fluid volume	Reduced pain from admission or pain free; Uses pain scale; O₂ saturation improved over admission baseline on O₂ therapy	Respirations equal to or less than on admission	O₂ saturation 90%; Resp 20–22; Vital signs stable; Crackles at lung bases; Mild shortness of breath with activity	Does not require O₂; Vital signs stable; Crackles at base; Respiration 20–22; Mild shortness of breath with activity	Does not require O₂ (O₂ saturation on room air 90%); Vital signs stable; Crackles at base; Resp 20–22; Completes activities with no increase in respirations; No edema	Can lie in bed at base line position; Chest x-ray clear or at baseline	No dyspnea
Potential for shock	No signs/symptoms of shock	No signs/symptoms of shock	No signs/symptoms of shock	No signs/symptoms of shock; Normal lab values	No signs/symptoms of shock	No signs/symptoms of shock	No signs/symptoms of shock
Potential for consequences of immobility and decreased activity; skin breakdown, DVT	No redness at pressure points; No falls	No redness at pressure points; No falls	Tolerates chair, washing, eating, and toileting	Has bowel movement; Up in room and bathroom with assist	Up ad lib for short periods	Activity increased to level used at home without shortness of breath	Activity increased to level used at home without shortness of breath
Alteration in nutritional intake due to nausea and vomiting, labored breathing		No c/o nausea; No vomiting; Taking liquids as offered	Eating solids; Takes in 50% each meal	Taking 50% each meal	Taking 50% each meal; Weight 2 lbs from patient's normal base line	Taking 75% each meal	Taking 75% each meal
Potential for arrhythmias due to decreased cardiac output, increased irritable foci, valve problems, decreased gas exchange	No evidence of life-threatening dysrhythmias	Normal sinus rhythm with benign ectopy	K(WNL); Benign or no arrhythmias	Digoxin level WNL; Benign or no arrhythmias	Digoxin level WNL; Benign or no arrhythmias	Digoxin level WNL; Benign or no arrhythmias	Digoxin level WNL; Benign or no arrhythmias

continues

Exhibit 1-A-3 continued

Location	Day 1 ER 1-4 hours	Day 1 Floor Telemetry or CCU 6-24 hours	Day 2 Floor	Day 3 Floor	Day 4 Floor	Day 5 Floor	Day 6 Floor
				Benchmark Quality Criteria			
Problem							
Patient/family response to future treatment and hospitalization	Patient/family expressing concern Following directions of staff	Patient/family expressing concerns Following directions of staff	Patient/family expressing concerns Following directions of staff	States reasons for and cooperates with rest periods Patient begins to assess own knowledge and ability to care for CHF at home	Patient decides whether he or she wants discussion with physician about advanced directives	States plan for 1-2 days postdischarge as to meds, diet, activity, follow-up appointments Expresses reaction to having CHF	Repeats plans States signs and symptoms to notify physician or ER Signs discharge consent
Individual problem:							
Staff Tasks							
Assessments/Consults	Vital signs q 15 min to 1 h Nursing assessments focus on lung sounds, edema, color, skin integrity, jugular vein distention Cardiac monitor Arterial line if needed Swan Ganz Intake and output	Vital signs q 15 min to 1 h Repeat nursing assessments Cardiac monitor Arterial line Swan Ganz Daily weight Intake and output	Vital signs q 4 h Repeat nursing assessments D/C cardiac monitor every 24 h D/C arterial and Swan Ganz Daily weight Intake and output	Vital signs q 6 h Repeat nursing assessments Daily weight Intake and output	Vital signs q 6 h Repeat nursing assessments Daily weight Intake and output Nutrition consult	Vital signs q 6 h Repeat nursing assessments Daily weight Intake and output	Vital signs q 6 h Repeat nursing assessments Daily weight Intake and output
Specimens/Tests	Consider TSH studies Chest x-ray EKG CPK q 8 hx 3 ABG if pulse Ox: (range) Electrolytes: Na, K, Cl, CO_2 Glucose, BUN, creatinine Digoxin: (range)	B/G	Evaluate for ECHO Electrolytes, BUN, creatinine			Chest x-ray Electrolytes, BUN, creatinine	

Exhibit 1-A-3 continued

Treatments	O₂ or intubate IV or heparin lock	O₂ IV or heparin lock	IV or heparin lock	DC pulse Ox if stable D/C IV or heparin lock			
Medications	Evaluate for digoxin Nitrodrip or paste Diuretics IV Evaluate for antiemetics Evaluate for antiarrhythmics	Evaluate for digoxin Nitrodrip or paste Diuretics IV Evaluate for pre-load/afterload reducers K supplements Stool softeners	D/C Nitrodrip or paste Diuretics IV or PO K supplements Stool softeners Evaluate for nicotine patch	Change to PO digoxin PO diuretics K supplements Stool softeners Nicotine patch if consent	PO diuretics K supplement Stool softeners Nicotine patch if consent	PO diuretics K supplement Stool softeners Nicotine patch if consent	PO diuretics K supplement Stool softeners Nicotine patch if consent
Nutrition	None	Clear liquids	Cardiac, low-salt diet	Cardiac, low-salt diet	Cardiac, low-salt diet	Cardiac, low-salt diet	Cardiac, low-salt diet
Safety/Activity	Commode Bedrest with head elevated Reposition patient q 2 h Bedrails up Call light available	Commode Bed rest with head elevated Dangle Reposition patient q 2 h Enforce rest periods Bedrails up Call light available	Commode Enforce rest periods Chair with assist 1/2 h with feet elevated Bedrails up Call light available	Bathroom privileges Chair × 3 Bedrails up Call light available	Ambulate in hall × 2 Up ad lib between rest periods Bedrails up Call light available	Encourage ADLs that approximate activities at home Bedrails up Call light available	Encourage ADLs that approximate activities at home Bedrails up Call light available
Teaching	Explain procedures Teach chest pain scale and importance of reporting	Explain course, need for energy conservation Orient to unit and routine	Clarify CHF Dx and future teaching needs Orient to unit and routine Schedule rest periods Begin medication teaching	Stress importance of weighing self every day Provide smoking cessation information Review energy conservation schedule	Cardiac rehab level as indicated by consult Provide smoking cessation support Dietary teaching	Review CHF education material with patient	Reinforce CHF teaching

continues

Exhibit 1-A-3 continued

	Day 1 ER 1–4 hours	Day 1 Floor Telemetry or CCU 6–24 hours	Day 2	Day 3	Day 4	Day 5	Day 6
Location			**Benchmark Quality Criteria**				
			Floor	Floor	Floor	Floor	Floor
Staff Tasks							
Transfer/Discharge Coordination	Assess home situation: notify significant other If no arrhythmias or chest pain, transfer to floor Otherwise transfer to ICU	Screen for discharge needs Transfer to floor	Consider home health care referral		Evaluate needs for diet and antismoking classes Physician offers discussion opportunities for advanced directives	Appointment and arrangement for follow-up care with home health care nurses Contact VNA	Reinforce follow-up appointment

Notes: ABG, arterial blood gas; B/G, blood gas; CPK, creatinine phosphokinase; DVT, deep vein thrombosis; No c/o nausea, no complaints of nausea; OX, oximetry; TSH, thyroid stimulating hormone; WNL, within normal limits.

Source: Reproduced with special permission from The Center for Case Management, South Natick, Mass. All rights reserved. CareMap is a registered trademark of the Center for Case Management.

■ 2 ■

The Early Years: The Evolution of Nursing Case Management

Karen Zander, MS, RN, CS

The mid-1980s marked the convergence of strong nursing beliefs and management methods for health care that became, like the American Revolution, a "shot heard around the world." Simply stated, that "shot" was a message that nurses were essential, if not the ultimate force, in countries in which resources allotted for health care might be limited by a variety of means. *Case management* became an umbrella term, usually meaning an array of methods to coordinate health services better so that both financial and clinical objectives could be reached. In the United States, clinical nursing took a leadership role in formulating new roles and tools to plan and manage a balance between cost and quality, more recently referred to as efficiency and effectiveness.

Case management existed in industry, social welfare, community services, and insurance companies before it emerged as a distinct strategy in acute care and related discharge follow-up activities. The two organizations that brought case management by nurses to the forefront in this new arena were New England Medical Center Hospitals (NEMCH) in Boston, Massachusetts, and Carondelet Saint Mary's Hospital (CSMH) in Tucson, Arizona. Ten years later, the NEMCH model tends to be credited with structuring the episode of care and the CSMH model is best known for its continued innovative work between the episode and into the continuum.

Both models grew out of nursing's response to patient/family needs at a large pattern or population level. Both organizations had visionary vice presidents of nursing who empowered their staffs to seek constantly better ways of giving care. They believed in patient-centered care and continuous quality improvement before those philosophies were in vogue. But most important, they created climates of learning with support, guided by sound theory. NEMCH's particular story is described in this chapter.

NURSING AS THE INDUSTRY CATALYST

It is true—case management and clinical pathways were introduced into acute care by nurses. Actually, clinical paths and case management were an outgrowth of work conducted in 1983 called "The Pratt 4 Project," a socio-technical-environmental analysis used by a fully sanctioned multidisciplinary study team to learn how NEMCH might "do more with less" within prospective payment.[1] Among other findings, the Pratt 4 study revealed:

1. Describing the work of a hospital by geographic unit was only a partial view of reality because patients traverse units while each discipline has its allegiances to non-unit groups, such as departments or service.
2. Physicians have low tolerance and commitment to process (discussion) meetings, because they are action people whose search for quality lies almost exclusively in determining and using accurate algorithms for diagnosis and treatment regimes.
3. Clinicians expect to "do battle" with each other and with unresponsive support services. They learn quickly how to circumvent every policy that does not get their patients what they need.
4. Defining the cost of care only in terms of resources ordered by a physician is an inadequate formula. Because the patient's mind/body is interdependent, so are the clinicians serving the patient.
5. Every department and discipline including physicians perceive that someone else has more control and, as a result, seek to maximize themselves to be able to do their work.
6. Administration generally does not understand clinical processes, which causes a schizm because clinicians define themselves as process-doers rather than outcome-producers.
7. Clinicians will require better planning/documentation tools and more reliable formal relationships among disciplines and departments if they are to produce the same or better clinical outcomes more efficiently.
8. Nursing care plans and even excellent primary nursing (which was firmly in place for 100 percent of patients) would not in themselves be strong enough to hold up in a diagnosis-related groups (DRG) world.

In 1985, NEMCH nurses took these findings seriously and proceeded to transform themselves and eventually their colleagues in other departments. In a budget-neutral initiative, without being aware of the use of case management in other businesses, nursing understood its own developmental stages of professional practice (Exhibit 2-1) and outlined a course of change.

Exhibit 2-1 Developmental Stages of Professional Practice

Components	1900 → 1969 Pre-Primary Nursing	Transition	1969 → 1985 1st Generation Primary Nursing	Transition	1985 → 1995 2nd Generation Primary Nursing/Case Management
Focal Point	Tasks with responsibility		Process with individuality		Outcomes (product) with accountability
Power Base	Dependent on extension of MD's expert and legitimate power	Parallelism	RN as expert	Collaborative practice with MDs, peers, and system	Referent power is shared goals
Role and Identity	Doer, reporter	Care Planner	Thinker, therapeutic nurse-patient relationship which includes families	Patient-teacher	Case manager → healer
Evaluation	Personal qualities & completion of responsibilities	Overall behavioral objectives for RNs	Competence	Outcome standards per patient; process standards for nurse	Effectiveness (within quality standards)
Quality Assurance	Problem identification	Target, anonymous audits	Nursing process	Comprehensive, personal and system audits (e.g., MIS)	Nursing product
Staff/Unit Organization	8-hour (shift) focus; use of team, functional, total patient care; interchangeable staff. Continuity sporadic	End of shift 'kingdoms'; continuity methods. Assignments of PN to patient	24 hr. focus per patient per primary nurse; use of geographic, modular, and other case assignment methods. LPNs, RNs, PN → Aides.	Flextime; formal associates	Length of stay focus per patient per primary nurse across episode of care: use of continuous and collaborative professional practice groups. PN/CM/LPNs, aides, RNs, MDs, other disciplines.
Management Structures and Processes	Highly centralized; attention to rules	Head nurse as manager	Decentralized; attention to group dynamics; staff nurses' clinical decision making and coordination	Staff nurse as manager	Mix of centralized and decentralized; attention to organization and system
Skills	"Instrumental Functions," bureaucratic; rule-passing	BSN	"Expressive functions" Participative interactions	BSN/MSN: inquiry; nurse-to-nurse learning	Group membership and leadership; management skills; clinical research; consultation; contracting

Source: Copyright © 1985, New England Medical Center Hospitals (NEMCH), Boston, Massachusetts. Developed by Karen Zander.

Before outcomes or disease management ever appeared in the literature, NEMCH nurses were using targeted definable, measurable, realistic, clinical outcomes per patient population to restructure practice. What was unique about NEMCH's approach to finding new ways of doing things was the possibility that outcomes based on assessment should drive process and that process could be more efficient in many cases. We had the same background and problems of nurses in other settings but put the elements of practice in a new relationship with each other, using the crisis of limits on length of stay as an ally rather than an enemy. We were convinced that nursing would be at risk in a DRG world and were motivated to explain first to ourselves and then others what nursing's contributions were to desired clinical outcomes (which we defined as true quality) and efficient care management. Two works we used in this endeavor were the Joint Commission on Accreditation of Healthcare Organizations' categories of outcomes for retrospective auditing (knowledge, health, activity, absence of complications)[2] and production operations' management theory.[3]

Nurses were the most likely candidates to introduce critical paths and case management because they are at the juncture where the system and the patient meet. Nurses have to either make the larger system work for the patient or they will directly experience the patient's anger, pain, and complications related to inefficient or ineffective activities. Also, through the applied scientific method they call the nursing process, nurses use nomenclature that breaks the medical diagnosis into workable, treatable parts (that is, into the nursing diagnosis), which in turn can make a conceptual bridge to outcome definition. In addition, accountability models such as primary nursing give nurses a background to begin a collaborative dialogue. Thus, with a sound structure in place, the nurses at NEMCH had the confidence to ask the following four questions of all disciplines:
1. What is the work required to get patients within certain case types to desired outcomes?
2. What is the best way to produce the work, including clinical decision making (academic, crisis, structured process) and a model/structure (people for care giving, responsibilities, relationships, documentation)?
3. Who is accountable for the results?
4. What do we need to restructure to better support our clinical processes?[4]

These were the same questions to be answered a decade later, always putting cost, process, and outcome in balance with the other. None could be investigated out of context of the other two components. Between 1985 and

1989, four designs of written documents (case management plans, timelines, critical paths, CareMap® medical record) for planning, managing, documenting, and evaluating multidisciplinary care toward outcomes evolved as more was learned about outcome-based clinical care within time frames. Each iteration of design created more confidence in the need and ability to move from open-ended care planning to structured care managing.

FROM CASE MANAGEMENT PLANS TO CAREMAP® MEDICAL RECORD

Contrary to popular opinion, critical paths did not appear out of the blue. In fact, they were a third attempt to have a user-friendly clinical planning and concurrent care management tool. The first attempt was a case management plan, the format shown in Exhibit 2-2. Case management plans were academically solid but unwieldy in practice without computerization, which was unavailable at that time.

In retrospect, case management plans were a transition from nursing care plans to the ultimate CareMap® tools, which currently create a foundation for documentation-by-exception. In between case management plans and CareMap® tools were time lines and critical paths, shown in Exhibits 2-3 and 2-4. Critical paths became the working document of choice by clinicians. In fact, both new and experienced staff nurses actually appreciated the critical paths. They were used as a reference, eventually available on a word processor on each unit, and began to replace care plans. Because of several factors, critical paths were unfortunately used almost entirely by nurses.

Use of critical paths was reinforced by a class and a programmed-instruction book on DRGs mandatory for all registered nurse (RN) orientation classes. Critical path use was evaluated during all performance appraisals. However, nursing documentation remained fragmented, including assessment, index of problems and outcomes, progress notes, care plan, and flow/treatment sheets. (CareMap® tools were the innovation designed to integrate these functions.)

Critical paths had obvious limitations that are still evident today and magnified if used only as a policing mechanism rather than the outcome production process descriptors they were meant to be. Their chief deficits are:

1. Critical paths emphasize tasks or interventions rather than outcomes.
2. Critical paths cannot replace any specific documents in the permanent medical record. Although they do constitute a multidisciplinary action plan, they have no built-in evaluation of results.
3. Variances from planned interventions listed on the critical path basically constitute a process audit, making clinicians wary of adapting processes

Exhibit 2-2 Excerpts from Time Line Overview

Emergency Room Day 1	Coronary Care Unit 2 3	Inpatient Cardiology 4 5 6 7 8 9 10	Outpatient Cardiology Visit 1 2
Health Outcomes			
1. DX: Alteration in comfort secondary to chest pain.	1. DX: Alteration in comfort secondary to chest pain.	1. DX: Alteration in comfort secondary to chest pain.	1. DX: Potential alteration in comfort secondary to chest pain.
Outcome:	Outcome:	Outcome:	Outcome:

Source: Reprinted from "Time Line: The Maps for Managed Care," by K. Zander, *Definition*, Vol. 1, No. 3, © 1986, p. 2.

(a necessary step in individualizing care) lest there be a variance to record.

Yet, those oversimplified critical paths had a positive impact on lengths of stay, especially by focusing interdisciplinary communication and care evaluation. The method grew as it gained internal recognition from finance, physicians, and other skeptical professionals. Once they became convinced that critical paths and also case managers built an infrastructure for *provider-controlled* case management, they became part of the program.

Unfortunately, the terminology used to describe all these innovations, although accurate, to this day becomes problematic for different groups. No

Exhibit 2-3 Case Management Plan Excerpt

Diagnosis:					Unit:		DRG:	
MDC:	Length of Stay:		Usual or Day (from admission day = 1): Health Outcomes					
DIAGNOSIS	OUTCOME (The patient . . .)	DAY VISIT	INTERMEDIATE GOAL (The patient . . .)	DAY VISIT	PROCESS (The nurse . . .)	DAY VISIT	PROCESS (The physician . . .)	

Source: Reprinted from "Case Management Plan: A Collaborative Model," by K. Zander, *Definition*, Vol. 2, No. 1, © 1987, p. 2.

Exhibit 2-4 Critical Path and Variance Record

Patient _____   Case Type _____
MD _____   _____
Case Manager _____   DRG _____
Date Critical Path _____   Expected LOS _____
Reviewed by MD _____
        Date

	Day 1	Day 2	Day 3	Day 4	Day 5	Day 6	Day 7
Consults							
Tests							
Activity							
Treatments							
Medications							
Diet							
Discharge Planning							
Teaching							

	Variation	Cause	Action Taken
Date			

(Reverse side of Critical Pathway form shown above)

Source: Adapted from *Managing Outcomes through Collaborative Care,* by K. Zander, ed., p. 12, © American Hospital Publishing, Inc., 1995.

Exhibit 2-5 Conversion to Paths and Case Managers

1982	Pratt 4 Project
	DRGs
1985	MD ordering practices and LOS information used to form 37 case management plans
	Case-type analysis conducted by nurse managers
1986	Senior staff nurses pilot case management plans
	Time lines and critical paths imagined
	Center for Nursing Case Management begun
1987	Definition of nursing domain by Stetler and DeZell
	Collaborative practices begun around core of nursing group practice with attending MDs
	Critical paths available on units
1988	108 RNs belong to 29 collaborative practices
	Critical paths merged with treatment record
1989	CareMap® medical record proposed but implemented outside NEMCH
	The Center for Nursing Case Management spins off from NEMCH as independent consulting firm
1991	Name changed to The Center for Case Managment, Inc., by co-owners K. Bower and K. Zander

term makes everyone happy! However, if we knew then what we know now, we would label:

1. critical paths, clinical paths
2. variance, exception or customization
3. managed care, care management
4. primary nurses, primary nurses or unit-based care coordinators
5. case managers, clinical case managers or expediters
6. case management, collaborative care

Unfortunately as well, there was no executive steering committee for this project, which ultimately limited its complete integration. The force of the conversion to new tools and roles outlined in Exhibit 2-5 was driven by NEMCH nursing administrators, managers, and senior staff working together. For example, staff nurses helped create and field test all versions of clinical paths, and managers/supervisors each wrote case-type analysis papers at the end of 1985 to propose clinical and operational changes to NEMCH administration. We had some cost-per-case data, but generally used length-of-stay data as a barometer or proxy of resources. Managers, as in the previous 10 years, received monthly management education to support them in their roles. The 1986 agenda included actual clinical validity studies of outcomes stated on the case management plans developed the previous year (Exhibit 2-6).

Exhibit 2-6 Learning Objectives To Be Met by December 1986

1. Develop a method for evaluating *individual sets of outcomes* per patient/family per primary nurse.
2. Investigate extending the case manager role beyond unit boundaries.
3. Identify a key issue for future research (i.e., variables affecting length of stay).

NEW ENGLAND MEDICAL CENTER HOSPITALS DEPARTMENT OF NURSING

1986 Management Seminars
Calendar

Month	Subject	Between-Seminar Assignment
January	Updating primary nursing consultation Overview of DRG projects	Read packet Discuss calendar with management team and your project-mate
February	Measuring the nurse-dependent complication and health outcomes	Use outcome audit
March	Involving MDs in the case management plan	Meet with MD and develop the MD section of case management plans
April	Measuring knowledge outcomes	Use outcome audit
May	Measuring activity outcomes	Use outcome audit
June	Case manager role: part I	Revise the time line for the total patient care continuum
July	Case manager role: part II	
August	Analyzing patient acuity/cost	
September	Case manager role: part III	Report of findings to date, including research questions
October	Anticipating 1987	Review MIS for revisions
November	Measuring the patient/family satisfaction outcomes	Use outcome audit
December	Methodologies for accountability: putting it all together	

Source: Courtesy of New England Medical Center Hospitals, Boston, Massachusetts.

At the time, NEMCH had a 65 percent RN, 35 percent nursing aide mix, and staff rotated 50 percent day–evening or day–night by contract. There were no clinical specialists hired as such on staff. Senior staff nurses, the group that trialed the case manager role, received mandatory monthly education (Exhibit 2-7) and carried a steady case load of primary patients to whom they gave direct care. As such, they always worked closely with physicians, social service, discharge planning, and utilization review. From their research diaries and their continuous feedback, case management "ground rules" were developed once everyone could agree on the basic expectations (Exhibit 2-8). Case management would look like the following description to the patient and family:

If you are admitted for an abdominal aortic aneurysm repair, you become a patient of a collaborative practice composed of two vascular physicians and four staff nurses who treat you throughout your entire episode of care. In fact, you probably are already followed by the physicians and the ambulatory nurse member of the group practice. Now that you are entering acute care, she will notify her group of your special needs and work with the physician to facilitate a smooth pre-op course. The group uses the Critical Path for DRG 100-Major Vascular Surgery (10–13 day length of stay) to plan, track, and evaluate your progress.

When you arrive on the inpatient unit, the inpatient nurse in the group practice becomes either your primary nurse or associate primary nurse. She will discuss your Critical Path with you and your family and will help you become familiar with the sequencing of events. She will give you direct care before the OR and after your SICU stay.

She will also coordinate your transitions with the OR/RR nurse member of the group practice and with the nurse member from the SICU. In fact, she will meet you before surgery, offer to take you on a tour of the SICU, and answer any questions you or your family may have.

The group practice communicate often with your surgeon and meet formally for about an hour a week to discuss their 30 active patients. Although these nurses are part of the regular staffing on each of their units, they take vascular patients within their primary caseloads and shift assignments. When any one of them is not on duty, their peers on their own units continue to follow the Critical Path in a way similar to following a nursing care plan.

When you are ready for discharge, she will again meet with you to reinforce your followup appointments in the ambulatory setting. With the surgeon and the rest of the group practice, she will assess

Exhibit 2-7 Management Seminar Series

NEW ENGLAND MEDICAL CENTER HOSPITALS DEPARTMENT OF NURSING
"Directions in Case Management"

OBJECTIVES
1. Identify key skills and structures essential to the case manager role.
2. Formulate management approaches that support the implementation of case management beyond the senior staff level.
3. Evaluate the implementation of the case management role for a specific case type, group practice, and unit.

Month	Content	Resources
January	Vertical Teams: Management Forum HMO Contracts/Managed Care Preliminary Findings from Case Management Diaries From Case Management Plans to "Critical Paths"	

February	Assessment:
	    Functional Assessment
	    Family Assessment
	Case Manager Consultation	

March	Formal Group Practices
	    Formation
	    Negotiation
	    Authority
	    Consultation
	Case Manager Consultation	

April	From Assessment to Goals
	    Nursing Diagnosis
	    Goal Setting
	    Contracting
	Case Manager Consultation	

May	Monitoring Progress and Resources
	    Critical Paths
	    Use of Rounds
	Case Manager Consultation	

June	Evaluating Case Managers Case Manager Consultation	
July	Education for Self-Care, Self-Meds Case Manager Consultation	
August	Use of the Phone Case Manager Consultation	
September	Working with the Health Care Team Case Manager Consultation	
October	Home Health Care Case Manager Consultation	
November	Identifying Case Manager Learning Needs Case Manager Consultation	
December	Evaluating Outcomes Objectively: Toward Peer Audit	

Source: Courtesy New England Medical Center Hospitals, Boston, Massachusetts.

Exhibit 2-8 Case Management Ground Rules

- Every designated patient will be assigned to a nursing group practice on or before entry to the system.
- Every group practice will assign a nursing case manager who works with an attending physician in evaluating an individualized case management plan (CMP) and critical path for each patient.
- A critical path is used to facilitate the care for every patient.
- Report will be based on critical paths.
- Negative variances from critical paths and/or CMPs require discussion with the attending physician, and a case management consultation when necessary.
- Every case manager must be a primary nurse or an associate when the patient is in his or her geographic area.
- The nursing case manager and physician case manager must communicate on a regular basis.
- Case managers will evolve/negotiate a flexible schedule that accommodates the needs of their patients and group practice as well as the needs of their units.
- Responsibility of the case manager begins at notification of patient's entry into the system and ends with a formal transfer of accountability to the patient, family, another health care provider, or another institution.

Source: Reprinted from Zander, K., Nursing Group Practice: The Cadillac in Continuity, *Definition,* Vol. 3, No. 2, p. 3, © 1988.

your achievement of the outcomes as well as analyze any variances from the Critical Path that you may have encountered. By doing this, they can better anticipate your future needs and can also improve the way our system works.

This first group practice demonstrated in several ways that "the whole is more than the sum of the parts." By viewing the whole episode of care as each of their responsibilities, they uncovered not only problems, but effective solutions. For instance several surgeries a week were being cancelled because patients who were already admitted and scheduled were not passing a Thallium-Persantine Scan (stress test). The group practice suggested that these scans as well as angiograms be done on an outpatient basis. They were able, through their nurse managers, to negotiate a set time for these scans, reserved by the vascular service. They then wrote a letter to patients explaining the importance of the scans and their scheduling. By this one change, they saved OR time, and eliminated unnecessary patient anxiety over surgery that might eventually not be performed. They have gained more control over their time and their environment.

Through enhanced communication between the nursing group and the physicians, they have cut SICU days from a range of 5–7 days to 3–5 days in the past year—without compromising standards. In addition, they have managed their caseload of patients through early intervention so well, that their patients (who tend to have complicated and chronic conditions with an estimated 70% on Medicare) do not frequent the Emergency Room.[5]

SKIPPING STEPS, LOSING THEORY BASE AS APPLICATION EXPANDS

As others observed the NEMCH experience, they rapidly wanted to implement some or all of the methods. Those who understood the underlying theories and kept up to date with NEMCH's developments as well as limitations fared better than those who did not. Some of the reasons that other institutions encountered problems that NEMCH did not were:

1. The case management plan stage in which outcomes and intermediate goals were attached to processes was skipped, instead moving directly to critical paths that have no written outcomes or intermediate goals.

2. Nursing rapidly proceeded to implement but in isolation from other disciplines, especially physicians.

3. Without a unit-based accountability model of either primary nursing or care coordination, no one took ownership of the path.

4. There was a failure to educate and gain a comfort level with management personnel before expecting staff to use a whole new role or system.

5. Clinicians were not reinforced in the clinical reasoning/scientific method that is at the core of a management plan or clinical path.

6. People assumed this could only be used in a tertiary care medical center, when actually both clinical paths and case management have very broad and often more successful applications in nonteaching settings.

7. Many still misconceived the variance aspect of a clinical path so that instead of it serving to individualize needs of patients and their families, it has become an obsessional exercise in "got-cha."

OUTCOME-BASED CLINICAL PATHS AS CORE

The symbol—good or bad—for case management has been the critical path. Improvements to it have been subtle on the surface but significant in use. Differences between the original critical paths and CareMap® tools are shown in Exhibit 2-9. See Exhibit 1-A-3 in Chapter 1 for a CareMap® content grid. When converted to a sign-off documentation system, the newer tools

Exhibit 2-9 Critical Paths and CareMap® Tools

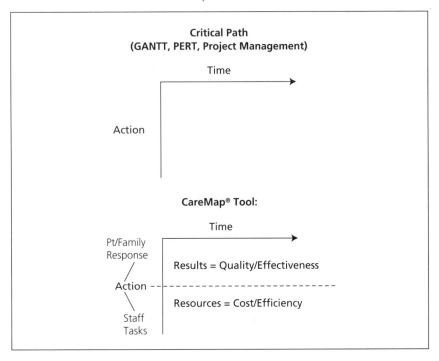

1. replace nursing care plans as multidisciplinary patient care plans

2. describe the contributions and accountabilities for outcomes of every department

3. show standards of care and standards of practice, and the timed, sequenced relationship between the two for a given case type, DRG, ICD-9 code, or constellation of problems

4. individualize care through analyzing and acting on variances

5. give each discipline the opportunity to streamline documentation by charting by exception (variance), with the CareMap® tool representing the "norm" (nonexception)

6. provide a data base for continuous quality improvement (CQI)

7. integrate the acuity systems, costing systems, and research

The ultimate tool will include utilization review/appropriateness criteria, outcome criteria, and quality process criteria recorded concurrently. Developing concurrent tools that require a single entry for each transaction after which the computer does the scheduling, linking, information sending, and tabulating is the work ahead. The concept of the clinical transaction driving all other information systems was not accepted in the 1980s.

A complete CareMap® system includes variance analysis, use of an outcome-time focus in all multidisciplinary communication, case consultation and health care team meetings for patients at more-than-acceptable variance, and CQI. The challenge, of course, is to create a dynamic system of complex care management from a static piece of paper. This can be accomplished with a series of CareMap® tools for different phases of treatment, the use of structured extensions or inserts, and the use of blank CareMap® tools for anecdotal documentation or for those patients who require a totally individualized map. When a patient's reason for remaining in the hospital changes in a major way (for example, remaining on a vent after a craniotomy), the CareMap® tool changes as well.

The ultimate result of a CareMap® system is that unnecessary variance is reduced to a minimum because of an increasingly accurate learning curve that helps clinicians predict, prevent, and manage. It is not unusual for collaborative groups to begin developing CareMap® documents for the more straightforward diagnoses, proceed to several varieties of that map, combine constellations of problems, and finally map care for the patient populations that were initially felt to be totally unpredictable.

Currently, CareMap® tools are used either on paper as references only, on paper as permanent documentation, or on computers. As institutions and clinicians become comfortable with CareMap® tool development, and as computer systems convert to CareMap® systems, higher percentages of patients will be managed by them (with daily or per visit screens). Similarly, variances are presently being handled differently depending on each agency's goals for implementing the system in the first place. Minimally, patient/family and community variances are recorded in the medical record (in the progress notes). A few institutions have decided to include clinician- and hospital-generated variances in the chart as well.

A CareMap® system implies more than using a new document to manage care. At the heart of the system is vigilant attention to patient/family outcomes, with increasingly more authority used at the multidisciplinary clinical level. However, the tool is only as useful as the people on whose practices it is built. The one major change in behavior required in a CareMap® system is the shift from passive "care following" to proactive care management toward agreed-on progressions of outcomes.[4]

NURSING CASE MANAGEMENT: A CLASSIC

As early as 1987, it became clear that nursing case management would be a classic model because it added value, consistency, quality, and accuracy to patient care, was adaptive to the environment, and both enhanced and defined the voluntary differentiation to a newly available professional level of nursing. Although initially discovered through primary nursing and care planning, it advanced the management of patient care into another quantum. In retrospect, its main strength was that it "spread" (i.e., could be applied) in a wide variety of settings with no or minimal consultation! What was projected as the vision in 1987 has actually occurred in some settings with very small modifications (i.e., CareMap® tools instead of case management plans, or nonstaff RNs being case managers). Those projections are given in the following paragraphs and described using concentric triangles in Figures 2-1 and 2-2.

As in all businesses, nursing links the classic anchors of structure, process, and outcome in a dynamic relationship of design, role, and feedback (Figure 2-1). *Design* is the way structural components (manpower, equipment, organization, time, etc.) are expected to support the actual production process. *Role* is the set of behaviors that is expected to transform the production process into an actual product. *Feedback* is the essential link between the outcomes of a system and the revisions and adaptations it must make to better do its work.

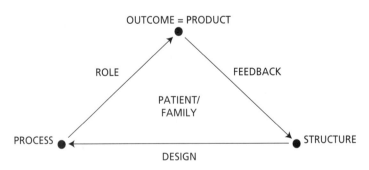

Figure 2-1 The Classic Triad: Inner Core. *Source:* Reprinted from "Nursing Case Management: A Classic," by K. Zander, *Definition,* Vol. 2, No. 2, © 1987, p. 1.

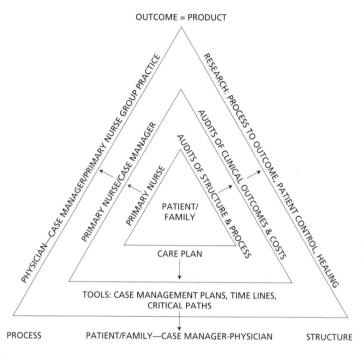

OUTCOME = PRODUCT

PHYSICIAN–CASE MANAGER/PRIMARY NURSE GROUP PRACTICE

RESEARCH: PROCESS TO OUTCOME, PATIENT CONTROL, HEALING

PRIMARY NURSE/CASE MANAGER

AUDITS OF CLINICAL OUTCOMES & COSTS

PRIMARY NURSE

AUDITS OF STRUCTURE & PROCESS

PATIENT/ FAMILY

CARE PLAN

TOOLS: CASE MANAGEMENT PLANS, TIME LINES, CRITICAL PATHS

PROCESS   PATIENT/FAMILY—CASE MANAGER-PHYSICIAN   STRUCTURE

Figure 2-2 Professional Advances of Nursing Case Management. *Source:* Reprinted from "Nursing Case Management: A Classic," by K. Zander, *Definition,* Vol. 2, No. 2, © 1987, p. 3.

Primary nursing was the first formal professional model in hospital nursing. The classic triad demonstrates that in a Primary Nursing Model, "design" is the nursing care plan, "role" is the Primary Nurse (and associate), and "feedback" is audits of structure and process, (i.e., charts, satisfaction, assignments, etc.).

Primary nursing is largely a unit-based model, implemented to achieve higher degrees of continuity and satisfaction for patients, their families, and their nurses. In addition, accountability for the outcomes of nursing care achievable while that patient is on a primary nurse's unit is a key principle of the model. The primary nursing tradition is one of nursing process, care giver as care planner, therapeutic primary nurse–patient/family relationships, communication, coordination, and collaboration among nursing staff and among disciplines. Indeed, the primary nurse must have a blend of clinical, process, and management skills.

Historically, nurses have always managed care. However, in hospitals, their perspective is usually the management of care for the crisis, the shift, or the stay in a given geographic unit. Nurses are still seen, and perceive themselves, as task workers. Thus their authority is limited and their image is weak. Yet, focused studies of nurses in practice reveal that nurses are very outcome oriented and effective in their interventions. In fact, one task may lead to three desirable clinical outcomes. However, the inherent strength of nursing seems to be lost in roles which have enormous responsibilities, but impoverished authority within the health care institution. Clearly, a stronger model that reformulates the role of the traditional primary nurse is needed. The model should keep professional nursing at the pivotal juncture of cost and quality and should empower the staff nurse so that he/she can truly be accountable for the clinical and financial outcomes of nursing care throughout an entire episode of illness.

In the past two years (1985–1987), New England Medical Center has experienced a rapid transformation in the definition and execution of the inpatient primary nurse role. In Nursing Case Management, the experienced primary nurse, in collaboration with the physician, activates a production process for each patient and uses a Case Management Plan to organize, direct, revise, and evaluate care. Although the primary nurse remains unit-based, the case manager's contact and authority extends to the whole episode of care.

In other words, the classic triad has undergone changes on each side. A transition or middle level emerges as shown in Figure 2-2.

Nursing Care Plans are being replaced by Case Management Plans for the entire episode of care of a case type. The typical patient problems, related intermediate and final outcomes, nursing interventions (process), and physician processes are outlined for the time interval in which they are expected to occur for each specific case type. They are both descriptive and prescriptive of standard practice, and serve as an informal contract between nurses, physicians, and patients that care will meet both quality and cost expectations.

TimeLines helped us understand the differences and similarities between nursing units treating the same patients through an episode of illness. Critical Paths are another tracking tool for the Primary Nurse Case Manager. They outline the key nursing and physician processes that are needed to reach outcomes during an entire episode of illness.

Just as in primary nursing, the case manager is a *direct care provider* during a significant phase of the episode of illness. While the patient is on his/her unit, the case manager is also the primary nurse.

When the patient transfers to other units, the patient receives a new primary nurse and the case manager continues contact, working collaboratively with the physician and the new primary nurse.

Inclusion of intermediate and discharge clinical outcomes is vital to the auditing of case management. Eventually, auditing of outcomes will occur on a daily basis by the case managers themselves, their peers, and their patients.

A third level of professional practice via Nursing Case Management is described in the outer triangle of Figure 2-2. Although our experience over the next year (1988) may change the strategy somewhat, the vision will remain as a goal: contracts, group practice, and research.

As software enables case managers to assess, individualize goals and interventions, document, monitor, audit, and price professional nursing, nurses will feel increasingly confident in informing patients and families of anticipated services. In addition, other changes in hospital departments will be important to the goal of transforming all of health care into truly patient-centered systems.

Already, formal nursing group practices of primary nurses who have the same patient on serial units are forming. Within the group it is determined who should have case manager authority and how the patient's outcomes can best be facilitated. Group practices are case-type based and, as such, represent a true collaboration between nurses from multiple units for the benefit of patient continuity and achievement of realistic outcomes. Group practices will eventually provide peer consultation, cross-training, and other professional benefits to their members.

As Case Management Plans become validated and revised, we learn much about causal relationships of process to outcomes. There is an enormous amount of research needed in many areas including potential problems, the prevention of complications, the acquisition of self-care skills, and the experience of being healed.[6]

CONCLUSION

Everything and nothing has changed since the early days of critical paths and staff nurse case managers. Fast-forward ten years later from 1985 and the evolution of the health care market necessitates new definitions. Even the term *market* implies that there are new buyers and sellers of goods, with many transactions and enticements. Figure 2-3 illustrates how care mapping and case management can be used by care providers to provide an infrastructure for capitation.

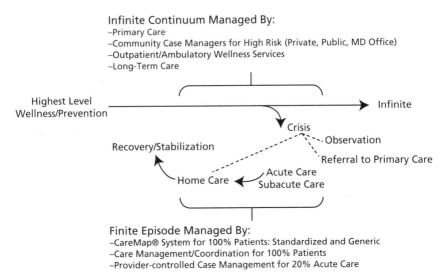

Figure 2-3 Mapping and Case Management Strategies for Capitation. *Source:* Copyright © 1995, The Center for Case Management, South Natick, Massachusetts. Developed by Karen Zander.

The three stages of market evolution have at their core the redistribution of risk for costs from traditional indemnity insurer, and to some extent the patient, to the provider. Those stages, simply defined, are:

1. Fee-for-service: provider(s) reimbursed for charges.
2. Prospective payment (DRGs): payment using a fixed price formula for specific procedures or conditions, largely those provided in acute care.
3. Capitation: the actual prepayment to a provider or insurer, and also the process by which a negotiated package of comprehensive and continuous health care services are provided on an annual basis regardless of actual use.

Two trends within capitation are creating more demand for mapping and case management than ever before. First is the shift from service as a process itself, regardless of results, to service that is evaluated for definable, measurable clinical outcomes. Second is the need to work together across settings. Segments of the industry formerly ignored or devalued by other segments will soon be partners under capitation agreements. The central problem in converting provider system to be savvy and powerful in capitation is that almost no provider is 100% into capitation, with some still having a majority of business in fee-for-service.

CareMap® tools as the core of the medical record and case management models provide an infrastructure upon which the micromanagement of patient care can occur. In preparation for capitation, they provide a vehicle for an administration to (1) support and translate new market strategies to clinicians, and (2) continuously reconfigure the business to adjust to the changing market.

The Center for Case Management (CCM) suggests the infrastructure in Figure 2-3 as the overall strategy for multiple provider agencies to use. It is comprehensive, flexible, focused, and realistic. It shows a line at the top representing the Continuum and a loop at the bottom representing the Episode. The Continuum is infinite and the Episode is finite. These words are more than semantics because they encompass the ability to adapt to different payment formulas by using different systems to manage different functions. Hand-offs between an Episode and a Continuum will be key to the way patient care and case management systems are developed and managed. These issues will be addressed as providers better understand overall disease management.

An Episode of care includes services given to a patient and family from first contact to the last contact for that specific set of symptoms or procedures; i.e., chest pain to cardiac rehab, diagnosis through hospice, MD office through surgery and recuperation. The Continuum encompasses a person's health and lifestyle. It may include chronic but stable states such as well-maintained diabetes, handicaps, or long-term care.

Capitation will cover large groups of people, sick or well. Most people in the Continuum will be able to manage their own optimal level of wellness using diagnostic, educational, and primary health services sparingly. Those in the Continuum are not experiencing the crisis of an acute situation or the exacerbation of a chronic illness, even though some may be receiving long-term institutionalized care or home care assistance. Obviously, the Continuum is not without cost and for about 10–20% of "covered lives" resources will be required to prevent a more expensive Episode. People in the Continuum most at risk will benefit from community-based clinical case management.

Community case management services will become increasingly available as they become reimbursed. They will be supplied by several competing entities as shown. CareMap® tools may or may not be used by these case managers. If they are, they will be largely patient-driven with a high degree of customization.

When either the community case-managed group or the self-managing group enters an Episode, they should be managed using CareMap® medical records either specific to a defined population or generic to conditions such as general surgery. CCM advised that all patients should have their care managed by a designated RN and MD accountable for outcomes, and that about 20% of these patients should also be case managed. CCM predicts, that under capitation, the Episode of care from crisis to recovery will take place in more rather than less settings and thus require Episode-length CareMap® tools and case managers more than ever.

Under fee-for-service, the micromanagement of care, as outlined and facilitated by CareMap® tools and case management, is helpful but not imperative for satisfaction, quality, and productivity goals. Decreasing length of stay or admissions may not even be desired by the providers.

In prospective payment methodologies, managing care within reimbursable limits and with good outcomes is paramount, especially within acute care. Other types of providers may not yet have financial incentives to revise their systems.

Capitation precipitates the need for partners in disease management across provider agencies. Reorganization will be required multiple times to adjust to different contracts covering varied patient populations. The only patient-centered, data-rich, stabilizing force will be the infrastructure described here.[7]

The future? CareMap® documents will be used as contracts, every bed will be a swing bed, every acute care room will have multifunction, every care giver will think like a rehabilitation specialist, and every agency will have a commitment to wellness. See me in ten years!

REFERENCES

1. Zander K. Revising the production process: when "more" is not the solution. *Healthcare Supervisor*. 1985;3(3):44–54.

2. Joint Commission on Accreditation of Hospitals. *Retrospective Patient Care Audits.* Chicago: JCAH; 1972.

3. Chase R, Aquilano N. *Production and Operations Management.* Homewood, Ill: Richard D. Irwin, Inc.; 1981.

4. Zander K. *Managing Outcomes through Collaborative Care.* Chicago: American Hospital Publishing, Inc.; 1995.

5. Zander K. Nursing group practice: the Cadillac in continuity. *Definition.* 1988;3(2):1–2.

6. Zander K, Bower K, Etheredge ML. *Nursing Case Management: Blueprints for Transformation.* Boston: NEMCH; 1987.

7. Zander K. Evolving mapping and case management for capitation. *New Definition.* 1995;10(2):1–2.

■ **3** ■

New Challenges and Opportunities in Integrated Health Care Systems

Joanne Ritter-Teitel, MA, RN

The lack of public and political consensus required to enact national health care reform results in an uncertain environment for the health care industry, particularly for hospitals. Yet, a state-by-state transformation of the health care system is underway, without national legislation. Local health care markets are achieving consensus regarding managed care and competition strategies to transform the delivery of American health care. As this transformation occurs, the next decade will bring striking and sometimes painful changes to hospitals.

Given the pressures to bring all the components of the delivery system together to create a single point of accountability, stand-alone hospitals are becoming extinct. Stand-alone hospitals are joining systems at a rapid pace.[1] A survey of hospitals conducted by Deloitte and Touche indicates 71 percent of respondents either belong to or are developing an integrated health care system.[2] As hospitals, clinics, primary care providers, and long-term care facilities create new partnerships, the shapes and sizes of integrated health care systems are as different as the communities they serve. During this period of rapid and turbulent change, nurse executives face a new mix of challenges and opportunities.

This chapter describes the use of the *integrated health care systems concept,* both in practice and in the literature. It provides a conceptual foundation for nursing practice and inquiry. A discussion regarding the challenges and opportunities for nursing is presented, as nurse executives design and coordinate services within this new organizational context—the integrated health care system.

DRIVING FORCES BEHIND INTEGRATED HEALTH CARE SYSTEMS

As the growing national debt and ability to compete internationally has caused concern, the American people and their employers are demanding a more cost-effective, coordinated system of health care that achieves good clinical outcomes. Responding to this demand, hospitals are reducing length of stay, shifting patient care services to ambulatory settings, and reducing the hospital work force. Unfortunately, these efforts are insufficient to reduce health care costs to the satisfaction of business and employers.

The health care marketplace is organizing around a managed care and competition strategy. Managed care describes health plans that closely monitor and control utilization of services and is projected to be the dominant form of health care reimbursement in the future.[3-5] Managed care organizations generally have a specific population of enrollees, a prepaid monthly premium, and a single entry point through a primary care provider. Managed care organizations use primary care providers as "gatekeepers" to identify actual or potential health problems early, reduce the use of costly specialists, and avoid expensive hospital care.

Price competition, managed or otherwise, has not been seen before in the American health care system. Competition is a purchasing strategy that managed care organizations use to obtain maximum value for consumers and employers, applying rules for competition derived from principles of macroeconomics. Competition becomes managed competition when a network of competing, nonoverlapping health plans operate under legislated economic incentives designed to encourage cost containment and efficiency and when national or state legislation guarantees universal access and coverage.[6]

A full discussion of principles of macroeconomics and competition are beyond the scope of this chapter. Briefly, competition stimulates health care providers to deliver cost-effective, high-quality health care in the most appropriate facility and by the most appropriate provider. The underlying dynamic in health care is similar to that in other industries; competition compels hospitals to deliver better value to consumers.[7]

Managed care expands the emphasis on cost-effectiveness to include quality outcomes, refocusing the health care team on wellness, disease prevention, and early intervention for cost-effective delivery of services.[8, 9] Costs, quality, and outcomes are important variables that must be balanced to serve the health care needs of the community. Potentially, an undesirable consequence of integrated health care system financial accountability is undertreating consumers in legitimate need of services.

Hospitals providing cost-effective quality health care are more attractive to managed care organizations. As the primary customer changes from the individual patient to the payer, hospital "operations as usual" no longer ensure profitability and, more important, survivability. According to Buerhaus,[10] hospitals that are inefficient and unprepared to develop competitive pricing structures risk their chance for continued survival.

It is difficult to predict the future in this turbulent, transitioning health care environment. As managed care and competition penetrate the local health care markets, there is increased pressure to reduce expensive hospital stays and the number of inpatient beds. Recent statistics published by the American Hospital Association indicate that, although outpatient visits continue to experience unprecedented vigor, hospital admissions have also increased by 2.4 percent.[11] Whether this trend will continue is uncertain; however, the increase in hospital admissions is offset by a reduction in average length of stay and so the downsizing of hospitals seems inevitable.

Nursing departments are often the largest cost center in the hospital. As such, they are targets of dramatic reorganization as hospitals join integrated health care systems and reduce the number of operating beds. Designing effective, efficient patient care systems and staffing strategies to care for more patients, while reducing the number of inpatient beds, presents a quagmire of challenges to hospital nurse executives.

Cost-effective health care, which achieves optimal clinical outcomes, is not sufficient for the present marketplace. The new economics require comprehensive coverage and a single point of accountability. As managed care and competition penetration increases, a parallel demand arises for a coordinated continuum of care, often over the entire life span. A coordinated continuum across settings and sites is thought to achieve even better clinical outcomes and cost efficiency than the previous fragmented fee-for-service system.

In preparation for this phase of health care transformation, hospitals are developing strategic alliances, partnerships, and networks with providers along the entire health care continuum. Membership in an integrated health care system enhances the hospital's ability to compete effectively for managed care contracts and survive in the marketplace by offering a full range of coordinated services.[12,13] In the most advanced health care markets (e.g., where managed care is the predominant form of reimbursement), integrated health care systems accept risk with a managed care organization and a capitated payment in return for providing complete health care services to members for whom the premium is paid.

Hospital nurses have vast experience with coordinating care and resources in fragmented, complex environments, collaborating with other members of the health care team and maximizing the health potential of individual patients. Previous challenges associated with severe nursing shortages and re-imbursement systems have made many nurse executives resourceful, responsive, and adaptable to new environments. This experience will be useful as hospital nurse executives in integrated health care systems respond to the familiar, yet unprecedented challenges.

Integrated health care systems represent an organizational structure that many believe will at least partially resolve the new challenges of the emerging health care environment.[14-16] Although the new health care economics, survivability, and profitability are the chief drivers of the evolution of integrated delivery systems, the simultaneous imperative for coordinated care and optimal clinical outcomes makes it quite possible that a healthier American population will emerge because of this health care delivery transformation.

DEFINITIONS

Integrated health care systems may be defined from three perspectives: organizational, social systems, and strategic management. These perspectives represent three important and distinct positions from which integrated health care systems are viewed. Integrated health care systems can be defined from the organizational perspective focusing on operating unit partnerships, the social systems perspective focusing on human and requisite relationships among system providers, and finally, the strategic management perspective focusing exclusively on system finances.

The Organizational Perspective

The definition from the organizational point of view dominates the literature. The current empirical understanding of this new organizational form is largely derived from a longitudinal study of 12 regionally based integrated health care systems, called the Health Systems Integration Study (HSIS). This study was conducted by the Center for Health Services and Policy Research and the J.L. Kellogg Graduate School of Management at Northwestern University. Unfortunately, the study does not address the contribution of, or consequences to, nursing. Despite this fact, the principal investigator, Shortell, and his colleagues have made fundamental contributions to the small but growing body of knowledge of integrated health care systems.

The investigators of the HSIS define integrated health care or organized delivery systems as:

> . . . a network of organizations that provides or arranges to provide a coordinated continuum of services to a defined population and is

willing to be held clinically and fiscally accountable for the outcomes and the health status of the population served.[17(p.447)]

These organizations may own or partner with an insurance or managed care company to create a responsible health care partnership.[17]

Social Systems Perspective

Integrated health care systems may also be defined from the social systems perspective. This definition focuses on the interaction and relationships among the members of the system. Stichler[13] views integrated delivery systems as

> . . . a collection of health care providers who work interdependently as an open system to respond to external forces and achieve outcomes that could not be achieved if they worked independently.[13(p.48)]

In the social systems perspective, integration is the result of resource sharing and interconnections among the work elements performed by different professionals.[18]

Strategic Management Perspective

The strategic management perspective defines an integrated health care system as a strategic business entity operating in a defined geographic area. Providers are joined together by a financial product that equitably allocates health care dollars.[12] According to this definition, the ideal system is an optimally configured health care corporation organized to maximize member providers' market shares by offering a full range of integrated cost-effective services to attract patients and employers.[12] This perspective focuses almost exclusively on economics and the bottom line of integrated health care systems.

DIMENSIONS

Integration, patient care coordination, and the extent of the continuum of care are important dimensions of all integrated health care systems.

Integration

Integration is an essential dimension of services offered by the integrated health care system. Integration characterizes the system to the extent that functions and activities are appropriately coordinated across operating units within the same organization and within other organizations in the same system.[19] Integration is a critical process that enhances the quality of health care delivery. Because of the potential to enhance access to services, reduce fragmentation, and avoid duplication, a compelling argument is made that optimal clinical outcomes can be achieved in highly integrated systems. This argument or its suppositions have not been proved empirically. To date, there is no evidence that patients are healthier when treated by an integrated health care system.

Clinical, provider system, and functional integration are three primary forms of integration.[19,20] It is these forms of integration that create the "systemness" required to have an effect on the health of the community that is served. Successful nurse executives recognize that integration is the process for achieving high-quality health care—not the outcome. The outcome is the net health status benefit to the community or population that the integrated health care system serves.

Clinical integration is the extent to which patient care services are coordinated across the various units of the system.[19,20] It can be both horizontal and vertical. Horizontal integration constitutes coordinating patient care services within and across care sites that are at the same stage of service delivery.[19,20] Hospital nurse executives who have instituted patient care strategies that coordinate care processes among nursing units within the acute care setting have begun to operationalize horizontal integration. Examples of these care management strategies include the implementation of nursing case management models and clinical pathways.

The new challenge on the horizon for nurse executives is vertical integration. Vertical integration is the coordination of patient care activities across care sites that are at different stages of service delivery.[19–23] If integrated health care systems are to achieve their objectives, nurse executives must vertically integrate patient care services. Patient care delivery systems are required to link and coordinate patient care processes across all sites, beginning with the primary, acute, and home care settings. Nursing case management models and clinical pathways may be successful strategies for achieving vertical integration. A number of nursing case management models successfully connecting patient care services at various stages of the care process have been described.[24–30] In addition, recent reports are describing successful attempts to link sites of care using clinical pathways.[30–33]

Conrad[20] asserts that coordinating patient care over time and across sites is the *sine qua non* of clinical integration. Integrating care across settings presents new challenges to nurse executives as providers from different organizations with different cultures, values, and perspectives come together to achieve consensus on how to coordinate care processes. Nurse executives must critically assess their own organization's performance and ensure that clinical integration strategies truly meet the new demands of integrated delivery systems and are not just a repackaging of previous strategies.

Functional or administrative integration is defined as the extent to which key support functions and activities are coordinated across care sites.[19,20] This involves grouping people, work, and responsibilities so that boundaries do not break at the patient care interconnections. Nurse executives who have created successful multiskilled workers and partners-in-practice models have operationalized functional integration at the hospital level. The new frontier for hospital nurse executives is the creation of innovative models at the system level. The most successful integrated health care system will build the bridges among care sites effectively.

Provider-system integration is defined as the extent to which providers are economically dependent on the system, use the system's services and facilities, and actively participate in its planning, management, and governance.[19,20] Provider-system integration has focused on physician-system relationships. As advanced nurse practitioners assume primary care provider and gatekeeper roles, provider-system integration will be more germane to hospital nurse executives.

Patient Care Coordination

Patient care coordination, at the individual and system levels, is another important dimension of integrated health care systems. Integrated systems demand a coordinating capacity to plan, deliver, monitor, and adjust individual patient care over time. In addition, clinical processes and care also must be coordinated at the macrosystem level, for specific aggregates of patients or populations. Nurse executives, who have implemented variance analysis strategies (see Chapter 10) to monitor and manage patient outcomes within the hospital setting, are agile and prepared to take on the new challenge of implementing patient care monitoring and coordination at the system level.

Continuum of Care

Another dimension of integrated health care systems is the extent of the continuum of care. Ideally, this continuum of services stretches from prenatal to postmortem care and includes primary, ambulatory, institutional inpatient, and home health care service lines (Table 3-1). A true health care system continuum provides skilled nursing care, subacute care, preventive care, mental health care, rehabilitative care, and long-term care services.[34] The most sophisticated integrated health care systems are closely linked with public health and social service agencies as well as educational institutions.

Table 3-1 An Integrated Health Care System Continuum

	Ambulatory Care			Institutional Health Services			Home Care	
Preventive Care	Primary Care	Specialty Care	Acute Care	Subacute Care	Nursing Home Care	High-Tech Care	High-Touch Care
Health education	Medical/ pediatrics/ ob-gyn	Ambulatory surgery	General	Surgical recovery centers	Skilled nursing facilities	Infusion therapy	Home health care
Immunization	Routine diagnostics	One-day medical	Specialty	Long-term rehabilitation	Intermediate care		Home aides
Research	Patient education	Imaging centers			Personal care		Outpatient hospice
Wellness programs	Urgent care	Sports medicine		Inpatient hospice	Alzheimer's units		Transitional care
School services							
Occupational health	Outpatient rehabilitation						

Source: Adapted from Jennings, M.C., and O'Leary, S.J., The Role of Managed Care in Integrated Delivery Networks, Journal of Ambulatory Care Management, Vol. 17, No. 1, p. 42, Aspen Publishers, Inc., © 1994.

According to Jennings and O'Leary,[9] the fundamental strategy for creating a business network is the belief that organizations that control the entire production process benefit economically. For health care systems, the fundamental strategy is much more complex and includes a responsibility for the community it serves. The health care strategy constitutes the extent to which the system can put together an integrated service continuum in a way that promotes continuity, coordination, and wellness in a cost-effective manner.

The integration and coordination of a diverse industry such as health care is a major challenge for all health care executives, including the hospital nurse executive. The nursing delivery models for integrating the entire continuum of care at the system level have yet to emerge.

SURROGATE TERMS

The integrated health care system's organizational form follows its function and as such, may be configured in a variety of models depending on the community or population it serves. As integrated health care systems emerge, an evolving continuum of system integration exists, ranging from loose affiliations health care systems that are more fully integrated. Just as stand-alone hospitals are fading, so is the familiar name. The various configurations of integrated health care systems are referred to by a variety of names.

In the fully integrated health care systems, providers, hospitals, and health insurance plans are balanced by common management and financial incentives so they can match health care resources with the needs of payers and patients.[35] The fully integrated health care systems are referred to as organized delivery systems, regional networks, integrated service networks, and community-based health care organizations. They are also commonly called vertically integrated systems.

A vertically integrated system, defined by Conrad and Dowling,[22] predates definitions of integrated health care systems. The attributes are essentially the same:

> . . . an arrangement whereby a health care organization (or closely related group or organizations) offers, either directly or through others, a broad range of patient care and support services operated in a functionally unified manner.[11(p.10)]

Although the traditional notion of vertically integrated systems relates to a full range of services, they might offer a range of services related solely to a specialized area such as cancer, cardiac disease, or mental health care.[22] In addition, vertical integration lacks the explicit reference to risk and clinical and financial accountability.

Regional networks are more fully integrated health care systems, where individuals who reside in rural communities receive primary, chronic, obstetric, and emergency care services locally, while obtaining diagnostic, secondary, and tertiary treatments at geographically distant locales.[14] Ackerman[21] refers to community-based health care organizations. He considers these as integrated health care systems that are regional in scope and that serve a geographically defined population. These systems offer a comprehensive continuum of care and ensure health care access to the community.

The more loosely aligned integrated health care systems are referred to as provider-hospital organizations, economically integrated primary care groups, hospital-owned practices, clinics without walls, group practices, and provider alliances. These models are considered by some to be transitional and eventually will mature into a more fully integrated system. Others believe the loosely aligned models are good ends in and of themselves and need not evolve into more complex organizations.[36]

As the health care marketplace continues to drive reorganization and transformation, new forms of integrated health care systems will emerge. The definitive position of the nurse executive of an integrated health care system and member hospitals has not been specified as yet in this rapidly changing environment.

ATTRIBUTES OF INTEGRATED HEALTH CARE SYSTEMS

HSIS reports identify several organizational attributes of integrated delivery systems.[17,37] While the purpose of the study is to evaluate integrated health care systems, the unit of analysis in the research reports is the hospital. This is an indication that although the participating organizations consider themselves an integrated health care system, they are not yet functioning as one. The findings of the HSIS should be interpreted cautiously. The identified attributes are:

- presence of a new management culture
- ability to conduct population-based needs assessments
- clinically integrated patient care management systems
- technology management systems
- continuous improvement processes
- information system linkages
- use of incentive systems

New Management Culture

Integrated health care systems are characterized by a management culture that emphasizes managing across boundaries.[17,37–38] Creating a health care system with no boundaries, in which care is seamless across the health care continuum, emphasizes a culture that manages across episodes of illness and, more important, across pathways of wellness.[17] Although nurse case management models and critical pathways are established strategies that successfully manage patient outcomes across pathways of illness, models to manage across pathways of wellness present new avenues and opportunities for nursing innovation.

Consistent with the goal of managing patient care across boundaries, nurse managers will also manage across departmental boundaries. Although only anecdotal evidence supports this prediction, all members of the nursing management team, from the nurse executive to first-line nurse managers, will have an increased scope of responsibilities as they manage departments and workers outside of the traditional nursing department boundaries. This includes the evening and night supervisors who, in this leaner system, may serve as the on-site administrators and nighttime pharmacists.

Some traditional nursing department head positions may be redesigned or vanish, and traditional distinctions between line and staff positions may become blurred. Unfortunately, a midlevel management downsizing goes hand in hand with the reduction of beds and staff. A positive consequence of downsizing is that often the remaining nurse managers and administrators have increased power and scope in their positions.

Physicians have more central management roles in integrated health care systems than in stand-alone hospitals.[35] Therefore, establishing collaborative and collegial relationships among physician and nurses is more important than ever before.

Ironically, four new boundaries have been identified in a seamless integrated health care system: (1) the authority boundary that determines who will lead and who will follow; (2) the task boundary that determines how the work is divided up; (3) the political boundary that defines individual and group interests; and (4) the identity boundary that defines group experiences of emotional connections and loyalties.[38]

Management of these new boundaries in integrated health care systems requires new competencies at all levels of the nurse management team. These include greater negotiation and conflict management skills, systems thinking, and team building efforts to administer the challenges of the seamless health care system effectively. It is incumbent on the nurse executive of hospitals in integrated health care systems to foster a management culture that values coordination, cooperation, understanding, and communication across all the operating units and providers.

Population-Based Needs Assessments

Understanding the needs of the community and region served is a required attribute for integrated health care systems to function effectively. This may involve an epidemiologic analysis of major employers, employees, and population groups within the area served by the system. According to Shortell and colleagues,[37] the core attribute of an integrated health care system is the focus on maintaining the wellness of the community and not on merely filling beds.

Understanding the needs of the community should not be difficult for most nurse executives. Nurse executives have always had a broad focus, responsible for the quality of care delivered within the entire institution. In the new context of integrated health care systems, nurse executives must help nurses understand their role as public servants and accept the challenge of public accountability.[14]

Patient Management Systems

Integrated health care systems are characterized by specific patient management strategies. The patient care management strategies involve clinical pathways for specific predictable clinical conditions; case management for complex, unpredictable patient conditions; and monitoring and feedback mechanisms. The goal of these structural complements to patient care management is to create integrated systems thinking through clinical consensus and caring processes for specific illness and wellness conditions.[20] Shortell and colleagues[37] assert that the patient care management system must extend from the patient's home, to the work site, and to the various operating units of the integrated health care system.

Nurse executives may make the strongest contribution to the success of an integrated delivery system in this area. Nurse executives have major responsibility for instituting the patient care management strategies in evolving systems including merging clinical specialties and service areas while maintaining the daily delivery of patient care services.[39]

Technology Management Systems

Integrated health care systems are characterized by technology management and assessment systems that use cost/benefit analysis methodologies to prioritize technology purchases.[37] No individual system can provide all the necessary technology needed to serve its population. Strategic alliances, partnerships, and outsourcing may be needed to meet the technology needs of the system. Nurse executives will certainly be involved in these decisions.

Continuous Quality Improvement

The findings from the HSIS indicate that integrated health care systems use continuous quality improvement processes.[17] These processes are particularly useful when they are conducted across care sites and departments; are used as a mechanism to communicate the system's management culture; provide individual employees with important staff level integration tools; and emphasize the underlying processes linking departments.[37] To keep the large bureaucratic integrated health care system responsive to the rapidly changing environment, the nurse executive should use continuous quality improvement strategies and self-managing work groups to resolve issues.

Creation of Information Linkages

Electronic linkages to clinical and financial data need to connect patient and providers across the continuum of care. In more sophisticated systems, this connection links the patient's home, work setting, and all care sites in the system. The clinical management information system in an integrated health care system is a tool that is used to address important issues of practice variation and resource utilization. It is the information backbone for developing and monitoring integrated patient care management strategies.[40] Nurse executives require computer skills and an understanding of how data-driven clinical and administrative decision-support systems are used to measure outcomes of care and support the operations of an integrated health care system.

Incentive Systems

Integrated health care systems use incentive programs that reward providers and managers for systems thinking and activity. Financial incentives are used to control costs and systems utilization.[35] Although not all incentives used by a nurse executive are financial, rewarding system thinking for managing change and the inevitable conflicts is important for successful nursing divisions in integrated health care systems.

Other attributes of integrated health care systems not mentioned in the HSIS are autonomous work teams, self-designed organizations, blurred boundaries, and teamwork at the executive level. The dynamic nature of the health care environment requires organizational attributes that enhance "structural fluidity" to maintain flexibility and responsiveness as these large, bureaucratic, integrated health care systems evolve.[41]

Some attributes of emerging systems can impede development into a fully integrated health care system.[1,17,37,41] These attributes are described as (1) the inability to move beyond the acute care paradigm of the hospital;[37,42] (2) the inability to reorganize across a service continuum rather than around functions;[41] (3) the inability to right-size the system, which includes determination of the appropriate size of the acute care hospital and the extent to which patient care can be appropriately integrated within a geographic area;[37] and (4) an inability to develop or invest in information systems that provide the glue linking the system parts.[37,41]

FORERUNNER HOSPITAL SYSTEMS

No health care system in the world has seen as many structural changes as has that of the United States.[42] Despite the seemingly chronic turbulence, the acute care hospital is undergoing yet another phase of rapid and fundamental change. The American health care system is transforming into a mosaic of partnerships, networks, and alliances.

Some of the earliest systems in health care, developed 15 to 20 years ago, were chains of acute care hospitals. Horizontally integrated hospital systems were designed to achieve economies of scale in joint purchasing, to operate efficiently by sharing information systems, corporate management, and clinical technology, and to enhance access to capital. These systems were formed as a defense against an increasingly hostile reimbursement environment and were health care systems that did not add to the net health status of the population they served. There was no incentive to improve the health of the communities served, and in an intensely personal human services industry, the primary moving force behind the creation of these early horizontally integrated systems was economic gain.[42]

The organizational form of hospitals has evolved from stand-alone facilities, to members of horizontal systems, and now, to participants in integrated health care systems. Traditionally, the hospital has been considered the centerpiece of the American health care system. There is no agreement as to its future position in integrated systems. Some experts believe that changes in the health care marketplace will push the hospital to the margins of the system, whereas others believe that the health care delivery system of the twenty-first century will remain centered around the hospital, albeit in vertically integrated systems where acute care beds play only a modest role.[43]

Some experts assert that future integrated health care systems are unlikely to be hospital-dominated and that hospitals will evolve into expensive cost centers in larger, more profitable systems.[1,3]

Membership in the top executive team of integrated health care systems is uncertain, particularly as it involves hospital nurse executives. Because nursing care is the primary service provided by hospitals, the transformation to integrated delivery systems requires the participation of the hospital nurse executive at the corporate decision-making table. The hospital nurse executive is a systemwide thinker by job design, with deep roots in community and primary care. Whether the hospital nurse executive is present as chief nursing officer of either the system or a member hospital depends on the organizational model. Regardless of the model, the nurse executive needs to be a member of the executive decision-making team.

MODEL SYSTEMS

Many innovative models of integrated health care systems have evolved, ranging from loosely to fully integrated. Each model seeks to place providers who align with each other into a better position to deal with today's health care marketplace.[16] One of the biggest challenges for integrated health care systems is to develop a primary care practice capability with appropriate backup support from specialists.[17]

The option to own versus the option to partner with the primary care practices and other network organizations is another challenge. Some health care strategists predict that integrated health care systems that form partnerships will out-perform those systems that own all the parts because they will deliver higher-quality care for less cost, will be more responsive to managed care organizations and patients, and will be less bureaucratic.[44] The variety of components in a vertically integrated health care system is so technically and culturally different that the diversity may be impossible for one executive team to manage.

Shortell[1] describes five models of integrated service delivery: generic, hospital-led, physician-led, hybrid hospital/physician-led, and insurance-company-led. These models are fully integrated health care systems on the integration continuum. Their features are summarized in Table 3-2.

Riley[16] identifies eight emerging models of integrated health care systems: the management service bureau, group practice without walls, the open and closed physician-hospital organization, the comprehensive medical service organization, the foundation model, the staff model, and the equity model. These models are loosely affiliated health care systems on the integration continuum. A description of each model is summarized in Table 3-3.

Table 3-2 Models of Fully Integrated Health Care Delivery Systems

Model	Description
Generic model	Has an enrolled population that has insurance coverage for a defined set of benefits. The enrolled population receives care from an integrated health care system that serves as the organizational hub for a variety of providers at all stages along the continuum of care. This model is reimbursed via arrangements ranging from fee-for-service to capitation.
Hospital-led model	The most popular model in existence due to the existing financial, organizational, and leadership resources and expertise of these systems. These advantages can be reduced by the inability of the system to change the acute care paradigm of filling hospital beds and feeding the cash cow (the hospital). Whether the model is affiliated with or owns an insurance product (e.g., a managed care organization) depends on the costs and incentives involved.
Physician-led model	Physician-providers own or lease hospital beds in the system. The physician-provider organization accepts clinical and fiscal responsibility for a group of enrolled lives, therefore is incented to be cost-effective. The disadvantage to this model is that physician groups do not have sufficient size, capital reserves, or organizational/managerial expertise to run an integrated health care system.
Hybrid hospital/ physician-led model	Combines the features of the hospital and physician-led models by creating physician-hospital organizations (PHOs) for purposes of aligning hospital and physician economic interests in pursuing managed care contracts. This model has many advantages through the combination of hospital resources and leadership expertise with the clinical component of physician-providers.
Insurance-company- led model	Likely to dominate in health care markets with no hospital- or physician-led systems. Insurance companies bring the advantages of actuarial expertise, claims administration, and marketing experience. They also provide a direct conduit of enrolled lives to providers in the system. A potential disadvantage has been identified as a lack of understanding of the provider side of health care and the intricate network of professional and institutional relationships that must be maintained.

ORGANIZATIONAL OUTCOMES

The organizational outcomes of integrated health care systems will be measured specifically by the improvement in the health and well-being of the population served relative to the costs incurred. As advances are made in outcome research methodologies, integrated health care systems will endure unprecedented accountability for cost and quality. In addition, the managed

Table 3-3 Models of Emerging Integrated Health Care Delivery Systems

Model	Description
Management service bureau	Physicians purchase practice services from a hospital subsidiary while retaining complete clinical and financial autonomy. Each physician contracts with the service bureau for desired services and pays fair market value for these services.
Physician-hospital organization (PHO)	The open PHO is open to all medical staff members. There is no selection or inclusion criteria for this model. The PHO has equal representation from the hospital and the physician groups. The PHO negotiates payer contracts; however, the physicians retain 100 percent ownership of their practices, controlling income and revenue streams. The closed PHO is membership selective and offered only to physicians that deliver high-quality, cost-effective care.
Comprehensive medical service organization (MSO)	Provides management services for payment of fair market price by physicians. An MSO purchases group practice assets, manages practices, and negotiates managed care contracts while the physician group maintains separate legal identity and retains ownership over its revenue stream.
Foundation model	A tax-exempt, nonprofit subsidiary of the health system that purchases physician practices. The physician practices retain separate corporate and legal structures but the revenue comes from the system. The foundation markets to and negotiates with payers.
Group practice without walls	Independent providers form a loose alliance (typically with no hospital involvement) to share overhead costs and negotiate payer contracts. Practice revenues are owned by individual physicians. A central administration staff negotiates with payers.
Staff model	Providers are direct employees of the system. Physicians are typically organized like a clinic with its own governance structure. The system markets to and negotiates with payers and owns all revenues.
Equity model	Providers are employees of the system but are given the opportunity to purchase equity in the system after several years. The system either owns or contracts with the hospital to provide inpatient services. The group practice markets to and negotiates with payers; the system owns all contract revenues.

care organizations will require objective demonstration of the health status of the community served by the system.

Assessing these complex systems requires a shift in thinking from the hospital level to the system level. For example, a care site, such as an acute care hospital, must not only be viewed in terms of its individual performance, but also in terms of how and what it contributes to the system as a whole. Effective outcomes research requires comparability and compatibility of appropriate data. The diversity of organizational operating units performing unique tasks raises challenging research methodology issues.

Clinical integration at the system level is only in the evolutionary stage. Devers and colleagues[15] are assessing integrated health care systems based on how patient care services are coordinated clinically across operating system units in the following ways:

- number of and extent to which clinical pathways are used in the system
- extent to which medical records are uniform and accessible across the system
- extent to which uniform clinical outcomes are collected and shared across all care sites
- extent of shared programming and planning efforts
- extent of shared clinical support services
- number of shared clinical service lines

As outcomes research methodologies become more sophisticated, it will be possible to identify areas of greatest leverage for achieving integrated care over the health care continuum. The challenge for nurse executives is to find appropriate ways to include nursing in these research efforts. Administrative billing data, often used for outcomes research, do not contain appropriate data to capture and measure nursing's marginal contribution to patient outcomes in an integrated system of health care delivery.

CHALLENGES AND OPPORTUNITIES FOR NURSE EXECUTIVES

Nurse executives in hospitals of evolving integrated delivery systems are confronted with unprecedented challenges within the hospital and within the evolving systems. Knowledge about the context, structure, and functions at the hospital level and the system level and the impact on nursing provides an important foundation for organizational decisions such as the design of case management models. Today's hospital nurse executive must strike a balance between the new values of the lean, and sometimes mean, integrated delivery system and the traditional values of nursing. Case management models have great potential to meet the new challenges of managed care and integrated health care systems.

Traditional concerns, such as rising health care costs, the growing elderly population, the technology explosion, and human resource issues are now combined with new demands for integration and coordination. At the macro-organizational level, fully integrated systems are complemented by case management models at the patient-care level. Hospital nurse executives will facilitate a familiar case management process; assessing, coordinating, and analyzing the delivery of health care. However, in a managed care environment, the emphasis will be on doing this for communities and populations of people. The expanded focus of integrated health care systems requires new partnerships, including those with health care teams from other organizations, occupational and school health programs, community committees, and social service organizations.

Nurse executives preparing for this system level of participation and those developing case management models require information related to sponsorship, governance, financing, organization, communication, and management.[14] The specific questions are summarized in Table 3-4. For example, a case management model in a system that is solely owned and operated, will be quite different from the model in the system that is in partnership with the

Table 3-4 Essential Issues and Questions for Hospital Nurse Executives

Issue	Questions
Sponsorship	Will the system have one type of owner or mixed group that includes public, private, and religious organizations?
	Will the system be owned or will there be a partnership?
	Will the partners develop a shared mission and how?
Governance	Will the system have one board or several boards that represent each care site within the system?
	In what way will the board(s) approach operating policies, fiduciary responsibilities, community participation, and clinical expertise at each care site?
Financing	Will there be one financial officer who shapes policy to negotiate on behalf of the system?
	What models will be used for evaluating patient care delivery systems?
	Who ensures financial viability for each care site within the system and the system as a whole?
Organization	Will the structure of the system be centralized or decentralized?
	How will each care site or organization within the system address planning, marketing, and clinical services?
Communication	What will be the mechanism for communication within the system?
	How will care providers and consumers in the system be integrated into the system in a way that facilitates communication?
Management	Will the management structure of the system allow each organization to continue its current management practices while treating system issues in a new fashion?
	Will the management structures change to serve the system?

Source: Adapted from Beyers, M., Health Care Networks: Public Policy and the Nurse Administrator, *Nursing Policy Forum,* Vol. 1, pp. 28–33, with permission of Nex-Wolfe Publishing, © 1995.

member organizations and care sites. Successful nurse executives will be well informed and articulate about the health care needs of the population served by the system, the organizational structure, the community, and the financial resources available. At the decision-making table, nurse executives may be involved in conducting and evaluating population needs assessments; creating new management cultures, information linkages, and patient management systems; and designing incentive systems. Although managing the bottom line is more important than ever, successful organizational outcomes will come from the service level at which clinical integration is a reality. It is at this level that nursing and case management models may make the most notable contribution.

CONCLUSION

Despite national debate, health care reorganization is occurring without national legislation. Accepting the charge to design and implement integrated health care systems creates unprecedented opportunities for nurses to address the health care needs of the American people by creating new care delivery models for patients and new practice environments for nurses.

Nurse executives must forge a future and create a strategic plan that charts a direction for hospital nursing at a new level: the system level. The plan must include clinical integration strategies and development of new technologies for improved information sharing and minimize fragmentation and duplication of effort. As a new frontier in health care emerges, nurse executives in integrated health care systems are trailblazers embroiled at the forefront, leading the way to an American dream—cost-effective coordinated health care that is accessible to all.

REFERENCES

1. Shortell SM. The challenges of health care reform: creating organized delivery systems. Presented at *Integrated Service Networks under Health Care Reform: Theory and Practice,* March 9, 1994, Washington, D.C.

2. Cerne F. The fading stand-alone hospital. *Hosp Health Networks.* 1994;2:28–32.

3. Higgins CW, Meyers ED. Managed care and vertical integration: implications for the hospital industry. *Hosp Health Serv Adm.* 1987;32:319–327.

4. Buerhaus PI. Managed competition and critical issues facing nurses. *Nurs Health Care.* 1994;15(1):22–26.

5. Iglehart JK. Rapid changes for academic health centers. *N Eng J Med.* 1995;332:407–411.

6. Enthoven AC. The history and principles of managed competition. *Health Affairs.* 1993;3(suppl):24–48.

7. Teisberg EO, Porter ME, Brown GB. Making competition in health care work. *Harv Bus Rev.* 1994;72:131–141.

8. Coile RC. *The New Governance Strategies for an Era of Health Reform.* Ann Arbor, Michigan: American College of Healthcare Executives; 1994.

9. Jennings MC, O'Leary SJ. The role of managed care in integrated delivery networks. *J Amb Care Manage.* 1994;17:39–47.

10. Buerhaus PI. Economics of managed competition and consequences to nurses: part II. *Nurs Econ.* 1994;12:79–80,106.

11. American Hospital Association. A dog day rebound. *Hosp Health Networks.* 1995;69(2):70.

12. Kania AJ. Hospital systems cluster programs and services. *Health Care Strategic Manage.* 1993;11(7):1,20–23.

13. Stichler JF. System development and integration in healthcare. *J Nurs Adm.* 1994;24(10): 48–53.

14. Beyers M. Health care networks: public policy and the nurse administrator. *Nurs Policy Forum.* 1995;1(1):28–33.

15. Devers KJ, Shortell SM, Gillies RR, et al. Implementing organized delivery systems: an integration scorecard. *Health Care Manage Rev.* 1994;19:7–20.

16. Riley DW. Integrated health care systems: emerging models. *Nurs Econ.* 1994;12:201–206.

17. Shortell SM, Gillies RR, Anderson DA, et al. Creating organized delivery systems: the barriers and facilitators. *Hosp Health Serv Adm.* 1993;38:447–466.

18. Charns MP, Tewksbury LJ. *Collaborative Management in Health Care: Implementing the Integrative Organization.* San Francisco: Jossey-Bass; 1993.

19. Gillies RR, Shortell SM, Anderson DA, et al. Conceptualizing and measuring integration: findings from the Health Systems Integration Study. *Hosp Health Serv Adm.* 1993;38:467–489.

20. Conrad DA. Coordinating patient care services in regional health systems: the challenge of clinical integration. *Hosp Health Serv Adm.* 1993;4:491–508.

21. Ackerman FK. The movement toward vertically integrated regional health systems. *Health Care Manage Rev.* 1992;17:81–88.

22. Conrad DA, Dowling WL. Vertical integration in health services: theory and managerial implications. *Health Care Manage Rev.* 1990;15:9–22.

23. Foxe WL. Vertical integration strategies: more promising than diversification. *Health Care Manage Rev.* 1989;14:49–56.

24. Bower KA. *Case Management by Nurses.* Washington, DC: American Nurses Publishing; 1992.

25. Ethridge P, Lamb GS. Professional nursing case management improves quality, access, and costs. *Nurs Manage.* 1989;20(3):30–35.

26. Migchelbrink D, Anderson D, Schultz P, et al. Population based care: one hospital's experience. *Nurs Adm Q.* 1993;17:45–53.

27. Rosenbloom AL. A public/private partnership providing an integrated system of health care for children: the children's medical services program of Florida. *Clin Pediatr.* 1993;32:597–600.

28. Schroeder C, Maeve KM. Nursing care partnerships at the Denver nursing project in human caring: an application and extension of caring theory in practice. *Adv Nurs Sci.* 1992;15(2):25–38.

29. Wolfe C. A model system: integration of services for cancer treatment. *Cancer Supplement*. 1993;72:3525–3530.

30. Zander K. Nursing case management: strategic management of cost and quality outcomes. *J Nurs Adm*. 1988;18(5):23–30.

31. Hampton DC. Implementing a managed care framework through care maps. *J Nurs Adm*. 1993;23(5):21–27.

32. Zander K. Care maps: the core of cost/quality-care. *New Definition*. 1991;6(3):1–3.

33. Zander K, McGill R. Critical and anticipated recovery paths: only the beginning. *Nurs Manage*. 1994;25(8):34–40.

34. DeMunro PR. Provider alliances: key to healthcare reform. *Health Care Financial Manage*. 1994;15:27–32.

35. Coddington DC, Moore KD, Fischer EA. Costs and benefits of integrated healthcare systems. *Healthcare Financial Manage*. 1994;15:21–29.

36. Hudson T. A model for integration? *Hosp Health Networks*. 1994;68(10):52–56.

37. Shortell SM, Gillies RR, Anderson DA, et al. The holographic organization. *Healthcare Forum J*. 1993;36(2):20–26.

38. Gilmore TN, Hirschhorn L, O'Connor M. The boundaryless organization. *Healthcare Forum J*. 1994;37(4):68–72.

39. Singleton EK, Nail-Hall FC. Charting the course for merger: key concepts for nurse executives. *J Nurs Adm*. 1995;25(5):47–54.

40. McMahon LF, Eward AM, Bernard AM, et al. The integrated inpatient management model's clinical management information system. *Hosp Health Serv Adm*. 1994;39:81–92.

41. Beckham JD. The architecture of integration. *Healthcare Forum J*. 1993;36:56–63.

42. Shortell SM. The evolution of hospital systems: unfulfilled promises and self-fulfilling prophesies. *Med Care Rev*. 1988;45:177–214.

43. Robinson JC. The changing boundaries of the American hospital. *Milbank Q*. 1994;72:259–275.

44. Johnson DEL. Vertical integration may be the most expensive strategy. *Health Care Strategic Manage*. 1993;11(10):2–3.

■ 4 ■

Developing a Successful Hospital Case Management System

David Bach, MD, Carolyn Hope Smeltzer, EdD, MSN, RN, FAAN, FACHE,
and Allen J. Baler, BA

Hospital case management is a system used to manage and coordinate a hospital's clinical care process to optimize quality, service, and clinical efficiency for patients. A typical hospital's case management system includes staff physicians, nurses, social workers, utilization review and discharge planning representatives, and admitting and medical records departments. This chapter describes the history of hospital-based case management, explores the key elements of successful case management systems, and proposes an action plan for creating an effective case management program in "traditional" hospital environments.

HISTORY

Hospitals have historically encountered many barriers to the development of effective case management systems. The fragmented U.S. health care delivery system created one of these barriers by limiting hospitals' ability to "manage" health care services they do not control. For example, the financial and organizational independence of physicians from hospitals has made it difficult for hospitals to integrate physicians, who are at the core of the clinical care delivery process, into case management development efforts. Similarly, the organizational independence of alternative care delivery sites (e.g., nursing homes, home care agencies) from hospitals has limited each hospital's ability to manage care outside the hospital's walls.

Traditional health care reimbursement systems created another obstacle to the development of case management in hospitals. Beginning with fee-for-service payment systems, and partially continuing with the diagnosis-related group (DRG) system of the early 1980s, health care reimbursement in the United States has financially motivated providers to overuse clinical resources.

This has limited the strategic value of case management for hospitals because case management tends to generate clinical efficiency and therefore reduce hospital revenues.

The growth of managed care in the early 1990s, for the first time in U.S. history, created both an opportunity and an incentive for hospitals to develop effective case management programs. Two particular features of managed care systems—channeling and capitation—have had particular impact in encouraging the growth of hospital case management.

Channeling is the process of directing patients to preferred providers (e.g., hospitals, physicians, nursing homes). Recently, managed care payers in many U.S. markets have begun channeling patients to a defined group of providers, called a panel. One of the most important criteria to determine inclusion or exclusion of providers from panels is utilization rates. Providers who profited from relatively high utilization rates in the past now face the specter of exclusion from payer panels—a potential loss of patients and revenue. The desire to join panels, coupled with the fear of being excluded, creates a strong incentive for providers to create clinically efficient care processes and has therefore increased the strategic value of case management for hospitals.

The second characteristic of managed care that promotes case management development is the growth of capitation-based payment systems. Capitation puts providers at risk for patient care costs by prospectively paying them fixed amounts of money to care for defined patient populations. Most providers today still receive the bulk of their reimbursement from fee-for-service-type arrangements. However, many providers now anticipate that they will be operating under capitation in the near future. This expectation of capitation has stimulated case management development in two important ways. First, it has encouraged the development of "integrated" delivery systems capable of accepting risk (as evidenced by the recent growth of physician-hospital organizations [PHOs]), thus implying the need for case management. Second, by markedly reducing the incentive for providers to overuse services and, in fact, motivating the pursuit of clinical efficiency, capitation has established the strategic value of case management for hospitals.

Given the new strategic imperative for case management, hospitals are now grappling with two critical questions: What is required for effective hospital case management? and, How do we get there? This chapter answers these two questions.

REQUIREMENTS FOR EFFECTIVE HOSPITAL CASE MANAGEMENT

Successful hospital case management requires a shared organizationwide mandate and vision for the role of case management in the care delivery process, accessible and reliable performance data, an appropriate organizational structure, aligned incentives between physicians and hospitals, and well-defined clinical care guidelines (Exhibit 4-1).

An Organizational Mandate

Effective case management requires a fundamental redesign in the way that hospitals operate and deliver care. This cannot be accomplished in the absence of a clear organizational commitment to case management and a willingness to redesign operating systems in line with the critical success factors for implementing case management. To be effective, therefore, case management must be seen as a critical strategic priority by both administrative and physician leadership in a hospital.

A Shared Organizational Vision

Case management means different things to different people. Physicians often believe that case management describes the physician's role in overseeing the care of patients. Insurance companies have largely defined case management as a nurse's role oriented toward reducing clinical utilization rates. The nursing community, largely guided by Karen Zander, has developed a vision of case management that also involves a designated nurse case manager chartered with implementing "critical paths." Social workers, utilization review nurses, quality assurance departments, and finance departments similarly have their own perspectives on what case management is and how its success should be measured.

For a hospital's case management system to be effective, it is critical that all constituents share a common vision of case management. Hospital staff need to understand the goals for case management, the respective roles for individuals involved in case management, and the criteria for measuring the program's success. The goals, structure, and success measures for a case management

---

Exhibit 4-1 Requirements for Effective Hospital Case Management

Organizational mandate for effective case management
Shared organizational vision
Meaningful performance data
Appropriate organizational structure
Cultural and financial alignment between physicians and hospitals
Clinical care guidelines

system may vary, of course, depending on individual hospital environments. However, in all cases, a common vision of case management is vital.

Meaningful Performance Data

Effective case management systems generally require extensive data and effective methods to get data. Compelling data are required, for example, to support clinical guideline development efforts, inform clinicians about current versus expected utilization patterns, and track clinical and operational outcomes. In addition, data from case management systems are needed to inform a variety of programmatic decisions for hospitals in areas ranging from pricing to physician credentialling to physician compensation.

Data are used in case management systems to answer two questions:

1. Where do we need to improve, and by how much?

Macrolevel measures of utilization and quality (e.g., total costs, length of stay [LOS], specialist referral volumes, ancillary test volumes, patient satisfaction, mortality rates) are the core of any case management program. They inform providers about where to focus their improvement efforts and how much they need to improve. These performance measures (versus aggressive benchmarks) should be profiled at many levels within a hospital including:

- individual physician groups
- individual physicians
- individual patient populations with either unique demographic (e.g., payer) or clinical (e.g., diagnosis) characteristics

These data must be presented in compelling ways, drawing attention toward core findings and motivating behavior change.

Accurate data collection and rigorous risk adjustment of macrolevel utilization data (which allow for comparisons among dissimilar patient populations based on patient demographic and/or clinical data) are needed to determine where to focus specific clinical improvement efforts and how much improvement to seek.

2. How can we change to improve our outcomes?

Data that can be used in this regard include:

- data identifying variations in the process of care for defined diagnoses within an institution (e.g., among various providers). For example, for surgical procedure Y, one could profile individual physicians based on percentage of cases performed inpatient versus out-patient, perioperative antibiotic choice, types of surgical instrumen-tation used, and time elapsed between incision and closure.

- data identifying variations between institutions in the process of care used for defined diagnoses. Here one can use data similar to that described above, as well as more high-level information (e.g., overall LOS, costs).

- data documenting providers' adherence to institutional clinical guidelines. This topic is described in more detail below.

- chart review data showing "potentially avoidable" service utiliza-tion by physician. For example, one case management department known by the authors gives physicians a monthly report on their "potentially avoidable" hospital days, by patient and by cause.

Information systems must have several data elements and the capability to generate the above-listed outputs. Key data elements include patient's demographics, principal diagnoses and comorbid conditions (by time they were identified) to allow for the creation of meaningful patient clusters, all clinical transactions (e.g., chest x-ray, rehabilitation consult) that were made for patients with accurate volumes and dates, definition of which physicians were accountable for which clinical transactions, and a cost allo-cation system that accurately identifies the cost of defined clinical transac-tions. Clinical data (e.g., from the laboratory or radiology) significantly im-prove an organization's ability to perform meaningful risk adjustments within and among patient cohorts. Note that all data should be collected for patients longitudinally, through multiple sites of care, to allow for meaningful profiling beyond the episode level.

An Appropriate Organizational Structure

Too often, even in advanced managed care markets, case management is viewed as either "the medical director's job" or "a nursing function." To be effective, case management must be conceived of as a core institutional func-tion in which all members of the care team participate.

Three organizational approaches in particular are effective ways to make case management part of the fabric of an organization:

1. Centralized accountability and authority

It often makes sense to create centralized accountability and authority for an institution's case management, generally with a respected physi-cian. In theory, centralized case management accountability and authority already exist in most organizations in either the medical director's office or the nursing department. In practice, however, few medical directors or nursing directors have either the organizational mandate or the resources available to effect practice pattern change. At minimum, the individual responsible for clinical resource management should be empowered both to influence operational functions in response to clinical needs (e.g., we need weekend coverage of service X, we need to open operating room [OR] 3 tomorrow morning) and to reward and punish physicians (e.g., through salary determination or credentialing). Case management functions (e.g., social work, utilization review) should report (at least in a matrix fashion) to this individual.

2. Product line organization and management roles

Hospitals have traditionally managed their operations by controlling departmental or patient care unit performance. Managers are given control over specific departments or patient care units. Budgets are oriented around specific departments and patient care units.

This perspective is not consistent with the needs of case management. Case management requires that operations are understood in terms of activities affecting specific patient groups, rather than departments or inpatient care units. An orthopedic surgeon, for example, is more interested in understanding the "whole costs" incurred by total joint replacement patients than costs available by examining a traditional health care organization's budget. Whole costs for a joint replacement patient include preoperative costs (including physician fees and laboratory testing fees) and operative costs including physician fees, OR supplies, and OR time. Inpatient costs include physician fees, postoperative nursing care, laboratory testing, and physical therapy; and postoperative costs including rehabilitation and/or home care. Similarly, the surgeon would want to evaluate care quality based on outcomes specific to patient groups (e.g., functional status of joint replacement patients) rather than institutionwide quality measures (e.g., medication error rate).

To make case management a core part of an organization, the traditional operations perspective (departments and care units) must be merged with the case management perspective (patient groups). Management structures and cost accounting systems and budgets should be partially redesigned around defined clinical groupings. Product line management positions can be created in which specific individuals are given both accountability and authority to manage the care of specific patient groups. Financial systems can be modified so that they track services and/or costs associated with specific patient groups (e.g., how many x-rays the average heart failure patient receives). These systems ideally should span the full continuum of patient care services. Similarly, budgets can be created so that overall revenues and costs associated with individual patients are tracked and managed.

3. Clear roles for members of the case management team

An effective case management program system involves several individuals including data analysts, social workers, nurses, and physicians. Case management is not, and cannot be, the function of a single individual.

Functions generally included in case management are clinical decision making, implementing the clinical care plan, identifying and fixing operational bottlenecks that prevent effective and efficient care, and collecting and disseminating data on clinical efficiency and quality.

Many compelling operating models for case management exist. The right model for an individual hospital depends on the program's goals as well as the hospital's history, culture, and market environment. Whatever model a hospital chooses to use for case management, however, individual roles of the case management team members must be clearly defined and any overlap in responsibilities must be meticulously avoided.

Cultural and Financial Alignment between Physicians and Hospitals

Physicians typically operate under a distinctly separate set of financial incentives and cultural norms than do the employees of most hospitals. Physicians generally bill for their services separately from hospitals and have financial incentives that are not consistent with those of hospitals.

Even the few but growing numbers of physicians who are employed by hospitals have little in common with their employers, and they share few incentives to support case management. Residents, and the content and structure of their training programs, although paid for by hospitals, are generally considered "out of bounds" for hospital administrators. Eliciting meaningful resident participation in case management efforts is therefore difficult. Generally, physicians are culturally more aligned with the "medical profession" and their specialist colleagues than they are with individual provider organizations.

One of the most important and challenging elements of case management, therefore, is creating cultural and financial alignment between hospitals and physicians so that true partnership between these two important constituencies can be attained. The next section of this chapter includes a discussion of how a

traditional hospital's physician culture can be changed to support the requirements of case management. Approaches that can be used to align financial
incentives between hospitals and physicians have been described extensively in
the managed care literature and are not included in this chapter.

CREATING AN EFFECTIVE CASE MANAGEMENT PROGRAM

There are several process steps that we have found useful in creating an
effective case management program in traditional hospital environments:

1. Create an organizational mandate for case management, beginning
   with physicians.
2. Invest aggressively in data support systems.
3. Blow up an ineffective and incomplete current "case management" system and use a physician-led process to create a new one (a completely
   fresh start is more effective than tinkering with a broken system).
4. Aggressively create and implement new clinical guidelines.
5. Track and publicize progress against defined goals.

The first step is the most challenging and important—creating an organizational mandate, led by physicians, for case management. To achieve meaningful and sustainable improvements in clinical practice patterns within an
organization, particularly in aggressively managed markets, the organization's practicing physicians and nurses must be motivated to "own" the efforts to redesign clinical care. These clinicians will make the day-to-day decisions that will either generate superior utilization or not. When nurses and
practicing physicians become strong advocates for case management, they
bring a wealth of innovative and practical ideas to the effort that make quantum improvements possible.

Most hospitals find that steps two through five described above are readily
achievable when an appropriate physician culture is present. As such, this
section of the chapter focuses on how to change a traditional hospital's clinical culture in keeping with the needs of case management.

The vast majority of U.S. physicians today have few financial or organizational incentives to support hospital-based case management efforts. Approaches to modify physicians' financial or organizational incentives (e.g.,
capitation or creation of PHOs) have been described extensively in the managed care literature and are not included in this chapter.

To change physician culture effectively, regardless of the financial or organizational realities under which physicians operate, an organization must develop a thorough communication plan (Exhibit 4-2), which includes the processes detailed in the remainder of this chapter.

Craft a Compelling Message for Physicians

Depending on a hospital's market and pre-existing physician culture, a variety of messages can be used effectively to enroll physicians in improvement efforts. Among the messages that various institutions have successfully chosen to engender physician participation are:

1. "We [the institution] are in trouble and we need you [the physicians] to help us."
2. "Our vision is to create the country's best health care institution; we need to work together to do this."
3. "We [both the institution and physicians] are in danger from managed care. We need to work together to respond effectively to this threat."
4. "We [the institution and physicians] have an opportunity to expand our market by becoming the most cost-effective network."
5. "Today, you [the physicians] have the opportunity to manage your own destiny, and take back control of the health care system. If you do not capture this opportunity, however, the market will redesign the system without you."

However framed, the message must compellingly motivate physician commitment to clinical efficiency improvement efforts.

Exhibit 4-2 Communication Plan

1. Craft a compelling message for physicians describing why their commitment to clinical improvement efforts is critical
2. Start by selling the message to formal and informal leaders in the clinical community
3. Get the message out, repeatedly, to the rest of the clinical staff
4. Use interesting data to support the case
5. Once physicians are committed to clinical improvement, work with the physicians to develop a joint approach to case management

Sell the Message to Leaders in the Clinical Community

In most physician communities, there is a core of leaders, both formal and informal, who command the respect of their physician colleagues. At times, nonphysicians who have earned credibility over time with physicians can be part of this core.

It is valuable to earn the allegiance of this core leadership group at the outset of a physician culture change effort. When bought into the process, this core group will both motivate their colleagues to join the effort and defuse tensions that may arise from other physicians who resist change.

Get the Message Out

A variety of physician and clinician forums, both formal and informal, exist within any institution. The message created to motivate nurse and physician participation in improvement efforts must be disseminated repeatedly through each of these forums. Often the best people to communicate the message in these forums are members of the core group described above.

Physician culture change does not occur as a result of a single presentation of a message, no matter how compelling that message might be. It occurs over time through physicians' subconscious experience of multiple inputs from multiple directions.

Use Interesting Data To Support the Case

The use of data to inform clinical decisions is a fundamental element of medicine. As such, compelling data on clinical practice patterns for individual physicians are among the most powerful tools an organization can use to modify physician behavior.

Two types of data are useful for changing physician behavior. The first type of data illustrates to physicians *how they compare* with their peers in overall efficiency (e.g., cost per covered life, days per thousand). This type of data motivates physician behavior change essentially by "grading" physicians and stimulating them to improve their grade. Over time, the data will include effectiveness in producing outcomes rather than just efficiency in delivering care.

The second type of data profiles physicians' clinical decision-making patterns to show *how they can change* to become more efficient (e.g., "you use drug A to treat condition C, but drug B would be better because . . . "). By informing physicians about characteristics of their practice styles, many of which they were unaware, these data create behavior change through education.

Work with Physicians To Develop a Joint Approach to Case Management

Physicians are generally trained to be independent practitioners, taking individual accountability for individual patients. Teamwork, systemwide thinking, and mutual accountability are not dominant elements of most physicians' professional experience.

As physicians gain experience working in groups during education efforts, solving problems together, and basing decisions on broad data rather than anecdote, their understanding and appreciation of the value of operational, system-based thinking grows. Once a positive experience in redesigning clinical processes has been accrued, physicians' commitment to institutionwide clinical process improvement, case management in particular, naturally tends to grow.

CONCLUSION

The escalation of U.S. health care costs and the increasing fragmentation of the health care delivery system have created a national mandate for managed care systems that both reduce costs and improve quality. A fundamental requirement for effective managed care is case management systems that coordinate and oversee the clinical process of care for defined patient populations.

Hospital case management is an important starting point in the United States' evolution toward managed care. Hospital case management both improves efficiency and quality for patient care provided in the hospital setting and catalyzes the integration of previously disparate elements of the health care delivery system.

As the U.S. health care delivery system becomes increasingly integrated, hospital case management will likewise evolve into integrated delivery systemwide case management. With that evolution, new demands and challenges for case management will develop, most likely challenging many of the ideas described in this chapter but also creating exciting opportunities for optimizing the quality and efficiency of patient care processes throughout multiple delivery sites.

BIBLIOGRAPHY

Bower K. *Case Management by Nurses.* Washington, D.C.: American Publishing; 1992.

Collard A, Bergman A, Henderson M. Two approaches to measuring quality in medical case management programs. *QRB.* 1990;16(1):3–8.

Curran C. An interview with Sue Hall Esleck. *Nurs Econ.* 1995;13:7–11.

Green S, Malkemes L. Concepts of new delivery models. *J Soc Health Systems.* 1991;2:14–23.

Ling K. Initiation and evaluation of managed care at Johns Hopkins Hospital. *Nurs Adm Q.* 1993; 17(3):54–58.

Mahn V. Clinical nurse case management: a service line approach. *Nurs Manage.* 1993;24(9): 48–50.

Meisler N, Midyette P. CNS to case manager: broadening the scope. *Nurs Manage.* 1994;25(11): 44–46.

Phillips C, Carson J, Huggins C, Wade B. Care manager/nurse manager: a blending of roles. *Nurs Manage.* 1993;24(10):26–28.

Rusch S. Continuity of care: from hospital unit into home. *Nurs Manage.* 1986;17(12):38–41.

Schull D, Tosch P, Wood M. Clinical nurse specialists as collaborative care managers. *Nurs Manage.* 1992;23(5):30–33.

Smith GB. A case management false start. *Nurs Quality Connection.* 1994;3(6):5–6.

Smith GB, Danforth D, Owens P. Role restructuring: case management. *Nurs Adm Q.* 1994;19(1):21–32.

Zander K. Responsive restructuring part I. *New Definition.* 1993;8(3):1–3.

Zander K. Case management series part III. *New Definition.* 1995;10(1):1–3.

■ 5 ■

Developing and Implementing Critical Paths in Case Management

Magdalena A. Mateo, PhD, RN, FAAN
Cheryl L. Newton, MSN, RN, CCRN, CNRN
Karen K. Kanatas, BSN, RN

The case management model for care delivery focuses on providing high-quality care and achieving positive patient outcomes within a designated time frame by effectively and efficiently using resources needed by the patient during an episode of illness.[1,2] Case management is a method of organizing and providing care with an emphasis on communication among health care team members.[3,4] The success of case management is enhanced when there is buy-in from a patient care multidisciplinary team, particularly in the development and use of critical paths (CP), an essential tool in case management.

DEFINITION AND USES OF CRITICAL PATHS

A CP is a guideline highlighting key events that must occur in a timely and predictable manner to achieve an appropriate length of stay (LOS).[5] It is a multidisciplinary tool used to meet the standard of care for a patient with a specific diagnosis.[2] Because the CP provides the framework and guides patient care, it needs to be individualized to meet the unique needs of the patient and revised as changes in practice or technology occur.[6]

Items on a CP include consults, tests, treatments, diet, medications, discharge planning, patient teaching, and interventions that should occur during a patient's episode of illness in order to achieve the standard outcomes within allotted LOS for the diagnosis-related group (DRG).[7] Critical paths can be used for identifying factors that contribute to early or delayed discharge, documenting the care provided to patients, and promoting staff and patient teaching.

Factors that Contribute to Early or Delayed Discharge

The CP serves as a guide to facilitate timely patient discharge by simplifying and standardizing a plan of care for a specific population and by continually monitoring variances and outcomes.[6] A variance is defined as a deviation or an activity that is different from the CP. Variances may be positive or negative and may or may not affect the patient's LOS. An example of a positive variance is that the patient is extubated sooner than anticipated. The end result of a positive variance may be that the patient is discharged earlier.

Variances can be categorized as patient/family, care giver, and environment. Patient/family variances are related to the patient or family situation (e.g., unavailable transportation, difficulty with compliance, or knowledge deficit). Care giver variances include discharge planning or inappropriate or delayed consultation by another health care service such as physical therapy. Environmental variances, also called hospital or system variances, result from inefficiencies within the system (e.g., difficulty with test scheduling, lack of needed equipment, or bed availability). Variances should be compiled and analyzed for similarities within the categories.[2] Changes in practice, services, or the CP may be identified as a result of this tracking.[2]

Documentation

Many institutions use the CP as a multidisciplinary documentation tool. Staff members document whether interventions and goals are met on the CP. Variances or unmet goals require further documentation in a narrative format. This type of charting is known as *charting by exception*.[8] Documentation of actions to correct variances should be performed in a proactive manner.[9] A proactive approach to monitoring variances enhances the possibility of addressing issues as they arise so positive outcomes are attained.

Although CPs can be used as documentation tools, CPs are only effective if they are used by a multidisciplinary team. Consider the following questions before deciding if a CP will be used as a documentation tool.

1. Is it replacing an existing form?
2. Will it meet the documentation needs of the institution, accreditation bodies such as The Joint Commission on Accreditation of Healthcare Organizations, and third-party payer requirements?
3. Will documentation result in duplication, thereby possibly contributing to a decrease in compliance?
4. Who will be documenting on the CP form?

5. Do institutional policies and procedures have to be revised to reflect the changes in the documentation process?

Patient and Staff Education

CPs can be valuable education tools for patients and their families, nurses, physicians, and other health care team members.[7] This can be done by developing two versions of the CP—one for patients and their families and another for health team members.

Patient education CPs are written in lay language at a reading level that a patient can understand. Our institutional policy at The Ohio State University Medical Center requires that patient education materials be at a fifth- to sixth-grade reading level. Each patient receives a copy of the CP and supplemental educational materials that may be appropriate. By using the CP, the patients can track their own progress and actively participate in their care. The patients' awareness of the plan of treatment and desired outcomes can help them prepare for the care they will require after discharge from the hospital.

Health team members can use the CP to monitor a patient's progress and to orient new employees to the care of a specific patient population. Staff members can gain experience by collaborating with the multidisciplinary team to decrease cost, by assuming accountability for the aspect of care for which their discipline is responsible, and by solving problems when a patient's course of stay deviates from a CP.

DEVELOPING CRITICAL PATHS

A multidisciplinary approach to developing and implementing a CP is desirable since various disciplines are involved in the care of patients. In addition to promoting collaboration among disciplines, a multidisciplinary approach enhances the use of resources in the pursuit of quality patient care.

Multidisciplinary Committee

A multidisciplinary steering committee can facilitate the development and implementation of a CP that is applicable to all health team members (physicians, nurses, social workers, physical therapists, occupational therapists, speech therapists, nutritionists, pharmacists, and respiratory therapists) who are involved in the care of a patient. This requires careful selection of people who have clinical knowledge, leadership skills, and the ability to influence others. Responsibilities of the steering committee may include: (1) gaining organizational support; (2) establishing a plan for promoting activities related to the development of CPs, including format, guidelines for use, and revisions; (3) orienting staff to the use of CPs; and (4) evaluating the use of CPs.

It is desirable to appoint or hire a person to oversee the case management project and direct the development of CPs. The role of the project director or project manager is to assist and guide the steering committee, coordinate and facilitate CP development, serve as an educational resource and staff support, and assist with variance data analysis.[6] The project director could also facilitate the acquisition of organizational support such as off-unit time for staff, secretarial support, computer software, and determination of meeting times convenient for all committee members.

Patient Population

Identifying patients to be case managed and for whom CPs need to be developed is one of the first decisions to be made. Types of patients could be identified by using DRG, ICD-9 codes, patient diagnosis, procedure, physician, or payer groupings. Patterns of patient flow through the health care system, institutional goals for case management, patient volumes, and fiscal reports provide background information to determine patient populations that could be case managed.

Medical records and fiscal departments can assist in assessing high-acuity, high-volume, and high-cost patients and can provide information about recommended LOS reimbursement by insurance carriers.[10] It is helpful to start with patient populations that have a predictable hospital course, such as patients who undergo coronary artery bypass surgery, laminectomies, and total hip replacements. A review of the medical records of these patients would reveal treatment approaches that have contributed to positive fiscal and patient satisfaction outcomes.

Developing versus Purchasing Available Critical Paths

Once target populations are determined, the next step is to decide whether a CP will be developed or purchased. Purchasing an existing CP is preferred as long as the CP can be adapted for use in the institution. It is not unusual that purchased CPs require revision because practices among institutions vary. However, adapting or revising existing CPs could still save resources and staff time.

A review of the literature is helpful in locating different types and formats of CPs. It may also be beneficial to network with colleagues or visit institutions using the case management model and CPs. Some CPs can be purchased from institutions and organizations such as The Center for Case Management, Inc. in South Natick, Massachusetts.

Computer software programs that can be used to format or print already developed CPs are also available. Adapting CPs to the needs of an institution and its patient population is necessary because of differences that exist in technology, funding, and clinical expertise.

Because each discipline plays an important role in the plan of care and discharge planning, it is helpful to examine practices, prospectively or retrospectively, of all disciplines. Delineating the contributions of disciplines is needed to minimize role conflict and to emphasize that each discipline has a unique contribution to the care of a patient and is accountable for its practice.

Individual sections of the CP include practices known to be associated with positive patient outcomes. An advanced practice nurse such as a clinical nurse specialist or nurse practitioner may assist with the development of the CPs by laying the groundwork for the team and by assessing and reviewing current practice as well as incorporating new trends.

Format

Critical paths provide the framework for planning patient care.[10] There are four components of CPs: (1) a time line along the x-axis and multidisciplinary interventions or key indicators along the y-axis; (2) a patient problem or needs list; (3) goals that progress to clinical outcomes; and (4) a variance record.[6,11] Refer to Appendix 5-A, Exhibits 5-A-1 and 5-A-2 for examples of CPs for a patient with cerebral vascular accident (CVA). The patient education CP (Exhibit 5-A-2 in Appendix 5-A) corresponds to the CP the health care team implements. There are several differences between the patient education and health care team CPs. The patient education CP is written in lay terms and uses illustrations. Supplemental educational materials are highlighted in italics so the patient can easily identify those handouts included in a stroke notebook. This notebook is given to the patient or family on admission. A specific section for patient notes and questions replaces the variance report that appears in the health care team's CP (Exhibit 5-A-1). Patients are encouraged to use this section for any questions they may have.

The episodic time line (day 1, 2, 3) can be based on hours in the intensive care unit, days on a general nursing unit, or weeks in a rehabilitation or subacute unit. Another way to format the time line is in terms of phases of the illness such as phase I, acute phase; phase II, intermediate; and phase III, recovery or rehabilitation. This type of format is especially useful for patients with chronic illnesses, for patients in the rehabilitation or subacute settings, and for weaning chronic ventilator patients.

Although the time line may vary depending on setting or patient type, a standard format is needed. The standard format allows for some consistency within the institution, thereby facilitating use of the CP and compliance among staff.

IMPLEMENTATION OF CRITICAL PATHS

Education programs including staff responsibilities are viable approaches to enlisting everyone's support in successfully implementing CPs. During education programs, participants could help identify strategies for monitoring and promoting compliance to the use of CPs. Audiovisual aides such as posters and flyers exhibited on the unit could be used to reinforce the information that is presented at education programs.

Conducting a pilot test of a critical path being used for the first time permits the assessment of its usability. Staff members need to be asked to use a newly developed CP before it is adapted, so categories that are problematic can be revised to conform with most of the patient population.

It is important at this time to develop guidelines for CP use. Two main issues that should be addressed in the guidelines are (1) what is the time frame in which the CP needs to be initiated, and (2) who can initiate a CP? It is beneficial that a CP be initiated within 24 hours of the patient's admission; however, there may always be exceptions to this. Initiation of the CP may be the responsibility of a case manager or any member of the health care team. Guidelines help prevent duplication of effort and delineate responsibility. The guidelines should also include information regarding documentation. Documentation on Exhibit 5-A-1 is done by the nursing staff. Each nurse caring for the patient is responsible for documenting on the CP during his or her shift. If interventions and outcomes are met, the nurse places his or her initials in the column next to the day. There is space for a full signature at the end of each day. If interventions are not met, an asterisk is placed next to the nurse's initials for that day and a narrative note is required. The nurse is also responsible for completing the variance report. The variance report is a brief summation of the problem and the action taken to correct the problem.

Education Program

Successful implementation is facilitated when there is buy-in from all team members. Presenting educational programs with a multidisciplinary faculty reinforces the importance of the involvement of all disciplines. It is essential to provide background information such as the evolution, concepts, and goals of case management, the roles of DRGs and third-party payers, and other reimbursement issues. The use of graphs and tables is beneficial when presenting information on LOS, cost, and trends in health care. Highlights or summaries of salient points presented during the education programs can be featured for display on the staff bulletin board and other visible places on the unit. It is important to include the benefits for staff and patients when CPs are used.

A specific curriculum may be developed for each discipline so the involvement of the staff is emphasized and their educational needs met. One method for encouraging the attendance of all staff is to make the educational programs mandatory and incorporate the program into new staff orientation.

In addition to general and background information, other topics that should be presented are (1) roles and responsibilities of the case managers and the multidisciplinary team; (2) use of CPs and variance tracking; (3) collaborative practice and team building; (4) effective communication and interpersonal relationships; (5) conflict resolution and problem-solving skills; (6) patient education; (7) use of resources in discharge planning; (8) time management techniques; and (9) variance tracking and analysis.

Pilot Test

Once a CP has been developed and the educational process completed, a pilot test is needed to assess the usability of the CP and ensure that it reflects current practice. As many staff members as possible should be involved to obtain feedback that can be used in revising the CP.

One way to evaluate the effectiveness and usability of a CP is to assess the number and types of variances. Sixty to 70 percent of patients should remain on the CP and follow the normal progression as opposed to "falling off the CP."[12] It is vital to review and revise a CP periodically to reflect changes in practice and trends in health care. For example, the LOS for a patient who undergoes a craniotomy may initially start at 13 days in the CP. However, after successful implementation of case management, the number of days may be reduced to seven as a result of better use of resources; therefore the CP needs to be revised to reflect the change.

ISSUES IN THE USE OF CRITICAL PATHS

Regardless of the preparation of the staff in using CPs, there are issues related to compliance with the use of CPs and deviation of a patient's course from the CP. Compliance means all patients that need to be on a CP are included, items are completed in a timely manner, and deviations from the CP are addressed promptly and documented on the variance tracking form.

Staff Compliance

Staff compliance with the use of the CP is crucial to successful implementation. Factors that foster compliance include the following: (1) use of the CP as a permanent part of the patient's chart/medical record, (2) familiarity of temporary staff with its use, (3) development of a standard template and uniformity of formats, (4) clarity of staff responsibilities related to continuity of CP use, and (5) a process for dealing with deviations from the CP.

When the CP is an approved document for the chart, double documentation is decreased, thereby increasing the possibility of compliance because staff members do not have to document on the approved medical record forms and on the CP. The use of temporary or floating staff members may be an issue unless they are included in the education programs on the use of CPs. When it is not possible to include temporary staff members in educational programs, guidelines can be developed so they can refer to these. Furthermore, a part of the brief orientation to a unit could include responsibilities with regard to CPs. This may help to decrease any anxiety the temporary or floating staff members may have.

Development of a standard template for the CP format is essential. Use of a standard format enhances compliance because it is easier for staff to follow and use. It is also helpful to keep CPs short and concise. Critical paths that are too long tend to be cumbersome, thereby resulting in decreased compliance.

Staff responsibilities with regard to maintaining continuity in the use of CPs are another issue. It is necessary to delineate staff responsibilities with regard to the initiation of the CP and completion of the form. Staff members also need to be informed about the process that will be used in dealing with noncompliance with CPs. The person responsible for following up with staff regarding noncompliance must be identified. The nurse case manager, an advanced practice nurse such as the clinical nurse specialist, or the nurse manager could fulfill this role. It is also important to give positive feedback to staff. This will encourage compliance in the use of the CP.

Deviation from the Critical Path

When a patient deviates or "falls off" the CP, a variance has occurred. A mechanism needs to be in place for dealing with variances. It may be the responsibility of the case manager to address and resolve variances. For example, if the intervention was to get the patient out of bed and that was not done, the case manager would need to determine why it was not done. Was the reason a change in the patient's condition or was it an issue of noncompliance by the nursing staff?

Although a variance may have occurred, many patients are able to remain on the CP with minor adjustments, but some variances may cause the patient to fall off the CP. A change in the patient's condition or a postoperative complication are two examples in which patients could fall off the CP.

There are several questions that need to be addressed. What happens to the patient who no longer is on the CP? How is documentation done? One solution to this problem is to have a generic or blank CP that can be individualized for that patient. Even though a patient falls off the CP, the CP can still be used as a guideline for directing care. Even if the care needs change, all aspects of care still need to be carried out for the patient. Length of stay can still be decreased if there are complications that require the patient to stay longer. Regardless, if the patient is off the CP, this does not mean that interventions should not be performed in a timely and efficient manner.

EVALUATION

With the development and implementation of CPs, an evaluation component needs to be included to determine whether CPs are being used as planned. Compliance of staff and the use of the CP in identifying critical indicators that affect patient outcomes need to be included as major aspects of evaluation. Other aspects are ease of use, completeness of information noted by staff, time when CP is initiated, currency of key indicators and interventions, and uses of the CP.

It is important to monitor the percentage of staff compliance to CPs so it can be determined if there is an increase or decrease in their use. The number of patients who could have been on a CP and those who actually were on a CP should be determined. For the patients who were not on a CP, it is necessary to find out the reason(s) for not having used a CP so strategies can be initiated to decrease this occurrence.

Types and frequency of negative and positive variances can be used to revise key indicators and interventions. Examining interventions and how they affect outcomes provides information that can be used in revising CPs.

CONCLUSION

The CP is a viable tool that can be used to promote multidisciplinary collaboration when a team approach is used in developing and implementing CPs and in monitoring variances as they occur. Therefore, it is ideal to foster a multidisciplinary approach when pursuing endeavors related to CPs. These include delineating responsibilities of each staff member in developing, completing, and following through with activities that contribute to the attainment of key indicators and monitoring variances to achieve positive patient outcomes. The steps performed in developing CPs are provided in Exhibit 5-1.

With shorter hospital stays, active participation of patients in their care is beneficial. The use of CPs as a tool to inform patients of their care facilitates

Exhibit 5-1 Steps in Developing Critical Pathways (CPs)

Establish a multidisciplinary core committee

Gain administrative support

Determine patients who will be case managed
Activities within the institution
Assess and analyze case mix: high-volume, high-risk, and high-cost patients
Review medical records and financial data on cost and charges
Activities beyond the institution
Review literature
Seek consultation
Obtain information or conduct site visits of institutions using CPs

Can CP be obtained/purchased?
Yes   No
If yes, can it be adapted for use?
If no, develop CP

Develop CPs
Groupings to be done
DRG

ICD-9 codes
Physician groups
Diagnosis
Procedure
Number of CPs to be developed
Identify staff who will assist
Uses of CP
Documentation tool
Patient/staff education
Format
Hour
Day
Phases of illness
Guidelines for use
Draft of CP
Medical records
Current practice
Standards of care
Trends
Core committee review
Revision of CP
Method for monitoring variances and patients who "fall off" the pathway
Preimplementation (pilot group)
Revision of CP
Creation of standard template

their involvement, can decrease their anxiety, and at the same time, can help them get ready for discharge.

A vital aspect of successful implementation of CPs is staff compliance. Strategies that can be used to promote staff compliance include:

- using a standard template for CP format
- keeping CPs short and concise
- giving positive feedback on use of CPs to staff
- integrating CPs into the documentation process
- assisting staff members to gain knowledge of CPs and their uses, and to realize their responsibilities by offering education programs
- encouraging staff to participate in all phases of CP development

REFERENCES

1. Weinman H. Case management: one physician's view. *Inside Case Manage.* 1994;1(3):5–7.
2. Marr JA, Reid B. Implementing managed care and case management: the neuroscience experience. *J Neurosci Nurs.* 1992;24:281–285.
3. Hampton DC. Implementing a managed care framework through CareMaps. *J Nurs Adm.* 1993;23(5):21–27.
4. Moser C, Cronk P, Kidd A, McCormick P, Stockton S, Sulla C. Upgrading practice with critical pathways. *Am J Nurs.* 1992;92(1):41–44.
5. Zander K. Nursing case management: strategic management of cost and quality outcomes. *J Nurs Adm.* 1988;18(5):23–30.
6. Hill M. CareMap and case management systems: evolving models designed to enhance direct patient care. In: Flarey D, ed. *Redesigning Nursing Care Delivery: Transforming Our Future.* Philadelphia, Pa: J.B. Lippincott; 1995:173–185.
7. Giuliano KK, Poirier CE. Nursing case management: critical pathways to desirable outcomes. *Nurs Manage.* 1991;22(3):52–55.
8. Hronek C. Redesigning documentation: clinical pathways, flowsheets, and variance notes. *MEDSURG Nurs.* 1995;4:157–159.
9. Sperry S. Opportunities and challenges: strategies for implementing multidisciplinary documentation forms. *Aspen's Advisor Nurse Executives.* 1994;9(9):1,3,4.
10. Smith GB. Hospital-based case management. *Continuing Educ Ohio Nurses 1995 Course Catalog.* 1995:45–70.
11. Zander K. CareMaps™: the core of cost/quality care. *New Definition.* 1991;6(3).
12. Villaire M. Putting critical pathways on the map. *Crit Care Nurse.* 1995;15:106–113.

Appendix 5-A
Sample Critical Pathways

Source: Courtesy of The Ohio State University Medical Center, Columbus, Ohio.

Exhibit 5-A-1 Health Care Team Critical Pathway for CVA Patient

Date:

Needs	Key Indicator	Day 1		Day 2		Day 3
Maintain Tissue Perfusion	1. Vital signs	VS q4h × 48 h T < 101 P 60–120 RR 12–24 BP 100–180/ < 110		VS q4h T < 101 P 60–120 RR 12–24 BP 100–180/ < 110		VS q shift T < 101 P 60–120 RR 12–24 BP 100–180/< 110
	2. Neuro ✓	q4h × 24 h		q shift		q shift
	3. Diagnostic tests	CBC with diff/ plts., PT/INR, PTT, Chem 7, CT scan, EKG, CXR, MRI		Carotid artery duplex scan, cerebral angiogram PT/INR, PTT		2-D Echo TEE PT/INR, PTT
Maintain Gas Exchange	4. Oxygen	Room air		Room air		Room air
	5. Incentive spiro- meter	q2–4 h as needed		Same		Same
Progress Activity	6. Activity	Up in chair BID Ambulate in room Fall risk assessment		Ambulate in hall BID		Up ad lib
Maintain Nutritional Intake	7. Diet	Heart healthy (low chol., low fat 4 g Na)		Same		Same
	8. I & O	q shift		Same		Same
	9. IV	Saline well or Heparin drip if needed		Same		Same
	10. Medica- tions	ASA, Ticlid, anti- hypertensives, Heparin		Same		Coumadin
	11. Bowel move- ment	Bowel sounds × 4 quads; abd soft		Same; bowel movement or LOC		

Exhibit 5-A-1 continued

Needs	Key Indicator	Day 1	Day 2	Day 3
Maintain Skin Integrity	12. Incision	Skin assessment Bleeding precautions	Check groin after angiogram Continue bleeding precautions	Remove bandaid 24 hours after angiogram Continue bleeding precautions
Provide Teaching	13. Teaching *Refer to Stroke Notebook and Patient Critical Path*	Orient to unit Orient patient to critical path Give patient *Stroke Notebook*	Reinforce activity progression; explain all tests and procedures	Instruct on care after discharge
Assess Home Needs	14. Discharge Planning	Social work, PT, OT, speech, pastoral care, and nutrition consults if needed	Consult Physical Medicine and Rehabilitation Services if indicated; identify support system and home needs	

Signature _____ _____ _____

_____ _____ _____

_____ _____ _____

continues

Exhibit 5-A-1 continued

Needs	Key Indicator	Day 4	Day 5	Day 6
Maintain Tissue Perfusion	1. Vital signs	VS q shift T < 101 P 60–120 RR 12–24 BP 100–180/ < 110	VS q shift T < 101 P 60–120 RR 12–24 BP 100–180/ < 110	VS q shift T < 101 P 60–120 RR 12–24 BP 100–180/ < 110
	2. Neuro ✓	q shift	q shift	q shift
	3. Diagnostic tests	PT/INR PTT	PT/INR, PTT	PT/INR PTT
Maintain Gas Exchange	4. Oxygen	Room air	Same	Same
	5. Incentive spirometer	As needed	Same	Same
Progress Activity	6. Activity	Up ad lib	Same	Same
Maintain Nutritional Intake	7. Diet	Heart healthy	Same	Same
	8. I & O	q shift	Same	Same
	9. IV	Discontinue or restart if needed	Same	Discontinue IV/ saline well
	10. Medication	Same	Same	Same
	11. Bowel move- ment	BM or LOC	Same	BM or LOC
Maintain Skin Integrity	12. Incision	Bleeding precautions	Same	Same
Provide Post- Op Teaching	13. Teaching	Refer to *Stroke Notebook* and patient critical path	Same	Review discharge order and instruction sheet
Assess Home Needs	14. DC planning	Initiate continuity of care (COC)	Continue working on COC	Complete COC

Signature   _____   _____   _____

_____   _____   _____

_____   _____   _____

Physician Approval: _____
                            Signature

Exhibit 5-A-1 continued

Variance Report			
Date & Time	Problem	Action	Signature

Date & Time	Positive Variance

Exhibit 5-A-2 Patient Education Critical Pathway for Stroke Patient

Date:				

Needs	Key Points	Day 1	Day 2	Day 3
Circulation	1. Vital signs (heart beat, blood pressure)	Every 4 hours *Your vital signs *Blood pressure	Every 4 hours	Every 8 hours
	2. Neuro ✓ (mental alertness)	Every 4 hours *Neuro ✓	Every 8 hours	Every 8 hours
	3. Tests	Blood tests *Chest x-ray *Head CT *EKG *MRI	Blood tests *Carotid artery duplex scan *Cerebral angiogram	Blood tests *2-D Echo *Trans Esophageal Echocardiogram (TEE)
Breathing	4. Oxygen	Room air	Room air	Room air
	5. Ability to use breathing instrument (incentive spirometer)	10 times each use, as needed every 2–4 hours	Same	Same
Activity	6. Activity	Up in chair 2 times a day Walk in room *Positioning handouts	Bedrest for 6 hours after angiogram Up in chair and/or walk after bedrest	Up in chair and/or walking in halls
Nutrition	7. Diet	Heart healthy diet as tolerated Do not eat or drink after midnight until angiogram is done *Heart Healthy Diet *Dysphagia (hard to swallow)	May eat after angiogram Nothing to eat or drink after midnight	Heart healthy diet 2 hours after TEE *Diet & Anticoagulation Therapy
	8. Fluid Intake and Output	Measure liquids taken by mouth, and from IV, and urine output *Bladder Care after a Stroke	Same	Same

Legend: *handouts to be given to you.

Exhibit 5-A-2 continued

Needs	Key Points	Day 1		Day 2		Day 3
	9. IV	IV for fluids or medicines as needed		Same		Same
	10. Medications	*Heparin *Aspirin *Ticlid		Review handouts		*Coumadin *Coumadin Calendar
	11. Bowel movement (BM)	*Bowel Care after a Stroke		If no BM, laxative of choice (LOC)		
Keep Skin Intact	12. Wound	None		Bandaid to groin after angiogram		Remove bandaid 24 hours after angiogram
Orientation to room and hospital	13. Teaching	Orientation to room and environment Orientation to critical pathway *Stroke Notebook *Nursing Case Management *What Is a Stroke? *Aphasia		*Dysarthria *Communication Skills		*Depression after Stroke
Care You Need after Leaving the Hospital	14. Planning your care after leaving the hospital	Resources available: occupational therapy speech therapy physical therapy social services pastoral care nutrition consult		Therapies that are needed will continue The social worker will review insurance coverage and discussion of options such as home health, rehabilitation facilities, and nursing home placement		Physical medicine and rehabilitation doctors will visit you. They will assess your rehabilitation needs.

continues

Exhibit 5-A-2 continued

Needs	Key Points	Day 4	Day 5	Day 6
Circulation	1. Vital signs (heart beat, blood pressure)	Every 8 hours	Same	Same
	2. Neuro ✓ (mental alertness)	Every 8 hours	Same	Same
	3. Tests	Blood tests to find out if your blood clots properly and the right amount of Heparin you need for your blood clot	Same	Same
		No other tests unless your condition changes	Same	Same
Breathing	4. Oxygen	Room air	Same	Same
	5. Ability to use breathing instrument (incentive spirometer)	10 times each use, as needed every 2–4 hours	Same	Same
Activity	6. Activity	Up in chair and/or walking	Same	Same
Nutrition	7. Diet	Continue heart healthy diet	Same	Same
	8. Fluid Intake and Output	Continue to measure liquids taken by mouth and by IV and urine	Same	Same
	9. IV	Stop saline well or give IV if needed	IV as needed	IV taken out

Exhibit 5-A-2 continued

Needs	Key Points	Day 4		Day 5		Day 6
	10. Medications	As needed Review medication handouts		Same		Same
	11. Bowel movement (BM)	Laxative of choice (LOC) if needed		Same		Same
Keep Skin Intact	12. Wound	None		None		None
Teaching	13. Teaching	*Rehabilitation after a Stroke*		*You Are Still a Sexual Person after a Stroke*		Release from the hospital and instructions sheet will be given to you by your doctor
Care You Need after Leaving the Hospital	14. Planning your care after leaving the hospital	*Dodd Hall Stroke Team* Rehabilitation staff to help you adjust after relase from the hospital				

Patient Notes and Questions	
Date & Time	Notes and Questions

■ 6 ■

Documentation To Achieve Patient Outcomes through Critical Pathways

Pamela E. Windle, MS, RN, CNA, CPAN, CAPA
Susan Houston, PhD, RN

The "buzz phrase" for the 1990s is *managed care—decade of quality.* With the shrinking health care dollar, increasing competition among health care institutions, and increasing federal regulations or restrictions, one method used by many facilities to control and reduce costs is case management. Case management provides a patient-centered program that embraces cost containment.[1] Today's focus is on affordable care that mandates achievement of quality standards and patient satisfaction. The managed care philosophy centers around a consumer-driven economy. Consumers include the patient/family, the physician, the third-party payer, and other health care providers.

Health care is rapidly changing and constantly moving toward a more patient-centered focus and enhanced outcomes. Most health care organizations have chosen downsizing or increasing patient volume to remain viable in a managed care era. In addition, case management and/or outcomes management (OM) programs can assist in improving outcomes while decreasing expenditures.

CASE MANAGEMENT/OUTCOMES MANAGEMENT

While at the New England Medical Center in the 1980s, Karen Zander was the pioneer in defining and implementing the case management model. Case management is a planned approach to patient care that delineates accountability for patient outcomes within specific time frames.[2] This model of patient care uses the nursing process to promote patient advocacy throughout the patient's entire hospital stay. Day-to-day nursing practice focuses on ensuring the normal course of a patient's illness, expected outcomes, and resource utilization by case type. The tools used to ensure adherence were nursing focused and included identifying problems with adherence, choosing the correct intervention, and determining expected outcomes over a specified length of stay. A critical path was developed, which then integrated crucial incidents and specific interventions taking place at a given time and day of hospitalization to achieve standard outcomes. The primary goals of the model were cost containment, reduction in length of stay, and consistent outcomes. In case management, a specific patient was identified by the case manager of the institution, and his or her care was managed to promote outcome achievement.

Outcomes management addresses the same goals as case management, except OM is quality oriented and broader in scope. It includes standardized practice for multiple disciplines applicable to both the uncomplicated and complicated patients. At St. Luke's Episcopal Hospital (SLEH), Houston, Texas, OM is defined as the use of outcomes assessment information to enhance clinical, quality, and financial outcomes through integration of exemplary practice and service delivery. The goals are to provide quality health care, decrease fragmentation, enhance patient outcomes, and ultimately decrease costs through outcomes assessment and research.[3] Outcomes management uses the knowledge gained through outcomes measurement to improve care practices and service delivery. A collaborative process involves all health care personnel (e.g., physicians, nurses, pharmacists, dietitians, social workers, discharge planners, outcomes managers, and management teams). The organization's philosophy is to provide high-quality patient care, improve outcomes, and decrease cost.[3] All team members must be aware of the organizational vision and must be willing to commit themselves to achieving the ultimate cost-efficient, outcome-driven patient care.

The OM model used at SLEH actualizes outcome-related efforts (Fig. 6-1). The first component of the model recognizes the institutional values and support required for a successful program. It was recognized early that the institution's dedication to the attainment of excellence in health care within a framework that is fiscally sound was necessary for inspirationalizing the work of OM. The next step in the OM model is to identify patient outcomes and/or variances requiring measurement and management within selected patient populations. The collection of outcomes data specific to patient populations is necessary for enhancing goal achievement and directing change toward improvement. The third step in the OM model requires the analysis of care practices and/or system processes that contribute to or impede the improvement of patient outcomes. The fourth step involves process, practice, and outcomes improvement activities. This step often involves systemic change, process enhancement, and the determination of care practices that yield best outcomes. The fifth step requires the continuous measurement of outcomes

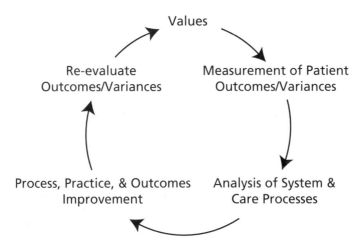

Figure 6-1 Outcomes Management Model. *Source:* Courtesy of St. Luke's Episcopal Hospital, Houston, Texas.

to determine the impact of change on the selected outcome(s). St. Luke's OM model emphasizes the measurement of patient outcomes, identification of barriers that impede the provision of quality cost-effective care, and implementation of the changes necessary to improve the future care of patients.

Outcomes management incorporates high-quality standards of care and identifies expected treatment practices with corresponding outcomes. Patient groups may include the fragile elderly; patients with long-term, medically complex, and severely compromised acute illnesses; and patients having surgical procedures such as open heart surgery, hip/joint replacements, A-V graft insertion, or laparoscopic cholecystectomy. Specific medical and surgical diagnoses guide in the formulation of critical pathways or other standardized tools. These pathways map out the patient's progression of care from admission to discharge, to determine the patient's needs as well as to guide care practices of multiple disciplines.

Outcomes management provides consistent documentation of outcomes experienced during the hospital episode and reflects the care delivered by multiple groups of health care providers. All providers document information pertinent to their care of the patient on the critical path. This provides a comprehensive picture of the total experience of the patient and serves as a multidisciplinary communication tool. Aggregate outcomes data may then show untoward outcomes and provide an opportunity for examining and developing continuous quality improvement. Ultimately, health care providers can then develop improved approaches to patient care by analyzing the patient's needs and establishing correct time frames and practice patterns, which eventually form the basis of managed care.[3]

BENEFITS

The tremendous benefits of OM to the organization are many. The most important goal is to have patients obtain their desired outcome(s) throughout the continuum of care, with an appropriate length of stay or visits and with appropriate use of resources. Common OM benefits include:

1. The promotion of collaborative practice, in which teams work together to achieve the desired patient outcomes. At SLEH, collaborative practice teams (CPTs) are developed based on the services (orthopedic, renal, pulmonary, cardiac, neurology, digestive, and obstetrics/gynecology). These teams work with other disciplines or departments to achieve the desired outcomes by examining the entire care process, monitoring what happens in one department and seeing whether it affects another department as well.
2. Coordination and review of clinical services. The team reviews the various services provided, which improves the patient's movement through the system. Outcomes managers facilitate the scrutiny of the total patient care process, from prehospitalization through postdischarge.
3. Appropriate patient referrals for resource utilization (i.e., home health services).
4. Achieving desired clinical outcomes for patients through standardized tools (e.g., pathways, protocols, guidelines). Constant evaluation from the CPTs is performed and discussed in the routinely scheduled meetings.
5. A timely patient discharge. Through education, patients and families receive support services and realistic expectations of needed home care.
6. Increased consumer satisfaction.

Outcomes management is not limited to an inpatient department; its principles can also be used in any setting of the hospital. An outpatient, ambulatory surgery, or perioperative setting can also apply the principles of OM. Critical pathways can be used that are defined in hours during the patient's usual length of stay in an ambulatory setting.[4] In the perioperative setting, OM is easily focused on care practices and supporting care processes. It addresses the patient's movement through the surgical experience, from the preoperative calls made before the scheduled surgery, up to and including postdischarge on the same day. It examines issues such as delays, availability of services and test results, unexpected changes to the actual surgical procedures, postoperative delays and complications, various reasons for discharge delays, and possible admission to the hospital.[4]

Outcomes management provides an avenue for any perioperative staff to be valued for their expertise in nursing knowledge and skills, their ability to allocate appropriate resources, and their collaboration with other departments. The overall goal is to achieve a positive outcome within the expected length of the perioperative experience. The perioperative documentation of the critical path is a reflection of identified patient/family needs, multidisciplinary interventions, and the patient's response to interventions. This documentation, with an OM approach, eases identification of variances and outcomes associated with the pathway and provides for an all-encompassing patient care documentation system. This documentation provides a meaningful avenue for the overall collection of data within the whole organization's OM program.[4]

DESIRABLE PATIENT OUTCOMES

Each organization must define what expected outcomes are desired or what ultimate goal or end result the health care team members want to achieve. Most expected outcomes are the anticipated results of a given specified intervention.[1] Examples of short-term patient outcomes are:

- The patient will be extubated 12 hours after open heart surgery.
- The patient will be able to ambulate unassisted one day postoperatively.
- The patient will be started on early feedings 12 hours postoperatively.
- The patient will be discharged safely at the expected time or day.

Patient outcomes become the responsibility of the multidisciplinary team. In the past, patient outcomes were focused through the physician's efforts. Through OM, the entire collaborative practice team makes an impact on the patient's outcome. The team is accountable and responsible for assisting patients and families in reaching the goal of safe health care in a quality-driven, cost-controlled atmosphere.

CRITICAL PATHWAYS

Critical pathways are developed to help achieve goal(s) or outcome(s). The path serves as a road map, care map, or clinical map.[5] It is a standardized outline for patient care, specifying what actions or critical incidents should occur during the patient's stay.[6] To develop a critical path, a patient population must first be identified. The selected patient population is often a diagnosis-related group (DRG) and should meet the criteria for a high-volume, high-risk, and/or problem-oriented group. Data regarding the selected patient population should be analyzed to determine the length of stay that is consistently attainable by at least 75 percent of the chosen population. Most pathways are developed from retrospective and concurrent chart reviews and/or past and current practices. Collaborative practice teams usually develop the final critical paths on a specific patient population identified. The ideal and actual practices are considered and discussed, recognizing that the ultimate goal of the organization is quality of care with decreased cost. The team reviews and refines each pathway and also tests it for validity.

As mentioned earlier, critical paths are road maps, which can also be written in lay language so patients and families can understand what is needed, what to expect during the hospital stay, and when to expect certain activities to occur. Generally, physicians know exactly what they want and would like to have happen for their patients, but the rest of the care givers providing direct care—whether nursing, pharmacy, respiratory, dietary, or other staff—may not be aware of the physician's plans and expectations. The critical path requires a consensus of all care givers, including physicians. As a result, when provided with a pathway many families take an active role in assisting the patient's progress through hospitalization.

Critical paths provide written criteria to guide care, based on standards of practice for any discipline. They delineate necessary critical incidences for a specific population, either on a day-to-day basis or hourly for ambulatory surgery patients, facilitating appropriate resource utilization and highlighting the expected practice standards. They do not replace a physician's orders, nor are they a substitute for clinical judgment. They outline services or clinical interventions while reflecting desired patient outcomes within a designated time period and still ensure the best utilization of resources.

The purposes/functions of critical pathways, as defined by SLEH,[3] are to:

- Identify expected outcomes
- Promote collaboration among disciplines
- Achieve continuity of care throughout hospitalization
- Use institutional resources appropriately
- Facilitate timely discharge of patients as defined by the institution
- Reduce omissions of necessary services and interventions
- Highlight care practices and associated expected outcomes

- Identify system barriers to patient progress.
- Identify variances and promote resolution of problems.
- Facilitate collection of aggregated outcome and variance data for further research.

After critical paths have been developed, reviewed, and chosen, all staff members and physicians are inserviced. For the care givers, the critical pathway serves as a "daily calendar" that allows each member of the team to know exactly what and when critical incidents should occur in a designated time frame. After pathways are implemented, they must become part of the documentation system within the organization. The bedside staff nurse or case manager can be responsible for initiating a pathway and continually documenting the patient's progress every 24 hours during the hospital stay or hourly during the ambulatory surgery stay. The staff nurse also seeks advice from the outcomes manager on potential high-risk patients or patients who do not progress according to the critical pathway.

Critical paths are useful tools in the management of episodic and aggregate patient experiences.[3] They focus on where the patient is during the hospital stay and what needs to happen to facilitate discharge at the expected time. Critical paths are easily integrated into a computerized documentation system. The operating room at SLEH is the first department to use computerized documentation. Data are easily retrieved and aggregated. This facilitates early identification of utilization review and can be designed as a method for data collection. Variances identified within and across each population can provide multipurpose quality indicators for quality improvement plans. Aggregated data also permit the benchmarking of health care workers against peer groups and practices both within and outside the organization.

Critical pathways in the perioperative service have improved quality care in the following ways: by allowing physicians and staff to share knowledge; by improving patient/family teaching plans; by allowing comparison of outcomes from various treatment processes; and by identifying and evaluating steps to improve the desired outcomes. Most of all, satisfaction from consumers and health care personnel has had an effect on the process of critical path implementation.[4] Exhibits 6-A-1 through 6-A-3 in Appendix 6-A are examples of specific critical pathways and associated outcome and variance data collected.

Variance

Variance is defined as any deviation from the activities or outcomes delineated on the critical pathway. Variances may be positive or negative. For example, a patient who progresses quickly and is discharged before the expected length of stay constitutes a positive variance. A prolonged length of stay, exceeding the critical path (i.e., development of an infection), would be a negative variance. Any event that alters the patient's progress toward the expected or standard outcomes is called a negative variance. Variances are examined when patient care or patient outcomes differ from what was predicted when patients move through the system. Three types of variances are identified:

1. *System variance:* a variance caused by the hospital departments/areas that prevents the patient's progress on the critical path. Examples include delayed laboratory results, delayed tests or procedures due to their unavailability in the organization, beds unavailable on the floors when patients are ready to transfer from intensive care units or post-anesthesia care units, or delayed transfers outside the hospital.

2. *Patient variance:* a variance generated by a patient, whether due to complications or aspects of patient status that affect patient outcome. Examples include developing complications, refusing to take medications, diet problems, continued nonrelief of pain, refusing treatments or tests, and failure to preadmit for ambulatory surgery (thus delaying surgery procedures due to delayed tests and procedures).

3. *Care giver variance:* a variance caused by any care giver that delays the patient's progress on the critical path. Care givers include nurses, physicians, physical therapists, x-ray technicians, respiratory therapists, and any other health care provider who interacts with the patient. Examples include misordering of diagnostic tests or treatments, mislabeling of a specimen, oversedation by the anesthesia department, delay in carrying out orders, and delay of procedure due to staffing issues and lack of awareness from team members.

Variance tracking is important, and documentation of variances should be done by the provider identifying the variance and should include the exact reason, where and when it occurred, and an identified course of action. Variance documentation should include the addition or deletion of treatments to the critical path. Because bedside nurses are in constant interaction with patients, they are the source for variance documentation approximately 90 percent of the time. Bedside nurses should possess a thorough understanding of variances and should document them accurately and completely.

Analysis of variances occurs either by reviewing the critical pathway or statistical analysis. Variances can be reviewed by the outcomes manager, nurse managers, or staff either on a daily or weekly basis. The occurrence of one variance might be insignificant, but continuous trending may show an increase of the variance, which necessitates follow-up. Immediate follow-up and an action plan can be developed in consultation with the outcomes manager. Reviewing aggregated variances involves the same process as reviewing individual variances but in the broader scope of the entire population. Addressing action plans to deal with variances is done via a multidisciplinary approach. The CPTs review what the variances are and decide on how to reduce or eliminate those variances. Action plans may be developed based on the statistical significance of the variance, the frequency of the variance, or any relationship of the variance to other variances or outcomes. Variance data provide necessary information and opportunities for development of continuous quality improvements throughout the organization. In Appendix 6-A, Exhibits 6-A-4 through 6-A-7 are examples of the SLEH reporting system.

The following case study represents an example with many variances:

> Scheduled for an 0730 surgery for anterior crucial ligament repair, Mr. Smith was instructed by his physician to report to the hospital for preadmission testing and evaluation two days before the day of surgery. Mr. Smith failed to do so. On the day of surgery, laboratory tests and an electrocardiogram (ECG) were performed and abnormalities were noted. Treatments were done to decrease his blood sugar and alter low potassium results. A cardiologist was consulted and asked to interpret the ECG findings. Consequently, Mr. Smith's surgery was postponed until 1300. During his postoperative recovery, Mr. Smith had hypotension, causing him to stay longer in the postanesthesia care unit (PACU). A continuous passive motion (CPM) machine was ordered for home treatment, but the PACU nurse failed to order the machine in a timely manner. Furthermore, the physical therapist was delayed in giving instructions regarding the CPM machine until 1.5 hours later. Finally, Mr. Smith's wife could not pick him up until 2100. Mr. Smith was finally discharged home at 2130. The following are the patient, system, and care giver variances that occurred:

Patient Variances
1. The patient failed to come for preadmission testing before surgery, which could have prevented the delay of surgery.
2. The physiologic occurrence of hypotension in the PACU caused the patient to stay longer for additional treatment.
3. The patient's wife was delayed in picking up the patient for home discharge.

System Variances
1. Delayed laboratory results caused the delayed interpretation of results.
2. Delayed cardiology consult caused delayed approval for surgery.

Care Giver Variances
1. Ordering of the CPM machine was delayed.
2. Arrival of the physical therapist for instruction and teaching in the use of the CPM machine was delayed.

All these variances delayed the patient's progress toward discharge and increased the hospitalization charges.

COLLABORATION

Outcomes management requires that boundaries be broken, effective communication techniques be developed, and active participation and interaction among and within departments be encouraged. Collaboration between departments is the key to success and is vital to the whole process. Through collaboration, *all disciplines* (rather than just the old, traditional work groups) involved can focus on maintaining and achieving the desired quality patient outcome.[7] What strengthens the collaborative relationship between disciplines is open communication and the continuous sharing of information related to patient outcomes and cost.

Role of the Physician

Like most people, physicians can be resistant to change. In this managed care era, physicians are urged to get involved, share with other disciplines in promoting positive patient outcomes, promote open communication and interactions related to patient progress, be willing to change practices for achievement of positive outcomes, be able to give and receive feedback from others, and support the overall values of the organization and outcomes management program. In the past, physicians were interested in addressing the effectiveness of the system or process, rather than looking at the larger picture of patient outcomes (thereby reducing the length of stay and cost of care for the patients).[2] In this new era, physicians must be adept at changing, for the good of their organization and clients and for the betterment of their own practice.

Role of the Staff Nurse

The key member of the health care team is the bedside nurse. The staff nurse is responsible for initiating the appropriate critical pathway, notifying the outcomes managers of patients who are not progressing according to the critical path, and observing that documentation of the pathway (as well as documentation of variances) occurs every 24 hours. Bedside nurses must be knowledgeable and remain current on new information regarding their patient population and support changes in practice based on the multidisciplinary team's recommendations.[8,9] Nurses demonstrate ownership of the critical path because not only are they part of the CPTs, they are empowered and desire more input and participation in the treatment process of their patients. Open communication is another important link to success.

Role of the Nurse Manager

The nurse manager needs to be able to work synergistically in teams, because collaborative work results in better outcomes. The nurse manager must portray management and leadership abilities. Possessing good people skills, the nurse manager is a negotiator and mentor. Financial skills are also necessary to assist in analyzing costs and benefits and maintaining a patient/family-oriented focus.[10] The nurse manager must be self-directed, goal oriented, and able to lead his or her staff toward a commitment to teamwork and successful outcomes-driven patient care. Open communication with all departments is also vital to success.

Role of the Outcomes Manager

The outcomes manager must always be visible to all health care professionals. He or she acts as a facilitator and provides assistance and support whenever redirection is needed. An outcomes manager must be clinically competent in his or her area of expertise and demonstrate understanding and patience with members of his or her team. Credibility is also an important element, to ensure trusting relationships and eliminate "turf battles." The outcomes manager must be goal oriented and develop partnerships, promote ownership, and provide working relationships with team members.

CONCLUSION

Nursing is a constantly evolving profession—what might be acceptable today may be unacceptable in the future. Each organization must determine which standards best fit its needs in this managed care era. The challenge for the future is the empowerment of integrated teams who can reengineer the process and practices of delivering patient care. Organizations must always be aware that something better may be just around the corner.

REFERENCES

1. Giuliano K, Poirier C. Nursing case management: critical pathways to desirable outcomes. *Nurs Manage.* 1991;22(3):52–57.

2. Zander K. Physicians, caremaps, and collaboration. *New Definition.* 1992;7(1):1–4.

3. Lindy C, Luquire R. Outcomes Management: How, What, Who, Why. Houston, Texas: St. Luke's Episcopal Hospital; 1992.

4. Windle P. An integrated documentation tool: critical pathways and desirable patient outcomes. *Nurs Manage.* 1994;25:80F–80P.

5. Etheredge ML. Critical paths: marking the course. *New Definition.* 1987;2(3):1–4.

6. Mosher C, Cronk P, Kidd A, McCormick P, Stockton S, Sulla C. Upgrading practice with critical pathways. *Am J Nurs.* 1992;92(1):41–44.

7. Downey-DeZell A. Case management plans: a collaborative model. *New Definition.* 1987;2(1):1–4.

8. Campbell C. Improving staff nurse participation. *Nurs Adm Q.* 1991;16(1):56–60.

9. Hastings C, O'Keefe S, Buckley J. Professional practice partnerships: a new approach to creating high performance nursing organizations. *Nurs Adm Q.* 1992;17(1):45–54.

10. Kerfoot K, Luquire R. Case management/outcomes management: the role of the nurse manager. *Nurs Econ.* 1993;11:321–323.

Appendix 6-A
Critical Pathways and
Examples of Reporting Tools

Source: Copyright © 1995, St. Luke's Episcopal Hospital, Houston, Texas.

Exhibit 6-A-1 SLEH Post-Anesthesia Care Unit Critical Pathway

GOAL: The anticipated goal of the critical pathway is to provide quality patient care in an efficient and cost-effective manner. This care will be accomplished through the following: 1. Immediate identification of potential problem. 2. Professional intervention through planned care of identified actual problem. 3. Reduction of anxiety level of both patient and significant other. 4. Provision of an injury-free environment.

	Adm.—30 Min.	1 Hour	2 Hours	3 Hours	4 Hours
Destina-tion	**Designated Area** Adult Pedi Isolation	**Mac/Blk** To DSC/floor/home	**Gen/Epi** To DSC **Cardioversion** To floor/telemetry/CV OP	**Spinal** To DSC/home **Epi/Gen** Home/to floor	**Spinal** To floor/ICU **Epi/Gen** ICU
Labora-tory	**Gen/Spinal/Epi/Mac/Blk** Lab work as ordered **Cardioversion** Lab work as ordered		**Cardioversion** EKG as ordered		
Activity/ Position	**Gen/Spinal/Epi** Bed rest, flat in bed **Mac/Blk** Bed rest, HOB **Cardioversion** Bed rest, flat in bed	**Gen/Spinal/Epi** HOB (per surg.)/ anesthesia turn PRN	**Cardioversion** HOB elevated		
Consults	**Gen** Anesthesiologist for vent. management Respiratory therapist for vent. patients **Cardioversion** Notify cardiologist of arrival	**Gen/Spinal/Epi** X-ray as ordered CPM as ordered Anesthesiologist for vent. management **Mac/Blk** S/O anesthesia	**Gen** Anesthesiologist for vent. management Respiratory therapist for vent. patients **Cardioversion** Cardiologist to release pt. from P.A.C.U.	**Gen/Epi** S/O anesthesiologist	**Spinal** S/O anesthesiologist

continues

Exhibit 6-A-1 continued

	Adm.—30 Min.	1 Hour	2 Hours	3 Hours	4 Hours
Nutrition	**Gen/Spinal/Epi** NPO IV maintenance as ordered **Cardioversion** NPO IV initiated/patient	**Mac/Blk** Ice as ordered IV maintenance	**Cardioversion** IV maintenance/heplock/ DC'd Diet as tolerated	**Spinal/epidural** PO fluids if not contraindicated or if ordered	
Medica-tions	**Gen/Spinal/Epi/Mac/Blk** Pain management Other meds	**Gen/Spinal/Epi/Mac** IV antibiotics IV steroids Other IV meds IV/IM analgesics Antiemetics PRN Epidural analgesia P.O. meds **Cardioversion** IV sedation	**Gen** PCA pump **Cardioversion** P.O. meds Topical meds IV meds/other		
Nursing General	**Check Post-op Orders** V.S. q 15 min./post-op assess/ check dressing/comfort measures/orientation/warm blanket(s)/O$_2$/pulse oximeter	**Gen/Spinal/Epi** Continue monitoring/ continue post-op orders Pedi family visitation	**Gen/Spinal/EPI/Mac** Wean off O$_2$ Weaning protocol for vent. patients ICU family visitation Routine DSC discharge protocol	**Gen/Epi** DC art. line DC central line if not needed VS q 30'	**Spinal** DC art. line
Spinal epidural	V.S. q 15 min./orient to routine/check level of anesthesia/check dressing Complete assessment/O$_2$/ pulse oximeter check dressing			**Spinal/Epidural** Complete sensation/ movement for lower extremities	

Exhibit 6-A-1 continued

MAC BLK	V.S. q 15 min./orient to routine/check level of anesthesia/complete assessment/check dressing/ O$_2$/pulse oximeter				
Cardio-version	Adm. V.S./assess/EKG monitor Cardioversion & intubation equipment O$_2$/pulse oximeter	**Cardioversion** V.S. q 15 min. x 1 hr. Observed site for redness	**Cardioversion** Wean off O$_2$		
Teaching	**Gen/Spinal/Epi/Mac/Blk** Assess learning needs/instruct pt. according to P.A.C.U. teaching protocol Barriers: Y___ N___ If yes check appropriately: ___Anesthesia ___Age ___Neuro status ___Language ___Others:___ **Cardioversion** Explanation of procedure	**Gen** DB & C/instruct patient on CADD pump **Spinal/Epi** Inform patient re: return of sensation & movement Allay anxiety **Mac/Blk** Demonstrate understanding of patient teaching	**Gen** Instruction & demonstrate to patient use of PCA pump **Cardioversion** Patient to notify nurse if any chest pain	**Gen/Spinal/Epi** Provide other instructions specific to surgical procedure	**Spinal** Instruct patient to get out of bed only *with* assistance
Discharge		**Mac/Blk** Discharge assessment/ instructions	**Gen/Epi** Demonstrate understanding of patient teaching **Cardioversion** Discharge assessment/ instructions	**Gen/Epi/Spinal** Discharge assessment/instructions	**Gen/Epi/Spinal** Discharge assessment/instructions

Exhibit 6-A-2 Critical Pathway Variance Report

Infant
Patient Variances
1. Low blood glucose (less than 40 mgm%)
2. Low temperature (less than 97.6F)
3. Respiratory distress (grunting, retracting, respiratory rate > 70 in first 2 hours).
4. Respiratory distress (grunting, retracting, respiratory rate > 60 after 2 hours).
5. + Coombs
6. Hyperbilirubinemia (dx - physiologic)
7. Negative cultures after 48 hrs.
8. Negative cultures after 72 hrs.
9.

10. Oxygen requirement < 3 hrs.
11. O2 saturation > 95%. Pulse oximeter dc'd after 4–8 hrs. O2 sat. > 95%.
12. O2 saturation > 92%
13. Antibiotics dc'd after 48 hrs.
14. Positive cultures, asymptomatic
15. Meconium aspiration
16. Meconium, none below the cords

Mother
Patient Variances
17. PROM
18. GBS+
19. Temp ≥ 100.4F
20. Chorioamnionitis
21. Hct. ≤ 30%
22. MgSO4 Therapy
23. Mat. glucose < 70 or > 130

Date	Unit	Variances (#)	Action Taken	Other Variances	Signature

Exhibit 6-A-3 DRG 014 (Stroke) Assessment Profile

Addressograph

St. Luke's Episcopal Hospital
DRG 014: Stroke

In the blanks below, place a "Y" (Yes), "N" (No), or "NA" (unable to test, ie:

Check one of the following:
___ Hemorrhagic (without craniotomy or coil embolization)
___ Ischemic: ___ Embolic ___ Thrombotic

Check one of the following:
___ Not entered in drug study
___ rtPA Study
___ Lubeluzole Study

Check the INITIAL anticoagulation order below:
___ No anticoagulation therapy
___ Heparin bolus/heparin infusion/warfarin started following day
___ Heparin bolus/heparin infusion
___ Heparin infusion (no bolus)

Admission NIH Stroke Scale Score: ___
Scale Weight (lbs) @ Admission: ___
Scale Weight (lbs) @ Discharge: ___

Decreased LOC):

Dysphagia Assessment Profile:
PO Diet: Dysphagia ___
Other ___
Pocketing food ___
Tubefeedings ___
Water Swallow Test:
Coughs on H₂O ___
More than 1 swallow to empty mouth ___
Wet voice after swallow ___
Drooling ___
Cranial Nerve VII (Facial):
Weakness ___
Incomplete oral labial closure ___
Cranial Nerve XII (Hypoglossal):
No tongue protrusion ___
No tongue lateral movement ___
No tongue upward movement ___
(No "L" sound) ___
Cranial Nerve IX & X (glossopharyngeal & Vagus):
No gag reflex ___
No "K" sound ___

Communication:
Expressive Aphasia ___
Receptive Aphasia ___
Global Aphasia ___
Dysarthria ___

PMH:
Previous stroke ___
Atrial fibrillation ___

Location of Stroke(s):
L cerebral ___
R cerebral ___
L cerebellar ___
R cerebellar ___
Subcortical ___
Brainstem ___

Discharge Information:
Home ___
Rehab Center ___
Subacute Care ___
SNF ___
Death ___

continues

Exhibit 6-A-3 continued

Date	Day 1:	Day 2:	Day 3:	Day 4:	Discharge Target Day 5:
Consults	Neurology; CNS (X4455) Social Service; Dietitian	Physical & occupational therapy	PM&R Consider speech pathologist		Consider Gastroenterologist (PEG)
Diagnostics	CXR; CT Scan; ECG Chem 7 & 12; CBC; PT/PTT Consider prealbumin	Carotid Doppler PT/PTT (if on anticoagulation)	PT/PTT (if on anticoagulation) Consider modified barium swallow	PT/PTT (if on anticoagulation)	PT/PTT (if on anticoagulation)
Treatments	Neuro VS q2–4 hours I & O; IV therapy	Neuro VS q2–4 hours Continency program (call 4455)	Neuro VS q2–4 hours Continency program prn	Neuro VS q2–4 hours Continency program prn	Neuro VS q2–4 hours Continency program prn
Activity	Bedrest	Up in chair 2–4 times/day Begin self-grooming/feeding	Up in chair 2–4 times/day Increase self-care	Increase OOB activity Identify max self-care potential	Increase OOB activity Self-care discharge plan
Nutrition	RN completes dysphagia assessment profile Consider dysphagia protocol	Soft diet Dysphagia diet _____ Tubefeeding	Soft diet Dysphagia diet _____ Tubefeeding	Soft diet Dysphagia diet _____ Tubefeeding	Soft Diet Dysphagia diet _____ Tubefeeding (consider PEG)
PT/Family Education	Stroke booklet & video	Nutrition/diet/dysphagia	Incontinence	Self-care needs/ADLs	Self-care discharge plan
Discharge Planning	RN gives NIH score to LMSW	LMSW completes assessment	Disposition planned	Support as needed	Discharge

Exhibit 6-A-4 General Surgery—Post-Anesthesia Care Unit Flow Sheet and Nursing Record

Initial assessment: Nurse signature

Neurological	Gastrointestinal	
___ Refer to NVS record	Abdomen: _____	2. GA: _____ Site:_____
Pupils: _____	Bowel sounds: _____	Rate: _____
Misc.: _____	NG Suction/drainage: _____	Healthy: Yes___ No___
Cardiovascular	_____	Arterial Line:
Rhythm _____ Lead_____	NCT Placement	Site: _____
Alarm On Yes___ No___	checked Yes___ No___	Healthy: Yes___ No___
Limits Set: Yes___ No___	**Integumentary**	Condition of Extremity
Pads & Leads	Pressure areas Yes___ No___	Involved _____
in Position Yes___ No___	Location _____	SBP Limits Set: Hi___ Lo___
NIBP Limits	Swelling Yes___ No___	Alarm On Y___ N___
Set: Yes___ No___	Location _____	Pulse Present Y___ N___
Alarm On: Yes___ No___	Redness Yes___ No___	Calibrates Well Y___ N___
Site: _____	Location _____	CVP_____ Site_____
Healthy: Yes___ No___	Pressure areas Yes___ No___	Healthy Y___ N___
Peripheral Pulses:	Location _____	**Safety Measures/**
RA Yes___ No___	Other _____	**Fall Precaution**
RL Yes___ No___	**Dressings**	Side Rails Up Yes___ No___
LA Yes___ No___	Yes___ No___ Other _____	Bed Low
LL Yes___ No___	Dry___ Moist___	Position Yes___ No___
TED Hose: _____	Saturated _____	Hand/Feet
Respiratory	Intact _____ Location_____	Restrained Yes___ Site___
Resp. Effort: _____	**Drainage Tubes**	N/A___
Depth: _____	JP: _____	Brakes on Yes___ No___
Airways: _____	Hemovac: _____	Prosthesis/
Breath Sounds: _____	Solcotran: _____	Valuables Yes___ No___
_____	Vacutainer: _____	Type_____
Pulse Oximetry _____	C.T.: _____	Location _____
Alarm On _____	Other: _____	ARMBAND Yes___ No___
O₂ Rx/Misc. _____	Suction: Yes___ No___	Location _____
_____	CmH2O	Isolation/Type _____
Vent. Alarm: On _____ Off___	Location of Tubes _____	**Psychosocial/**
NA___	**Position**	**Emotional Status**
Renal	Side: ___Rt. ___Lt. ___	Anxious_____ Calm _____
DTV: _____ Time:_____	Supine___ Prone___ HOB___	Smoker _____
Foley: _____ Secured:____	FOB___ Other _____	ETOH HX: _____
Urine color/character: _____	**Invasive Lines**	Drug HX: _____
_____	1. GA: _____ Site:_____	**Physical/Psychosocial**
Bladder	Rate: _____	**Impairments**
Distended: Yes___ No___	Healthy: Yes___ No___	Physical Impairment _____
		Pertinent History _____
		Psychosocial _____

continues

Exhibit 6-A-4 continued

Patient/Family Teaching	
Time	Nursing Progress

Exhibit 6-A-4 continued

Post-Anesthesia Care Unit Variance Report

	POP___ POS___ SDA___ Floor___ IMC___ ICU___ Other___
	Goals: Met____ Unmet____ Type of anesthesia: _____
	Variances: Delay: Yes____ No____
	Patient: _____ (See back) Length of delay_____
	System/Caregiver: _____

Reason:

___ Rm (floor) not ready   ___ RN unable to take report
___ ICU bed not ready   ___ Awaiting sign out
___ DSU not ready   ___ Awaiting M.D. consult
___ No room (floor) avail.   ___ Awaiting procedure/TX to be
___ No ICU bed avail.   done
___ No IMC bed avail.   ___ No transport help
___ Change of shift   ___ RN too busy to transport
                                  ___ Others _____

ADDRESSOGRAPH

Nurse signature _____

Patient Variances

Respiratory
___ Obstructed Airway/Respiratory Arrest
___ Reintubation
___ Decreased Oxygen Saturation
___ Respiratory Depression
___ Prolonged Intubation

Cardiovascular
___ Hypotension
___ Hypertension
___ Chest Pain
___ Arrythmia(s)

Eurologic
___ Deficit Not Present Pre-Op

Additional Variances
___ Excessive Drowsiness
___ Pain Management
___ Excessive Nausea/Vomiting
___ Temperature < 94° or > 101°
___ Bleeding
___ Low Urine Output
___ Spinal Anesthesia—Slow To Move
___ Observation
___ Others

Unplanned Admissions
___ Outpatient to Floor Reason: _____
___ To an ICU   Reason: _____

Exhibit 6-A-5 St. Luke's Medical Tower, Ambulatory Surgery and Endoscopy Center, Outcomes Management/Critical Pathways Variance Worksheet

PREOP	TIME IN:		PATIENT READY (TIME):			TIME OUT:	
UNIT:	INTERNAL	DISCUSSION/EXPLANATION	COMMENTS	CODE	DELAY # OF MIN		
Patient		Arrived late		18			
		Noncompliant with Preop procedure (NPO)		19			
		Requiring additional bowel prep		36			
		Difficult IV start		77			
		Knowledge deficit		83			
Care Giver		Physician arrived late		88			
		Workup delay (H&P/consent)		39			
		Plastic prep delay		40			
		Staff unavailable: Preop ❑ O.R. ❑ Endo ❑		8			
		Anesthesia/Interview ❑ Epidural ❑ Eye Block ❑ Unavailable ❑		1			
System		Registration/Insurance delay		20			
		Lab/additional testing required		9			
		Last minute scheduling change		5			
		Previous case delay: Physician Late ❑ Difficult Case ❑		16			
		Other/Explain:		17			
R.N. SIGNATURE			MET ❑				ADDRESSOGRAPH

Exhibit 6-A-5 continued

O.R./ENDO	TIME IN:	PROCEDURE START TIME:	PROCEDURE END TIME:		TIME OUT:
UNIT:	INTERNAL	DISCUSSION/EXPLANATION	COMMENTS	CODE	DELAY # OF MIN
Patient		Difficult-Induction ❏ Emergence ❏		28	
		Not candidate for LOCAL/MAC/IV sedation		79	
		Knowledge deficit		84	
		Unexpected return to O.R.		87	
		Adverse drug/procedure response		86	
Care Giver		Physician not available: On phone ❏ Seeing patients ❏ Late ❏		11	
		Anesthesia delay due to-Late ❏ Not scheduled ❏ With another patient ❏		27	
		Cases not pulled ❏ Supplies incomplete ❏ Not available ❏		47	
System		X-ray delay-Not scheduled ❏ Late ❏ Films not available ❏		26	
		Instrument/equipment malfunction		29	
		Incomplete/Incorrect pref list-Details missing ❏ Wrong procedure ❏		80	
		Procedure added after patient identification		78	
		Case longer than posted time		41	
		Staff unavailable: Positioning ❏ Cleaning ❏ Tech ❏		78	
		Other/Explanation:		17	
R.N. SIGNATURE			MET ❏		

ADDRESSOGRAPH

continues

Exhibit 6-A-5 continued

R.R.	PRIMARY TIME IN:		PROGRESSIVE TIME IN:	DISCHARGE TIME:		ASA#
UNIT:	INTERNAL	DISCUSSION/EXPLANATION	COMMENTS	CODE	DELAY # OF MIN	
Patient		No ride home ☐ Waiting for S/O ☐		6		
		Nausea		30		
		Pain control		32		
		Sleepy		33		
		Hyper/Hypotension		34		
		Respiratory Depression		75		
		Epidural delay		35		
		Patient request to stay longer		44		
Care Giver		Waiting for anesthesia sign-out		24		
		Waiting for surgeon/physician ☐ Waiting for clarification of orders ☐		82		
		Physician order to stay longer		43		
System		Waiting for PT		38		
		Discharge/Admission delay due to staffing problems		3		
		Transfer delay due to SLEH shift change		50		
		Transfer delay due to: No private room ☐ No bed ☐ Room not clean ☐		49		
		Delay less than 15 minutes		99		
		Other/Explain:		17		
PRIMARY R.N. SIGNATURE			PROGRESSIVE R.N. SIGNATURE		ADDRESSOGRAPH	MET ☐

Exhibit 6-A-6 Texas Children's/St. Luke's Episcopal Hospital Newborn Care

Transition
(6–8 hours)
Admission Day
DRG: 385–391

MATERNAL
ADDRESSOGRAPH

NEWBORN
ADDRESSOGRAPH

Mother:
Age: _____
Prenatal care started @ _____ wks
Childbirth Education _____
WBD: _____
WBE: _____
Date of Delivery: _____
Vag _____ C/S _____
IDDM _____ Yes _____ No
GDM _____ Yes _____ No
Total labor length _____ hrs
2nd stage _____ hrs
Antibiotic prophylaxis
_____ Yes _____ No
Steroids prior to delivery
_____ Yes _____ No
Smoker _____ Yes _____ No
PPROM _____ Yes _____ No

Ethnicity:
Blk _____
Hisp _____
Cauc _____
Asian _____
Other _____

Neonate:
WBE: _____
Admit Date: _____
Discharge (Date/Time) _____
Apgar Scores: _____ @ 1"; _____ @ 5"; _____ @ 10"
Sepsis Risk Factors _____ Yes _____ No
Sepsis Work-Up _____ Yes _____ No
Phototherapy _____ Yes _____ No
Asymptomatic of Infection _____ Yes _____ No
Normoglycemic:
Date: _____
Time: _____
PO feeding:
Date: _____
Time: _____
Full PO feeding established by
12 hr   24 hr   48 hr

continues

Exhibit 6-A-6 continued

Aspect of Care	Reproductive/Maternal	L & D		Unit	Unit
	Antepartum	Mother	Neonate		
Respiratory/ Newborn	Antepartum Positioning	Antepartum Positioning	Silverman Blow-by O2 ☐ Suction mouth/nose for meconium T ____ TH ____ Intubated ☐ Meconium below cords ☐ Oxyhood ☐ Bag Mask ☐ Pulse oximetry ☐ IMV ☐ Cord gas/ABG	Cardiorespiratory monitor ☐ O2 via hood ☐ @ ____ % to maintain O2 sat 85%–95% ☐ Pulse oximeter Oxygen Weaning Protocol ☐ Silverman score q 30 min x 2; then q 1 h til respiratory distress resolved ☐ D/C Oxygen @ ____ D/C Pulse Oximeter @ ____ Other ____ Respiratory Distress and O2 requirement resolved ☐ Mg Level ☐	
Safety	FHR Activity: Bedrest, Bedrest with BRP, PRN	Positioning	Radiant warmer Hat Heart monitor	Radiant Warmer, ISC @ 36.5C for admission ☐ Continue radiant warmer ☐ Isolette ISC ☐ Manual ☐ (as ordered) Open Crib (order) ☐ Identification per policy ☐ Temperature stable 97.6 to 99.5 ____ hrs. of age	
Integumentary	Dry	Dry	Dry Evaluate	Neonatal Skin Care Plan ☐ No skin breakdown ☐	

Exhibit 6-A-6 continued

Infection	Membranes Intact vs. Ruptured	CBC w/Diff. ___ RPR HBsAg UA V/S	Vit K ☐ Eye Prophylaxis ☐ CBC w/Diff/pH ☐	Handwashing/policy ☐ Begin sepsis workup as ordered ☐ RPR ☐ Blood type ___ Rh ___, Coombs ___ Record Maternal HBsAg ☐ VS q 1 hr x 6; then q 4 h ☐ Vitamin K ☐ Eye prophylaxis ☐ Triple Dye cord p bath ☐ Alcohol cord q diaper ☐ Antibiotics as ordered ☐ Chest x-ray ☐ NB Screen prior to discharge or @ 7 days of age ☐ H/H on admission ☐
Nutrition/ Fluids Electrolytes	Mg ___ Terbutaline ___	NPO IV Therapy I & O Type of IV Fluids D5IR x ___ # bags D10W LR x ___ # bags	NPO D10W Chemstrip IV Bolus	Strict I/O ☐ Daily weights ☐ Chemstrip or Whole Blood Glucose on admission ☐ Notify HO/NNP if glucose ≤ 40 ☐ Electrolytes as ordered ☐ NPO ☐ IVF ___ @ ___ cc/h Feed ___ ___ ca/oz Restricted @ ___ ml q ___ PO OG NG

continues

Exhibit 6-A-6 continued

Aspect of Care	L & D — Mother	L & D — Neonate	Unit ___	Unit ___
			Ad lib feeding ☐ Breastfeed on/off monitor ☐ Supplement BF ___ Other ___ Normoglycemic ☐ All nutrition PO ☐ Urine output 1cc/kg/hour	
Consults MD Neo Social Services NNP	Mother NNP MD Social Services Child Life	Infant Pedi Neo		
Psychosocial Family ___ Y ___ N Tour	Boarding Support Separation	Opportunity for patient to see, touch and/or hold infant		(Evaluate needs from Patient/Family Data Sheet ☐) Assist holding/touching ☐ Provide comfort/support to infant during and after tests/handling ☐ Provide information to parents about infant's condition and plan of care ☐ Provide info on skin-to-skin ☐ Other: ___

Exhibit 6-A-6 continued

	Teen AMA	Teens	Positioning Containment Facilitation _____ procedures	
Developmental				Initiate developmental assessment/interventions ☐ (see Developmental/Age Appropriate Plan of Care for Premature/High Risk Infants)
Education	POC DX Tour Educ. material	1. Expectation for delivery & neonate 2. Normal NB recovery 3. Level III Breastfeeding	TCH Parent Handbook	Initiate TCH/SLEH Teaching Guidelines for Newborn Infant ☐
Discharge Planning	ID Caregivers Patient/Family Data Sheet		Transfer to Nbn. Level II Level II	Identify care givers for home. Admission needs assessment evaluated ☐ Consults: _____ Initiate Neonatal Admission Assessment ☐ Triage to appropriate level of care: Transfer to Level III or II ☐ Transfer to NBN ☐

Exhibit 6-A-7 DRG 014: Stroke Intermediate Outcomes Worksheet

Privileged and confidential medical peer review communication generated pursuant to ad hoc review under V.A.T.S. 4495b, dec. 5.06; T.R.C.P. 166b(3)(d).

Record by number below the applicable intermediate outcomes:

Physiologic Outcomes

1. Activity Intolerance: Unable to tolerate more than 2 hours of physical activity.
2. Decreased LOC: Lethargy or lower LOC that persists despite attempts to arouse for participation in ADLs.
3. FUO: Fever of unknown origin *not* present at time of admission.
4. UTI: Urinary tract infection *not* present at time of admission.
5. Pneumonia: Diagnosis of pneumonia made by x-ray, *not* present at time of admission.
6. Atelectasis: Diagnosis of atelectasis made by x-ray, *not* present at time of admission.
7. Skin breakdown, pressure related: The occurrence of new skin breakdown, *not* present at time of admission.
8. Ventilator dependency: Inability to wean from mechanical ventilation within 24 hours of initial wean attempt.
9. MBS aspiration: Aspiration witnessed on modified barium swallow.
10. Cerebral edema: Evidence of cerebral edema on CT scan.

11. Transformation: Evidence of ischemic stroke transformation to a hemorrhagic lesion as documented by CT scan. (Initial CT scan must have reflected either ischemic stroke findings or have been negative.)
12. Disoriented to time.
13. Disoriented to time and place.
14. Disoriented to time, place, and person.
15. Seizures: New onset of seizures occurring following admission for stroke.
16. Urinary incontinence.
17. Bowel incontinence.

Psychosocial Outcomes

18. Code status: Family considering change in code status, but remain undecided for greater than 24 hours.
19. D/C indecisiveness: Patient and/or family undecided about discharge disposition for greater than 24 hours.
20. Patient D/C refusal: Patient refuses discharge plan but is incapable of independent living.

Provider Outcomes

21. Delayed nutrition intervention: Nutrition withheld for the first 72 hours following admission.
22. Inadequate nutrition intervention: Failure to administer sufficient calories and/or protein to meet patient's needs; (can only be recorded by the nutrition support dietitian).

System Outcomes

23. No bed on 17 Tower.
24. No bed on 22 IMC.
25. No bed on 22 Tower.
26. No insurance coverage for rehabilitation.
27. Delay in insurance verification greater than 24 hours; (include name of insurance carrier).
28. No medicaid SNF bed available.

Exhibit 6-A-7 continued

Date	Unit	Variance	Recorder	Date	Unit	Variance	Recorder	Date	Unit	Variance	Recorder

continues

Exhibit 6-A-7 continued

Indicator	Descriptor	Score	Score	Score
LOC:	Alert, keenly responsive.	0	0	0
	Drowsy, but arousable by minor stimulation to obey, answer, or respond.	1	1	1
	Requires repeated stimulation to attend, or lethargic or obtunded requiring strong or painful stimulation to make movements.	2	2	2
	Responds only with reflex motor or autonomic effects, or totally unresponsive, flaccid, reflexless.	3	3	3
LOC Questions:	The patient is asked the month and his/her age; only the initial answer is graded.			
	Answers both correctly.	0	0	0
	Answers one correctly.	1	1	1
	Answers both incorrectly, or unable to speak.	2	2	2
LOC Commands:	The patient is instructed to open or close his/her hand or eyes. Only the initial response is graded; credit is given if an unequivocal attempt is made but not completed.			
	Obeys both correctly.	0	0	0
	Obeys one correctly.	1	1	1
	Answers both incorrectly.	2	2	2
EOMs:	Normal.	0	0	0
	Partial gaze palsy. Score is given when gaze is abnormal in one or both eyes, but where focused deviation or total gaze paresis is not present.	1	1	1
	Forced deviation or total gaze paresis not overcome by the oculocephalic maneuver.	2	2	2
Visual Fields:	Test for hemianopia using moving fingers on confrontation with both of patient's eyes open; double simultaneous stimulation is also performed. Use visual threat where LOC or comprehension limit testing. Score 1 only if clear cut asymmetry is found; complete hemianopia (2) is recorded for dense loss extending to within 5 to 10 degrees of fixations.			

Exhibit 6-A-7 continued

No visual loss.	0	0	0	0
Partial hemianopia.	1	1	1	1
Complete hemianopia.	2	2	2	2
Facial Palsy: Normal.	0	0	0	0
Minor.	1	1	1	1
Partial.	2	2	2	2
Complete.	3	3	3	3
Motor Arm: Patient is examined with arms outstretched at 90 degrees if sitting, or at 45 degrees if supine; request full effort for 10s. If consciousness or comprehension are abnormal, cue the patient by actively lifting his/her arms into position as request for effort is orally given. Grade only the weaker limb.				
Limb holds for full 10s.	0	0	0	0
Limb holds position but drifts before full 10s.	1	1	1	1
Limb cannot hold position for full 10s, but there is some effort against gravity.	2	2	2	2
Limb falls; no effort against gravity.	3	3	3	3
Motor Leg: While supine, patient is asked to maintain each leg at 30 degrees for 5s. If consciousness or comprehension are abnormal cue the patient by actively lifting the leg into position as the request for effort is given orally. Grade only the weaker limb.				
Leg holds 30 degree position for 5s.	0	0	0	0
Leg falls to intermediate position by the end of the 5s period.	1	1	1	1
Leg falls to bed by 5s, but there is some effort against gravity.	2	2	2	2
Leg falls to bed immediately with no effort against gravity.	3	3	3	3
Plantar Reflex: Normal.	0	0	0	0

continues

Exhibit 6-A-7 continued

Indicator	Descriptor	Score	Score	Score
	Equivocal.	1	1	1
	Extensor.	2	2	2
	Bilateral Extensor.	3	3	3
Limb Ataxia:	Finger-to-nose and heel-to-shin tests are performed. Ataxia is scored only if clearly out of proportion to weakness. Limb ataxia is charted as "absent" in the hemiplegic; do not chart it as "untestable."			
	Absent.	0	0	0
	Ataxia is present in one limb.	1	1	1
	Ataxia is present in two limbs.	2	2	2
Sensory:	Test with pin; when consciousness or comprehension are abnormal, score sensory normal unless deficit is clearly recognized (ie: grimacing, withdrawal). Only hemisensory losses are counted as abnormal.			
	Normal, no sensation loss.	0	0	0
	Mild to moderate; patient feels pinprick is less sharp, or is dull on affected side, or there is a loss of superficial pain with pinprick, but patient is aware of being touched.	1	1	1
	Severe to total sensation loss; the patient is not aware of being touched.	2	2	2
Neglect:	No neglect.	0	0	0
	Visual, tactile, or auditory hemi-inattention.	1	1	1
	Profound hemi-inattention to more than one modality.	2	2	2
Dysarthria:	Normal.	0	0	0
	Mild to moderate; patient slurs at least some words, and, at worst, can be understood with some difficulty.	1	1	1
	Patient's speech is so slurred as to be unintelligible (in the absence of, or out of proportion to any dysphasia).	2	2	2

Exhibit 6-A-7 continued

Language:	The patient is asked to name the items on the naming sheet and is then asked to read from the reading sheet. Comprehension is judged from responses to each of the commands in the preceding neurologic examination.			
	Normal.	0	0	0
	Mild to moderate, as follows: Naming errors, work-finding errors, paraphasia, and/or impairment of comprehension or expressive disability.	1	1	1
	Severe: Fully developed Broca's or Wernicke's aphasia (or variant).	2	2	2
	Mute or global aphasia.	3	3	3
	TOTAL SCORE:			

■ 7 ■

Outcomes Assessment through Protocols

Nancy Shendell-Falik, MA, RN
Katherine B. Soriano, MS, RNC

Spiraling health care costs have mandated a new approach to the traditional system of patient care delivery. A major catalyst for change is the significant challenges posed by an evolving, reformed reimbursement system. In the past, hospitals were paid retrospectively for the care they provided to patients. Reimbursement was maximized by increasing the services offered. This fee-for-service system was then replaced in 1983 by a prospective payment system based on diagnosis related groups (DRGs). The DRG methodology was a fixed cost per case reimbursement system, which required concentrating on shortening the length of stay and controlling resource utilization for a hospital to be successful. Unfortunately, these systems were not effective in controlling escalating health care costs.

In the fee-for-service system, providers were paid for the care rendered to patients. The more opportunities for a physician to see a patient, the more dollars generated. Thus, in the fee-for-service environment there was no incentive to reduce cost. Similarly, the DRG method lacked incentives for providers to keep patients out of the hospital, control length of stay, or eliminate overuse of services. This is related to the fact that a hospital's reimbursement was determined by a blending of costs. The blended rate was based on the hospital's specific cost and a standard cost for a particular case. Therefore, a significant portion of the inefficiencies incurred were reimbursed to the hospital. Again, this illustrated an environment in which there was no motivation to decrease cost.

Acknowledgment: Appreciation is expressed to Kathi Kendall Sengin, MSN, RN, CNAA, Vice President, Nursing; Marguerite K. Schlag, EdD, RN, Director, Nursing Education; Maureen Bueno, PhD, RN, CNAA, Director, Nursing Systems, Outcomes Management and Research; Joanne McCollian, MSN, RNC, Head Nurse, Obstetrics; Eileen Naviello, BSN, RNC, IBCLC, Outcomes Manager; Mary Herbermann, MPH, RN, Director, Home Care; and Robin Adams, Secretary, for their support.

Thus, managed care and capitated payment initiatives have been developed and demonstrate the influence of the purchasers of health care services to curtail costs. Both managed care and capitation shift the financial risk from the payers to the providers of care. These shifts are hastening the pace to find effective solutions to manage health care delivery. Current issues in health care reform have refocused energies on the need to balance health care cost and health care quality. Health care reform calls for control of resources and better management of treatment for patients across the health care continuum.[1] The pressures on providers and payers in a fiscally constrained environment are increasingly evident.

As health care reform and components of managed competition infiltrate the health care system, health care providers will face legitimate challenges in responding to priorities that dictate the delivery of appropriate, cost-efficient, quality patient care.[2] The survival of health care institutions depends on a delivery system that efficiently uses resources and manages length of stay while monitoring progress toward identified outcomes.[3] Case management offers a strategy to succeed in balancing cost and quality in today's increasingly complex and dynamic health care arena. Case management is an integration of services for the achievement of specific clinical, financial, and satisfaction goals.[4] Use of protocols as a case management tool to predict the critical targets a patient will achieve within specific time intervals, coupled with efficient use of resources, is one method to measure patient outcomes. This chapter focuses on assessing various outcomes achieved through protocols in case management systems.

PROTOCOL OVERVIEW

The challenges facing hospitals to remain competitive in an era of health care reform and uncertainty were the impetus for the development of a system to promote cost-effective quality care. Although not new, case management is a means of responding to such complex demands. Case management is the coordinated multidisciplinary approach to patient care whereby a case manager bears the responsibility of directing the patient's hospital course to achieve identified goals within established time frames. This is accomplished through thoughtful communication and collaboration while ensuring effective resource utilization.[5]

For case management to be successful, the development of tools to help manage the patient's hospital experience is necessary. Such tools for managing care provide the multidisciplinary team with desired outcomes and identified time frames in which they should be accomplished. Terminology for such tools includes, but is not limited to the following:

- case management protocols
- case management plans
- practice protocols
- clinical protocols
- practice guidelines
- critical paths
- critical pathways
- CareMaps®

A critical pathway, one of the most common tools, is a schedule of activities that should occur within a structured time line.[6] Evolution of the critical pathway at The Center for Case Management resulted in the concept of a CareMap®. A CareMap®, quickly emerging as a favored tool, is a cause-and-effect grid that identifies expected outcomes against a time line for similar case types of patients.[7] Additionally, the CareMap® includes a way to link the process to outcomes and total quality management by use of an outcomes index that includes indicators for measuring quality.[8]

"The functions of a CareMap® tool include coordinating the interdisciplinary plan of care over an episode of illness, focusing care delivery on outcome management, providing central documentation for the medical record and establishing the standard against which to measure care delivered to a specific patient within an identified population."[9] For the purpose of this chapter, the term *protocol* is used to describe the multidisciplinary plan of care for a specific case type that identifies outcomes to be achieved within determined time frames and provides multidisciplinary documentation in the patient record. Protocols provide a method to decrease variation and manage patients through the health care continuum by ensuring quality and cost-effectiveness.

The demand for innovative strategies in patient care is a direct result of the heavily managed care market. Because managed care will be the primary insurance mechanism, it is evident fiscal pressures will continue to escalate. Payers are now demanding that providers strike a balance between an appropriate level of consumer benefit and gaining control over the seemingly uncontrollable increase in health care cost.[10] Protocols are one way to ensure operational efficiency in conjunction with high-quality, patient-centered care.

PROTOCOL DEVELOPMENT AND IMPLEMENTATION

The determination of which protocols to develop is an important decision. High-cost, high-risk, high-volume, and variable physician practice criteria are key considerations in the process. Data that are severity and risk adjusted provide critical insights to determine priorities for choosing a target population. Severity and risk adjustment systems produce data to ensure comparison and benchmarking of outcomes (e.g., length of stay, mortality, morbidity, costs, charges) for similar patients at like institutions. It is important that there is an apples-to-apples comparison when analyzing performance between institutions and establishing best practice protocols. In a managed care environment, case types should be selected through data analysis and determination of areas of greatest opportunity for financial savings.[4] Fiscal accountability promotes a commitment by the health care team and hospital administration to use protocols as one approach for effective performance in a managed care system. The effective use of protocols will facilitate the achievement of certain goals.[4,11] These include the following:

- deliver high-quality patient care in an environment with restricted financial and human resources
- provide consistency in the care of patients within a similar case type
- decrease fragmentation of care by anticipating care activities
- identify and eliminate practice patterns that are excessive or inefficient
- build collaboration among all members of the health team

Multidisciplinary participation is crucial to the successful development and implementation of practice protocols. It is important that all disciplines involved in the care of a particular case type have input and share in the decision-making process during protocol development. This collaboration facilitates a broad-based understanding and promotes the highest-quality patient care from a given disciplines perspective. Additionally, the process promotes renewed respect for other disciplines and builds collaborative relationships.

Physician leadership cannot be underestimated. At Robert Wood Johnson University Hospital (RWJUH), a 418-bed academic medical center located in central New Jersey, practice protocols have been developed. Physicians have taken a role in the forefront to facilitate protocol development and implementation. Once the case type or patient population has been selected, physicians with expertise in providing care to those patients are asked to participate.

A hospital administrator coordinates the protocol development process. This includes activities such as determining and securing resources for the team, monitoring progress, and preparation of meeting minutes. The administrator guides, coaches, and ensures support for the process.

Successful outcomes in protocol development require a thorough understanding of existing practice patterns. This can be accomplished through a comprehensive chart review in which current standards of practice and variances among practitioners can be identified. Validation of practice can be accomplished through interviews of every member of the health team. Evaluation of the most current literature and review of professional organization standards are also important activities. Collectively, these activities provide a baseline for analysis of practice patterns. It is also useful to compare standards of care and practice at other institutions that care for similar patient populations. These findings can then be compared with those of benchmark institutions in an effort to identify either barriers or opportunities for improvement. Although knowledge gained from benchmarking against other institutions' practice is crucial, protocols should be built internally from derived standards of care that lead to improvements in the effectiveness and outcomes of patient care.[2] External guidelines may be the catalyst in the multidisciplinary team's ability to consider eliminating unnecessary testing or procedures without affecting the quality of care. Challenging existing practice must be encouraged to search for new opportunities for innovation.

In the obstetric and pediatric services at RWJUH, the increase in managed care companies requiring a 24-hour length of stay after vaginal delivery was the impetus for the early discharge protocol. Although many practitioners had differing perspectives, no one could argue that the need to have a coordinated and structured approach to these patients was critical to ensure a safe and timely discharge. Thus, a protocol development team of professional staff involved with the care of mothers and infants was initiated. This protocol team included members from obstetrics, pediatrics, hospital administration, nursing, lactation services, utilization management, outcomes management, quality management, and home care. Through multidisciplinary collaboration, the goal of developing a protocol representing the best practice for early discharge of mothers and babies was realized. The completed protocols are illustrated in Appendix 7-A, Exhibits 7-A-1 through 7-A-7.

Completion of the written protocol, which reflects best practice, is only the first step in effecting change. The next challenge is operationalizing this into clinical practice. During this phase, the value of continual communication and commitment to create desired outcomes is critical.

Throughout the protocol development phase, frequent progress reports should be given to the multiple disciplines that will be affected. During the months of creating the early discharge protocol, updates were provided to the obstetrical suite committee, a multidisciplinary group focusing on operations of the perinatal service. Also, regular feedback was provided to pediatricians via two monthly committee meetings. This meeting structure keeps communication open and flowing during the period of development. On completion of the protocol, a presentation was made to the involved medical staff for support and approval. A formal presentation was given at the obstetrical and pediatric business meetings, which are committees of all obstetricians and pediatricians, respectively, who practice in the hospital.

Broad-based education of all involved disciplines occurs in the departments that are involved in the care of a patient within a particular case type. Staff are taught that protocols represent the current practice patterns that promote efficient, high-quality care. Nursing and ancillary staffs held around-the-clock meetings to educate those who care for mothers and babies to review the protocol and implications for practice. Differences between past practice patterns were discussed and the rationale for changes shared. This dialogue fosters a spirit of understanding, which is imperative for success.

System processes and practice patterns must be evaluated to continually improve patient outcomes and facilitate efficient and appropriate resource utilization. At a minimum, protocols are reviewed annually to ensure existing practice represents the current standard of care and that potential opportunities for innovation and efficiency are explored. Suggested revisions for change are reviewed by the protocol development team, and if implemented, the revised protocol is presented to the appropriate medical staff and hospital departments.

VARIANCE ANALYSIS

On implementing the protocol, monitoring of variances is initiated. A variance is defined as a deviation from the expected patient and family goals or outcomes.[12] Variances are both positive (those that foster progression toward anticipated achievable goals) and negative (those that hinder such progression). Both positive and negative variances provide invaluable information that enhances the intricate and complex relationship between actions and outcomes. Successful interpretation of data provides the multidisciplinary team with new and exciting directions to improve the delivery of care. "Variance analysis shows how and why clinicians differ from the norm as well as where an institution might improve its service."[12(p.1)] A crucial component of variance analysis is establishing an institution's individual standard from which comparisons are made.

Variances can be broken down into several components: those that are attributed to the patient, clinician, or system. Collectively these types of variances affect the total health care experience either positively or negatively. An example of a positive variance is a patient who is having her second or third child and demonstrates a solid knowledge base and realistic expectations. This patient is able to rely on previous experiences for guidance. In this example, the patient successfully progresses toward identified goals within established time frames. A negative patient variance may occur when a mother fails to demonstrate adequate feeding skills from breast or bottle or has a postdelivery complication such as hemorrhage. These two scenarios impede progression toward the goal of early discharge.

Variance in clinician practices may at times be more difficult to identify, analyze, and ultimately change. A negative physician variance may be a practitioner who does not discharge patients in accordance with the established time standard, therefore encouraging patients who are ready to be discharged in the morning to remain until evening. Although, this practice may not be immediately problematic, the long-range ramifications are evident. Continual education of clinicians about managed care and the institution's response is of paramount importance. A positive physician practice that influences the variance is a practitioner who emphasizes childbirth education and counsels patients on physical, psychosocial, and emotional preparation. This translates into a patient and family who are better prepared for childbirth.

System variances may involve the allocation of scarce resources in the most cost-effective manner to keep pace with a competitive, heavily managed care market. During the protocol development phase, it was noted by lactation and nursing staff that the goal of providing a lactation consultation to all breast-feeding mothers would be difficult. This was related to having one part-time certified lactation consultant who worked three days per week, thereby missing an opportunity to provide consultation to a significant number of breast-feeding mothers and infants. Identification of this variance led to a true performance improvement initiative. To expand this vital service, the decision was made to support lactation education, training, and certification of selected professional nurses. Today, this service is provided on a daily basis.

After careful collection of positive and negative variance data, systematic interpretation of information must ensue. The variances are compiled on a monthly basis and categorized and trended over time. This allows system processes and practice patterns to be evaluated to improve patient outcomes and facilitate efficient and appropriate resource utilization. Data analysis provides the critical link between outcomes and performance improvement. Such findings influence and guide our practice to ensure quality care across the health care spectrum. Institutional commitment is integral to the success of data collection, interpretation, and evaluation.

OUTCOMES

In general, variance analysis findings reflect the inpatient hospital experience. To move beyond this limited time segment, evaluation of outcomes must recognize the interdependence of health care providers as they work together to overcome sickness and promote health.[13]

Defining outcomes is a complex task involving a multidisciplinary analysis of the consumer, the provider, the payer, and the system individually and in its entirety. This task is a difficult one in that there is no one clear definition of outcomes. An outcome is the result of "what happened" during a state of illness or wellness. Outcomes assessment refers to the measurement, monitoring, and feedback of outcomes.[14] According to Nelson,[15] outcomes are the ultimate indicator of quality. The term *outcomes management* was pioneered by Paul Ellwood in the 1980s. Outcomes management is a process of initially determining desired outcomes and then defining the process to achieve them, always cognizant of the delicate balance of the cost/quality ratio.[16,17]

Maternal and newborn length of stay, newborn readmission rates, and patient satisfaction are the outcomes measured in the early discharge of mother and infant. In comparing data from 1993 and 1994, the numbers of patients qualifying as an early discharge rose from 5.6 percent to 18 percent. Analysis of 1995 statistics reveals a projected 32 percent early discharge rate when current year-to-date data are annualized.

The second outcome measure, unplanned readmission, is defined as an infant delivered at RWJUH who is readmitted to the institution within 31 days. Before the early discharge protocol implementation during 1994, the readmission rate was 0.3 percent compared to 0.0 percent after implementation. Thus, these evaluation data indicate that a well-planned change in practice via a protocol can have a positive effect on patient care in today's health care environment. To date, there is no significant change in obstetric patient satisfaction. This may be related to the practice of random sampling of all discharged patients from RWJUH. To this end, a specific survey addendum for obstetric patients is in the developmental stages to understand accurately the impact of early discharge on patient satisfaction levels.

Who or what, in fact, are the driving forces behind outcomes? The consumer, the provider, or the payer? Several themes emerge regarding this matter. Because outcomes are a measurement of "what happened," a report card so to speak, outcomes belong to the recipient of the process, the patient.[17,18] A different approach to forces driving outcomes clearly links them to the payer and the financial impact of reimbursement on health care.[1] This encompasses the comparison of outcomes data by managed care companies to receive the best, most comprehensive care for their money. Providers are astutely interested in outcomes data to maintain a competitive edge in the managed care market. Effective outcomes assessment is the logical goal in determining ways in which health care organizations can improve care while maintaining fiscal responsibility.

Identifying consumer outcomes may be more simplistic, although difficult to measure in that a patient's primary concern is solely related to personal experience. Desirable outcomes include the absence of complications, increase in feelings of wellness, and increase in satisfaction with the providers and prescribed course of treatment. Outcomes for consumers extend far beyond the immediate state of illness or wellness. These include functional status, quality of life, and role performance.

Outcomes related to the patient's perception of care have to do with surveying the patient's responses in regard to access and satisfaction of care and the functional and perceptual benefits of health care interventions.[2] For example, a patient who is hospitalized for a scheduled Caesarean section is not primarily concerned with remaining in the hospital for an expected length of stay or that specific goals are met on a particular day as outlined in the protocol. To this consumer, outcomes reach far beyond the immediate pre- and postoperative course, focusing on things such as short- and long-term physical, psychosocial, emotional well-being and the ability to integrate the newborn into the family system. For the consumer using any health care service, the perception of functional status is an individual one that extends throughout the life span. Patient-reported outcomes are the ultimate indicator of "best treatment" as consumers continue to play an integral role in health care reform.

One illustration of an enhanced system for patient care management across the continuum is demonstrated in the follow-up of early discharge mothers and infants. During the protocol development process, an objective review of payers was conducted. This highlighted that although payers were anxious to discharge patients early, some did not have a system in place for providing home visits. Home visits are supported as the vital link in the transition from hospital to home by the professional standards of the American College of Obstetricians and Gynecologists and the American Academy of Pediatrics. Thus, opportunities to provide this service for patients whose insurance companies did not was undertaken.

Although RWJUH boasts an active home care department, perinatal expertise of home care personnel was not a developed strength. Through the collaborative efforts of all professional staff, a goal of providing home visits by seasoned perinatal nursing staff was envisioned. Total involvement of all individuals within the institution and home care department was essential.

A pilot program was initiated in which a staff nurse from the perinatal service would visit early discharge mothers and babies within 72 hours of leaving the hospital. The home care department absorbs the cost of the nurse and bills the insurance company for the home visit. Thus, all obstetric patients who are discharged in accordance with the early discharge protocol are offered a home visit if their insurance company does not provide it. Nurses who participate in the early discharge home visitation program have a minimum of two years recent obstetric nursing experience and lactation certification or education. Additionally, orientation is provided by the home care department related to home care standards, community resources, and family safety.

This program is supported via a newly created documentation record (Exhibit 7-A-8 in Appendix 7-A) focusing on assessment of the mother and infant as well as the environment. This innovation clearly enhances the continuity of patient care from the hospital to home with a focus on positive patient outcomes resulting from care received.

Providers and payers are acutely aware of the intimate link between outcomes, quality, and the highly competitive reimbursement system. Key characteristics for desirable outcomes in the hospital setting include:

- decrease in length of stay
- decrease in cost per patient day
- decrease in readmission rates
- decrease in resource utilization
- increase in throughput of the system

Outcomes related to utilization and resource management focus on traditional utilization statistics such as lengths of stay and denied days, whereas resource management focuses on the utilization of ancillary services.[2] Benchmarking in terms of local, regional, and national standards enables hospitals to view themselves comparatively and see where service improvements may be made to be positioned strategically in the health care arena. Obviously, payers understand the challenge to maintain high-quality care in a fiscally responsible manner. To be competitive in this new era of health care, insurance companies are challenged with "grading" acute care settings, then guiding subscribers in informed decision-making processes.

CONCLUSION

The new millennium of managed care challenges the consumer, provider, and payer to reconfigure traditional ways of providing care. These innovative approaches must traverse the continuum of care from illness to wellness. This change demands breaking down barriers that once fragmented the health care system by viewing the consumer in isolation. This new vision of health care reenergizes the focus on wellness promotion and illness prevention across the life span. The emergence of a comprehensive, integrated health care system that focuses on outcomes and economics is the wave of the future.

The development of standardized protocols to monitor patients' episodes of illness and well-being are quickly emerging as the standard of care in a heavily managed care, capitated environment. Careful analysis of data gleaned from such protocols allows institutions to correlate patient process to patient outcomes. Enhancement of quality depends on the caliber of information the institution compiles, as well as the management of this information both internally and externally. The need for information system management to reflect accurately the input and output of the system is of paramount importance. Institutions must decide what types of information will have the most positive effect on the cost/quality ratio.

Sophisticated variance analysis tracking allows institutions to gather vital data. This is accomplished via state-of-the-art computer technology specifically designed to monitor information such as clinical management, specific variances, and lengths of stay. A national data base to link data collected from a variety of sources may lead to a multidisciplinary approach to information management.[19]

An expansion of outcomes management to encompass the outpatient setting and preventive health care forums would further enhance the ability to link process and outcomes across the health care continuum. Such direction would simplify the communication of increasingly complex health care needs among payers and providers. The link between outcomes and performance improvement along with the synergistic relationship between the two cannot be underestimated.[20] This should be a focus of strategic planning for institutions nationwide as outcomes and quality influence and guide our practice.

REFERENCES

1. Cohen EL, Cesta TG. Case management in the acute care setting: a model for health care reform. *J Case Manage*. 1994;3:110–116.

2. Rosenstein AH. Financial risk, accountability and outcome management: using data to manage and measure clinical performance. *Am J Med Quality*. 1994;9:116–121.

3. Clark CM, Steinbinder A, Anderson R. Implementing clinical paths in a managed care environment. *Nurs Econ*. 1994;12:230–234.

4. Zander K. Case management series. IV: who could be case manager? *New Definition*. 1995;10:1–4.

5. Shendell-Falik N. ProACT™ for pediatrics: work redesign and nursing case management. In: Flarey DL, ed. *Redesigning Nursing Care Delivery: Transforming Our Future*. Philadelphia, Pa: JB Lippincott; 1995: 162–172.

6. Zander K. Care maps: the core of cost/quality-care. *New Definition*. 1991;6:1–3.

7. Zander K. Toward a fully-integrated Care Map® and case management system. *New Definition*. 1993;8:1–3.

8. Zander K. Quantifying, managing and improving quality. I: how care maps link CQI to the patient. *New Definition*. 1992;7:1–3.

9. Hill M. Care Map® and case management systems: evolving models designed to enhance direct patient care. In: Flarey DL, ed. *Redesigning Nursing Care Delivery: Transforming Our Future.* Philadelphia, Pa: JB Lippincott; 1995:173–185.

10. Hayward C. Planning for the hospital of the future. *Adm Radiol.* 1994;13(2):26–30.

11. Girard N. The case management model of patient care delivery. *AORN J.* 1994;60:403–415.

12. Zander K. Using variances concurrently. Ill. *New Definition.* 1992;7(4):1–4.

13. Kelly KC, Huber DG, Johnson M, McCloskey JC, Maas M. The medical outcomes study: a nursing perspective. *J Pro Nurs.* 1994;10:209–216.

14. Davies AR, Doyle MAT, Lansky D, Rutt W, Stevic MO, Doyle JB. Outcomes assessment in clinical settings: a consensus statement on principles and best practice in project management. *Joint Commission J Quality Improvement.* 1994;20(1):6–16.

15. Nelson EC. Using outcome measures to improve care delivered by physicians and hospitals. In: Heithoff KA, Lohr KN, ed. *Effectiveness and Outcomes in Health Care.* Washington, DC: National Academy Press; 1990:201–211.

16. Ellwood PM: Outcomes management: a technology of patient experience. *N Eng J Med.* 1988;318:1549–1556.

17. Moss MT. The rebirth of quality: managed care and managed cost in perioperative nursing. *Nurs Econ.* 1995;13:54–57.

18. Howe RS. Inside case management: emerging trends, tools, and techniques. *Inside Case Manage.* 1995;1(10):1–8.

19. DesHarnais S, Marshall B, Dulski J. Information management in the age of managed competition. *Joint Commission J Quality Improvement.* 1994;20:631–638.

20. Reinersten JL. Outcomes management and continuous quality improvement: the compass and the rudder. *QRB.* 1993;19(1):5–7.

Appendix 7-A
Examples of Protocols and Documentation Records

Exhibit 7-A-1 Early Discharge/Vaginal Delivery Protocol

Categories	Date: 0–12 hrs	Initials	POD Date: 13–24 hrs	Initials	POD #1 Date: Discharge	Initials	POD #2 Date: Post Discharge	Initials	POD #3 Date:	Initials
Tests	CBC, Prenatal labs on chart, Rhogam screen									
Consults	Social Service, Lactation, Birth Certificate, Dietary				Lactation Consult if necessary		Home health care Assess physical environment, postpartum assessment			
Fundus	Fundus firm at midline Lochia scant—heavy									
Respiratory Status	Respirations regular and easy									
Nutrition	Regular diet									
Activity	OOB with assistance x 2 then ad lib Shower									

continues

Exhibit 7-A-1 continued

Categories	Date: 0–12 hrs	Initials	POD Date: 13–24 hrs	Initials	POD #1 Date: Discharge	Initials	POD #2 Date: Post Discharge	Initials	POD #3 Date:	Initials
Wound/ Episiotomy	Peri care Surgigator		Initiate sitz bath							
Fluid Status/ Elimination	D/C IV fluids Stool softener PRN Voiding without difficulty I&O x 3 voids		Laxative PRN Voiding without difficulty							
Nursing Interventions	Admission Primary RN Assessment OM Assess mother infant bonding		Appropriate breast, bottle feeding Rhogam		Rubella					
Medications	Pitocin PO analgesics Sleeping pill Stool softener/ laxative IRON/vitamin supplement									

Exhibit 7-A-1 continued

Teaching	Orient to unit and Newborn crib Feeding/ positioning Handwashing Self care		Newborn bath and safety class Car seat info/ return demo	Discharge Instructions Gift packs Infant car seat F/U appoint- ment Home Visit Referral	Reinforce teaching of infant and self care
Discharge Plan	Notify MD of need for home visit Assess knowl- edge and discharge needs			Arrange appropriate home visit Discharge criteria	Arrange additional home visits Lactation consultant follow-up

continues

Exhibit 7-A-1 continued

Initiated (Date/Initials)	Diagnoses (RT Related to) Breastfeeding	Date Discussed w/pt. and/or Family	Expected Outcomes	Achieved Outcomes (Date/Initials)
	• Alteration in comfort RT • Breast engorgement ___ Frequent feeding: at least q 2–3 hrs. ___ Wake baby to feeding during day ___ No supplements/pacifiers ___ Warm compresses/showers • Sore nipples ___ Proper positioning ___ Express colostrum prior to LATCH/ after feeding ___ Lanolin ___ Air nipples ___ Initiate in LDR • Alteration to nutrition RT Breastfeeding ___ Well balanced meal ___ Fluid intake		Patient will anticipate potential engorgement by P.P. day 3/4 and verbalize comfort measures. Patient will verbalize minimal soreness by discharge. Verbalize understanding of dietary modification RT breastfeeding.	
	Latch:			
	Audible sucking:			
	Type of nipple:			
	Comfort:			

Exhibit 7-A-1 continued

Hold:		
Educational Literature:		
Supplies:		

Brief Variance Notes (Please fully describe in-progress notes.)

Initials	Signatures	Initials	Signatures

Source: Courtesy of the Robert Wood Johnson University Hospital, New Brunswick, New Jersey.

Exhibit 7-A-2 Early Discharge: Vaginal Delivery Multidisciplinary Plan of Care

MD: _____

Outcomes Manager: _____

Primary Nurse: _____

Date to Begin: _____

Significant Past OBSTETRICAL MEDICAL HISTORY

VAGINAL DELIVERY

Initiated (Date/Initials)	Diagnoses (RT Related to)	Date Discussed w/pt. and/or Family	Expected Outcomes	Achieved Outcomes (Date/Initials)
	• Alteration in oxygenation RT PP hemorrhage ___ uterine atomy ___ increased lochia/clots ___ distended bladder ___ straight catheterization ___ vital signs q 2x4, q 4-2, q shift		• Absence of hemorrhage, dizziness, and weakness upon discharge	
	• Alteration in comfort RT vaginal delivery ___ positioning ___ analgesics ___ episiotomy ___ hemorrhoids ___ ice pack		• States pain is in tolerable range by discharge	

Exhibit 7-A-2 continued

_____ peri care
_____ surgigator
_____ sitz bath

- Breast engorgement/tenderness RT
  _____ bottle feeding
  _____ supportive bra
  _____ ice packs
  _____ avoid warm water to breast

- Alteration in elimination RT vaginal
  delivery
  _____ I&O x3 voids

Date	Time	Amount
1.		
2.		
3.		

  _____ straight catheterization
  _____ bowel movement _____
  _____ bowel sounds

- Alteration in protection RT PP infection:
  _____ temp q 2x4, q 4x2, q shift
  _____ foul smelling lochia
  _____ purulent drainage
  _____ abdominal or perineal pain/tenderness

- Minimize engorgement and decrease breast swelling

- Return to pre-pregnancy function by discharge

- Absence of infection

Source: Courtesy of the Robert Wood Johnson University Hospital, New Brunswick, New Jersey.

Exhibit 7-A-3 Management of Health Post-Partum Self-Care Teaching

Patient's ability to learn _____

_____

Communication deficit _____
Language spoken _____

TOPIC	

Oxygenation
  Splinting C&DB
  Incentive Spirometry	

Ambulation	
Comfort Ice pack	
Rubber ring	
Positioning	
Pain medication	
Breast engorgement	
Nutrition Balanced diet/fluid intake	
Protection Handwashing	
Surgigator	
Peri care: Sitz bath, Peri care aids	
Abdominal incision care (if applicable)	
Breast care	
Normal involution Lochia fundal massage	
Coping Emotional changes	

Initials	Signature and Title	Initials	Signature and Title

Patient's Signature _____

Source: Courtesy of the Robert Wood Johnson University Hospital, 1996. Developed by: Eileen Naviello, BSN, RNC, IBCLC and Joanne McCollian, MSN, RNC.

Exhibit 7-A-4 Early Discharge/Nursery Protocol

Categories	Date: 0–12 hrs	Initials	POD Date: 13–24 hrs	Initials	POD #1 Date: Discharge	Initials	POD #2 Date: Post Discharge	Initials	POD #3 Date:	Initials
Tests	Type & Coombs Dextro stix, Rhogam screen, prenatal labs		Check type and coombs, hearing screening, birth defects registration if necessary		PKU prior to discharge Bilirubin if needed		Home visit repeat PKU Bilirubin results to pediatrician			
Consents	Circumcision and Hepatitis consent									
Consults	Social Service, Lactation									
Cardiac Status	Skin color Cyanosis Heart rate Heart sounds									
Respiratory Status	Respirations regular and easy 40–60 minutes Lusty cry									
Nutrition	Good suck/ swallowing LATCH on/ swallowing Sterile water Formula Breast milk		Tolerate feeding				Lactation consult if necessary			

continues

Exhibit 7-A-4 continued

Categories	Date: 0–12 hrs	Initials	POD Date: 13–24 hrs	Initials	POD #1 Date: Discharge	Initials	POD #2 Date: Post Discharge	Initials	POD #3 Date:	Initials
Activity	Radiant heat warmer, moves all extremities		Open crib		Open crib		Assess home environment			
Wound/ Circumcision			Circumcision							
Fluid Status/ Elimination	Voiding Meconium Soft abdomen I&O		Voiding Meconium Soft abdomen I&O		Voiding Meconium Soft abdomen I&O		Voiding Transitional stool Soft abdomen			
Nursing Interventions	Nursing Assessment by RN Assessment by OM Thermoregulation Mother–Infant bonding		Assess bleeding Post circumcision x 4 hours Baby photo Bonding appropriately		Bonding appropriately Assess jaundice Discharge mother and baby in wheelchair Discharge to car seat		Assess Jaundice Follow up phone call/ home visit make appropriate calls to pediatrician			
Medications/ Immunizations	Vitamin K Erythromycin Ointment Triple Dye		Hepatitis Vaccine				Alcohol to cord			

Exhibit 7-A-4 continued

Teaching	Initiate teaching checklist Hand washing Breast feeding/ positioning Bottle feeding Burping Car seat safety	Bathing Safety Teaching checklist	Complete teaching checklist	Reinforce all teaching
Discharge Plan	Discharge teaching initiated with parent	Meets discharge criteria	Discharge instructions to parents	

Source: Courtesy of the Robert Wood Johnson University Hospital, New Brunswick, New Jersey.

Exhibit 7-A-5 Nurses' Admission Assessment: Newborn Nursery

Sex _____ Identification Bands Checked _____

Birth Day _____ Time _____ am
                                                                                  pm

Admission Date _____ Time _____ am
                                                                                  pm

DR Complications _____

Apgar _____   _____ 1 minute   _____ 5 minutes

Weight _____ gms   _____ lbs.   _____ oz.

Length _____ cm   _____ in.   Head _____ cm _____ in.

Chest _____ cm   _____ in.   Abd. birth _____ _____ in.

Color_____   Cry _____   Tone _____

Apical _____   Resp. _____   Quality _____

Temp. on admission   _____   Time _____

                      _____   _____

                      _____   _____

                      _____   _____

                                          am   am
                      Void @ _____ pm   Stool @ _____ pm

Admission Bath Given _____ am
                      _____ pm

Dr. _____ Notified _____ am   Message taken by _____
                      _____ pm

Comments _____
_____
_____
_____

Admitting Nurse _____

Variance Note: _____

_____

Initials	Signatures	Initials	Signatures
_____	_____	_____	_____
_____	_____	_____	_____
_____	_____	_____	_____
_____	_____	_____	_____
_____	_____	_____	_____

Source: Courtesy of the Robert Wood Johnson University Hospital, New Brunswick, New Jersey.

Exhibit 7-A-6 Early Discharge: Vaginal Delivery Multidisciplinary Plan of Care

MD: _____

Outcomes Manager: _____

Primary Nurse: _____

Date to Begin: _____

Significant Delivery Information

VAGINAL DELIVERY

Initiated (Date/Initials)	Diagnoses (RT Related to)	Date Discussed w/Pt. and/or Family	Expected Outcomes	Achieved Outcomes (Date/Initials)
	• Alteration in oxygenation RT PP extrauterine life ____ respirations 40–60/minute ____ heart rate: R/O murmur ____ flaring/retracting ____ bulb syringe in crib ____ v/s q 15x4 then q 4 hours		Establish and maintain patent airway	
	• Alteration in elimination RT extrauterine life ____ I&O ____ stools		Baby will be voiding and passing stool upon discharge	

continues

Exhibit 7-A-6 continued

Initiated (Date/Initials)	Diagnoses (RT Related to)	Date Discussed w/Pt. and/or Family	Expected Outcomes	Achieved Outcomes (Date/Initials)
	• Alteration in protection RT infection/thermoregulation ___ temp rectal x 1 ___ temp q 15 hours until bath ___ temp q 4 hours until D/C ___ triple dye to cord ___ eye drainage ___ radiant warmer until after bath ___ hat ___ double wrap		Baby will be free of infection upon discharge	
	• Alteration in nutrition RT extrauterine ___ tolerates feeding ___ weight daily at 6 AM ___ sucking/swallowing ___ spitting/regurgitation ___ fontanels		Maintain adequate nutrition	

Source: Courtesy of the Robert Wood Johnson University Hospital, New Brunswick, New Jersey.

Exhibit 7-A-7 Management of Health: Parent Teaching/Infant Care Checklist

TOPIC	Demo	Date	Initials	Father Present	Return/Demo	Comments
NUTRITION (*Circle*) Breastfeeding/bottlefeeding Positioning techniques						
Burping techniques						
Regurgitation						
COMFORT Bathing						
Diapering						
Dressing						
PROTECTION Umbilical cord care						
Circumcision care						
Reading thermometer						
Axillary temperature						
Car seat safety						
Immunizations reviewed						
Bulb syringe use						
Positioning in crib						
Handwashing						

continues

Exhibit 7-A-7 continued

Initials	Signature and Title	Initials	Signature and Title

Comments: _____

Source: Courtesy of the Robert Wood Johnson University Hospital, New Brunswick, New Jersey. Developed by: Eileen Naviello, BSN, RNC, IBCLC and Joanne McCollian, MSN, RNC.

Exhibit 7-A-8 Visiting Nurse Documentation Record

Name _____
Case Number _____ Date _____
Address _____
Telephone _____ ER Name _____ Phone _____
Directions _____
_____
_____

Members in household	Sex	Age or DOB	Immunizations Current	Current Health Problems

Life Stressors: Physical Abuse _____ Sexual Abuse _____ Domestic Abuse _____
Elder Abuse _____ Child Abuse _____
Comment: _____
_____
_____

Exposure Habits: Tobacco _____ Alcohol _____ Drugs _____ Other _____
Comment _____
_____
_____

Safety: Emergency Response _____ Smoke Detector _____ Medical Safety _____
Home Safety Book Given _____
Lactation Consultant
  Breasts   _____   Feedings   _____
  Nipple   _____   Supplementation _____
  Position   _____   Infant   _____
  Latch-on   _____   Mother   _____
Comment: _____
_____

Community Resources/   Local Welfare _____ Medicaid _____ Food Stamps _____
  Support Groups: Planned Parenthood _____ WIC Program _____
                       Other _____
Comment: _____
_____
_____

Advanced   Do you have a living will or Durable Power of Attorney? Yes ___ No ___
Directive Where do you keep it? _____
           Who is your Health Care Representative? _____
Insurance   Name _____
Information: Address _____
             Policy Number _____ Group Number _____

continues

Exhibit 7-A-8 continued

MOTHER'S FORM

Name _____ DOB _____

DD _____ Allergies _____

Type of Delivery   G   T   PT   A   L

Vaginal   _____

vbac   _____

episiotomy/laceration   _____

c/section   _____

tubal   _____

complications   _____

temp _____   pulse _____   resp _____   bp _____

PHYSICAL	N	ABNORMAL	COMMENTS
chest	_____	_____	_____
breasts	_____	_____	_____
nipples	_____	_____	_____
abdomen	_____	_____	_____
fundus	_____	_____	_____
perineum	_____	_____	_____
lochia	_____	_____	_____
extremities	_____	_____	_____
bowels	_____	_____	_____
bladder	_____	_____	_____

TESTS	ASSESSMENTS		PSYCHOSOCIAL	COMMENTS
CBC	incision	_____	fears	_____
	epis/perineum	_____	depression	_____
	breasts	_____	bonding	
	activity	_____	behaviors	_____
	nutrition	_____	coping	
	environment	_____	mechanisms	_____
	social	_____		
	medication	_____		
	hemorrhoids	_____		

Exhibit 7-A-8 continued

TEACHING	Yes	No	Comments
incision care	____	____	_____
universal precautions	____	____	_____
self care/normal involution	____	____	_____
infant care	____	____	_____
feeding breast/bottle	____	____	_____
safety	____	____	_____
nutrition activity	____	____	_____
car seat	____	____	_____
family planning	____	____	_____
handwashing	____	____	_____
universal precautions	____	____	_____
waste disposal	____	____	_____
signs and symptoms (including infection)	____	____	_____
Follow-up M.D. App't	____	____	_____

NARRATIVE _____

_____

_____

_____

_____

_____

INITIALS	NURSE'S FULL SIGNATURE	TITLE
_____	_____	_____

NA—Not Applicable
T— Teach
D— Demonstration
RD—Return Demonstration
N— Narrative
R— Review

continues

Exhibit 7-A-8 continued

BABY'S FORM

Name _____ DD_____ Age_____ Room_____

temp _____   pulse _____   resp _____

PHYSICAL	N	ABNORMAL	COMMENTS
head	_____	_____	_____
fontanels	_____	_____	_____
eyes	_____	_____	_____
mouth	_____	_____	_____
chest	_____	_____	_____
heart	_____	_____	_____
abdomen	_____	_____	_____
genitals	_____	_____	_____
color	_____	_____	_____
umbilicus	_____	_____	_____
tone	_____	_____	_____
reflexes	_____	_____	_____
moro	_____	_____	_____
suck/rooting	_____	_____	_____
grasp	_____	_____	_____

TESTS   ASSESSMENTS
PKU
Bilirubin   environment   _____

             feeding   _____

             crying   _____

             sleeping   _____

             voiding   _____

             stooling   _____

Exhibit 7-A-8 continued

TEACHING	Yes	No	Comments
circumcision care	____	____	_____
bathing/water temp	____	____	_____
cord care circumcision care	____	____	_____
breast feeding	____	____	_____
bottle feeding	____	____	_____
safety	____	____	_____
car seat	____	____	_____
Follow-up M.D. App't Date	____	____	_____
signs and symptoms (to notify M.D.)	____	____	_____

NARRATIVE _____

_____

_____

INITIALS   NURSE'S FULL SIGNATURE   TITLE

_____   _____   _____

NA—Not Applicable
T— Teach
D— Demonstration
RD—Return Demonstration
N— Narrative
R— Review

Source: Courtesy of the Robert Wood Johnson University Hospital, New Brunswick, New Jersey.

■ 8 ■

Improving Quality through Nursing Case Management

Ann Scott Blouin, PhD, RN
Jodi A. Lewis, MS, MBA, RN
Nancy A. Malone, MBA, MPH, RN
Katherine E. Metz, MBA, RN

Case management has received considerable attention during the past decade in the literature and among health care providers in a variety of settings. The proliferation of anecdotal commentaries on quality improvements has prompted many health care organizations to begin serious study on the linkages between improved quality, outcomes measurement, and the implementation of case management. Although the growth of case management programs has been fueled by heightened financial constraints, there is continued evidence that case management can achieve incremental as well as overall quality improvement.

QUALITY OF CARE: GROWING INTEREST IN A CHANGING ENVIRONMENT

Widespread interest in the issue of quality health care delivery began to develop during the late 1960s with the rapid growth of health care expenditures. With the expansion of private health insurance during the postwar era and the enactment of the Medicare and Medicaid programs, substantially more health care dollars expended were paid by third parties. As these expenditures rose, providers were challenged to demonstrate to public and private payers that good value was received for the increasingly significant outlays. The overall concern with quality was directed at whether the funds spent on the provision of care were actually benefiting patients.[1]

Current interest in quality also stems from the continued increase in health care expenditures. However, attention now focuses on how quality of care is affected by cost containment efforts. The Medicare prospective payment system and similar limited reimbursement strategies, in combination with major advances in diagnostic and therapeutic technology, have significantly changed the speed and scope of health care delivery. Health care providers have been challenged by substantial changes, and continued uncertainty requires new managerial techniques to ensure future financial viability. Rapid turnover of patients, shortened lengths of stay, and increased patient complexity dictate the need for the efficient delivery of patient care services through methods such as case management.[2]

Health care organizations must examine how and why resources are organized and used, and embrace the concept of change, avoiding a business-as-usual approach. This is necessary if providers wish to position themselves to provide high-quality care while controlling costs, maintaining financial viability, and retaining the ability to invest in the future. Managed care, competition, constrained resources, and stringent regulations have created the imperative to balance the quality of care and the cost of services while encouraging a better understanding and closer evaluation of what is quality care.[2]

QUALITY DEFINED

Given that health care is generally viewed as a dynamic and developing enterprise, the quality of that enterprise is also dynamic. Hence, defining quality under such circumstances has remained a major challenge, particularly because many definitions for quality exist. Most definitions incorporate the concepts of appropriate processes of care and patient outcomes, with the former, properly applied, maximizing the latter. Newer definitions incorporate the concept of resource scarcity and stress outcomes within available resources. Included in these concepts are the technical or scientific aspects of care and interpersonal or humanistic elements of care.[3]

Traditionally, quality of care has been defined in terms of the technical delivery of services. This definition is changing to incorporate the expectations, desires, and opinions of patients, their significant others, and society in general. In addition, the clinical dimensions of the definitions of the quality of care have expanded to include care provided by nonphysician professionals. Such developments continue to challenge how we perceive and define quality of care.[3]

Many organizations and individuals have articulated definitions of quality of care. The Joint Commission for Accreditation of Healthcare Organizations has defined quality of care as "the degree to which health services for individuals and populations increase the likelihood of desired health outcomes and are consistent with current professional knowledge."[4] Lohr et al.[3(p.17)] state that health care quality is "a multidimensional concept reflecting a judgment that the services rendered to a patient were those most likely to produce the best outcomes that could reasonably be expected for the individual patient and that those services were given with due attention to the patient-physician relationship."

Although definitions of quality vary, Donabedian[1(p.15)] concludes that "the balance of health care benefits and harms is the essential core of a definition of quality." Therefore, as long as we can specify the actual or potential benefits of the care provided to a patient, we can evaluate the quality of that care. However, the ability to specify such benefits and harms is not always possible, nor without difficulty.

Donabedian[5] recommends using seven attributes of health care to define its quality: efficacy, effectiveness, efficiency, optimality, acceptability, legitimacy, and equity. Efficacy is the ability of health care, at its best, to improve health and well-being and is established through controlled clinical research. Effectiveness is the degree to which achievable results or improvements in health are realized in relation to what has been established by the studies of efficacy. Efficiency incorporates the concept of cost and is a measure of the cost of the given improvement. When two strategies are equally efficacious and effective, the more efficient strategy is the less costly one.[5]

Optimality incorporates an examination of the benefits and costs of care and strives for the most advantageous balance. In essence, the concept of optimality recognizes the consequences of making continued additions to care. Although the additions may be useful, beyond a certain point the balance of benefits and costs becomes adverse. Acceptability incorporates the patient's perception and value of the first three attributes, as well as the elements of accessibility of care, the patient-practitioner relationship, and the amenities of care. Patient preferences can significantly alter estimates of effectiveness, efficiency, and optimality. In addition, such preferences introduce significant variation among patients, making it difficult to determine what constitutes the best quality. Legitimacy, however, takes into consideration social preferences, and equity examines fairness in the distribution of care and its effects on health.[5]

As discussed above, care quality contains many components or attributes. Some attributes are reinforcing, such as effective care, which is usually legitimate and acceptable, whereas other attributes are in conflict. Hence, a balance must be obtained. Quality of care is judged in relation to standards derived from the science of health care. These standards establish efficacy, individual values and expectations that determine acceptability, and social values, and expectations that determine legitimacy. In assessing and ensuring quality, health care professionals must take into consideration both individual and societal preferences. Challenges arise when societal preferences are in disagreement with the individual in terms of what is optimal and equitable.[5]

CARE GIVER VERSUS PATIENT PERCEPTIONS OF QUALITY

In the traditional health care delivery paradigm, providers are considered to be the technical experts who know what is best for patients. Therefore, the very nature of services provided have in effect been controlled by provider perceptions of the needs of their consumers.[6] Health care professionals cite improved communication, fewer complications, reduced length of stay, reduced mortality and morbidity, reduced readmission rates, and improved patient satisfaction as quality outcome measures. Studies also show that care givers consider such indicators as the ratio of nurses to beds, the percentage of board-certified physicians on staff, the presence of discharge planning services, and the level of technology as top indicators of hospital quality.[7] These perceptions are generally consistent among physicians, nurses, and allied health professionals. Unfortunately, however, care givers are unable to predict patient perceptions of quality, and the literature shows that there is little or no relationship between patient perceptions of quality of care and those of the care giver.[6]

An additional, patient-focused definition of quality states that it "can be thought of as the goodness of the match between patient total need, the need for health and health care that is effective, and the set of services delivered."[8] The patient's view of what is important in the care he or she receives may be seen as one aspect of quality, and patient satisfaction has increasingly come to be used as an indicator of quality. Although Donabedian[9] considers client satisfaction as a judgment of the quality of care and not a part of the definition of quality, it is, however, the best representation of certain components of quality: client expectations and valuations.[10]

Patient perceptions of quality are formed by encounters with existing care structures and by their system of norms, expectations, and experiences.[10] From the patient's perspective, the overall quality of health care is determined by the entire package of characteristics including perceived health outcomes resulting from care and the patient's evaluation of the entire experience of seeking and receiving care. This experience includes accessibility, timeliness, and efficiency of services, the way providers interact and communicate with the patient, and the direct and indirect costs of illness and care.[8]

Davis and Adams-Greenly[11] identified four basic needs of customers: the need to feel important, the need to feel welcome, the need to be understood, and the need for comfort. Several studies have looked at what patients expect from care givers. In ambulatory settings, Ware et al.[12] identified eight dimensions of satisfaction: the art of care, accessibility, convenience, physical environment, financial state, availability of care giver, continuity of care, and efficiency/outcomes of care. Additional research indicates that most patients value the technical quality of their health care, followed by cleanliness, supportive and friendly attitudes, and physical comfort.

Nelson and Larson[13] suggest that from the customer's point of view, there are three different types of quality characteristics: "take-it-for-granted" quality attributes, expected quality attributes, and exciting quality attributes. Take-it-for-granted quality attributes are those a hospital must possess to be acceptable, such as competent staff. Expected quality attributes are those attributes that are necessary and expected, such as caring and concerned nursing staff, food quality, and positive health outcomes. Exciting quality attributes are those that are welcome but not perceived as necessary, such as extra accompaniments, supplies, or environmental features.

Quality of care is a multidimensional concept for which many definitions exist. As a result, the challenge will continue to be to look beyond the semantics and find a way to clearly define, measure, and improve quality attributes that are recognized and valued by consumers and providers, as well as payers. This is significant within a case management framework because effective case management programs must demonstrate measurable quality improvements in the face of these varied perceptions and expectations.

THE COST/QUALITY RELATIONSHIP

Within the context of a rapidly changing health care environment, providers are confronted with the imperative of maintaining or improving quality while reducing costs. The quality of health care is dependent on appropriate objectives of care and the selection of appropriate ways to achieve those objectives.[14] Often, efforts to improve productivity and reduce costs have been equated with a reduction in quality. Research examining the relationship between quality indicators, such as medical-surgical death rates and postoperative complication rates, has found no trade-off between high-quality care and efficiency. In essence, high-quality care can, in fact, equal cost-effective care.[2]

As noted by Donabedian,[14] quality and costs are interrelated, and this relationship is characterized by diminishing returns over time. As one adds increments of cost, corresponding improvements in health eventually become notably smaller. Ultimately, additions in cost produce no further improvements in health, or improvements too small to justify additional expenditure. Also, using additional resources beyond a certain point could, in theory, have a negative effect on quality through the use of unnecessary or potentially harmful interventions.

Of interest are the noted diminishing returns. The provision of quality care in general costs money; however, additional expenditures do not guarantee better quality or improved health status. As a result, if it is not known with certainty when additional expense yields little or no improvements, then it cannot be known with certainty the point at which cost controls will negatively affect quality of care.[3]

Further research in this area and the application of appropriate clinical management strategies such as case management provide the potential for simultaneously achieving the imperatives of quality care and cost reductions. Aiken[15] advocates a strategy that avoids across-the-board cuts and targets reductions in services that offer little return in terms of improved health in comparison to the investment or to areas where care has produced no notable positive benefits. Such a strategy incorporates changes to the process of care, in turn leading to improved outcomes and lower costs.[15]

THE ROLE OF CASE MANAGEMENT

Nursing case management is a model of patient care delivery and the management of resources that enables the strategic management of cost and quality by clinicians for an episode of illness or throughout the continuum of care. According to the American Nurses Association:

> Case management is a system of health care delivery designed to facilitate achievement of expected patient outcomes within an appropriate length of stay. The goals of case management are the provision of quality health care along a continuum, decreased fragmentation of care across settings, enhancement of the client's quality of life, efficient utilization of patient care resources, and cost containment.[16]

Quality is prescribed in written detail, concurrently managed, and collaboratively evaluated. Case management evolved as nurses, managers, and administrators asked difficult questions about clinical and administrative practices within the context of a changing health care environment. Such an environment has been viewed as nursing's best opportunity to produce gains for key constituencies including patients and families, care providers, health care organizations, and payers.[17]

The evolution of case management is driven by the belief that quality is not a vague ideal but can be defined based on the use of particular clinical process and outcome standards that resolve identified patient care problems. Therefore, quality in health care is a product, not a service. Another important driver of the case management evolution is the premise that the cost of producing a range of expected outcomes can be understood and revised on a case-type basis.[17]

Case management and the continuous quality improvement process are connected closely in terms of both philosophy and process. Case management enables the simultaneous consideration of both quality and cost, and within this framework, all practitioners are monitored for quality, resource use, and impact on length of stay. Further, the simultaneous movement toward the philosophy of continuous quality improvement and quality improvement teams matches the ability to use case managers' variance analyses to track results of managing patient care via critical pathways and clinical guidelines.

It is during the development of the managed care plan that the optimal treatment plan is identified or developed. Such a plan streamlines care by identifying appropriate objectives of care and a process for how to achieve these objectives without compromising quality. Development of the plan of care is typically a multidisciplinary process, and if executed correctly, these collaborative guidelines are developed and agreed on by a group of relevant practitioners by whom the guidelines were established.[18] These plans are designed to describe the single best treatment plan for a specific patient problem. By implementing and following these guidelines, quality issues and concerns are tracked and identified. Essentially, the plan and process provides for the collection and evaluation of potential quality issues, which can be identified through variances or complications. These variances may or may not indicate the need to modify the plan. The process enables a focus on quality by continually assessing and identifying opportunities for improvement.[18]

Assessment of quality improvements affected by nursing case management assumes quality can be defined and captured by objective elements. Zander[19] outlines six constructs for quality measurement and nursing case management: (1) Quality can be defined, (2) the critical pathway is the instrument for defining and measuring quality, (3) the time frames stated in the critical pathways prompt the definition of outcomes and benchmarks along the way, (4) when the critical pathway is multidisciplinary, there is a tangible definition of quality that is consistent for all health care providers, (5) the more clearly clinicians define interventions and outcomes of patient care, the more adminstrators will support the innovation of case management, and (6) a tight definition of quality drives a clear assignment of accountability.

Juran[20] notes that "improvement means the organized creation of beneficial change; the attainment of unprecedented levels of performance. A synonym is breakthrough. All quality improvement takes place project by project and in no other way." The planning and development of a case management system is an organized change directed at improving quality and efficiency in patient care and cost. An analogy can easily be conceived between Juran's concept of quality improvement "project by project" and case management's improvement case type by case type.

EVIDENCE IN THE LITERATURE

The recent literature demonstrates that case management decreases fragmentation and duplication of services and provides efficient management of care, accomplished through monitoring, coordination, and intervention. Gibson et al.,[21] Tahan and Cesta,[22] and Wimpsett[23] note that case management improves multidisciplinary communication and increases team collaboration. Collaborative planning stimulates role clarification and coordination and maximizes the contributions of all the members of the health care team. Tahan and Cesta[22] show that case management increases collaboration and opens lines of communication among nursing, medicine, and ancillary departments and reduces duplication or fragmentation in the care provided.

According to Smith,[24] patient health goals are more specific, realistic, and measurable. These goals are related to the patient, rather than to the staff. Flynn and Kilgallen[25] and Vautier and Carey[26] note that case management reduces duplication in charting, improves documentation of desired patient outcomes, and increases physician, staff, and patient satisfaction.

According to Gibson et al.,[21] a considerable impact has been made in decreasing total inpatient admissions, mean length of stay, and total charges. Wimpsett[23] states that case management demonstrates a decrease in inpatient days, delays, and surgical cancellations, as well as duplication of testing and supplies. Sinnen and Schifalacqua[27] discovered that on specific patients within identified case types an average decrease in length of stay of 22 percent was realized and total hospital charges decreased an average of 6 percent after the implementation of case management.

Rogers et al.[28] noted fewer hospital admissions and shorter stays, and the diagnosis-related groups (DRGs) for which patients were readmitted under case management required, on average, 1.5 fewer hospital days. Consequently, managing patient care effectively requires fewer, less costly resources for shorter periods to achieve expected outcomes. Rogers et al.[28] also noted that community-based case management tends to prevent patient health problems from becoming more complex. According to Erkel,[29] however, within the context of maintenance care, case management consistently increases the use of community-based services but also increases the cost of maintenance care to specific populations without necessarily improving health outcomes.

Many hospitals have reported positive impacts on a variety of quality performance measures after the implementation of nursing case management. At Intermountain's LDS Hospital in Salt Lake City, after implementing changes in the administration of prophylactic antibiotics for surgical patients via standardized clinical guidelines, the postoperative infection rate dropped from 1.8 percent to 0.4 percent, a decrease of 78 percent and savings of about $700,000.[30] Henry Ford Medical Center in Detroit reported definitive improvements in patient satisfaction after the implementation of case management protocols.[30] Mercy Hospital Anderson in Cincinnati, Ohio, discovered a 50 percent reduction in readmissions and emergency department use after implementing clinical guidelines.[31] Further, case managers are able to identify pre-existing systems problems and their root causes due to careful variance analysis. Many hospital executives believe the decreased problems or fewer variances patients experience result in higher levels of patient, physician, and staff satisfaction, leading to an improved reputation in the community.

As the emphasis continues to shift from inpatient care to outpatient, home care, long-term care, and subacute settings, the case manager's focus will shift to patient advocacy and prevention of variance across the continuum of care. Green and Malkemes[32] report that Harper Hospital in Detroit found patient satisfaction, overall quality, and cost management improved across the continuum of care with the use of case management. Critical pathways coordinated across varied settings can lead to improved colleague communication and collaboration, efficient and effective discharge planning, as well as improved patient and family education about the patient's illness and preparation for home care.

Overall, the literature demonstrates the broad benefits of case management, including decreased fragmentation, increased access to services, streamlined care and resource availability, and improved patient and family response to education. Additional benefits include standardization of the plan of care, improved interdisciplinary collaboration and communication, decreased readmission rates, increased involvement of the patient and family in care, and increased patient awareness of financial and quality implications. Finally, case management enables the effective measurement of quality and cost outcomes.

Early reports of nursing case management's achievements in reduction of length of stay and other cost-related factors are important, particularly in this era of increasing fiscal constraints. A concomitant interest will swell, and evidence in the literature will continue to grow, as the playing field of price-based cost competition levels, forcing payers to differentiate between care facilities on the basis of quality.

THE ROLE OF LEADERSHIP

Leadership's role in delivering quality improvement through case management is critical in program design, through establishment of structure and systems as well as selection of indicators against which to judge the success of the case management initiative. Patient populations, procedures, DRGs, or other targeted categories should be selected based on quality improvement data in addition to significant financial trends. High-volume, low-contribution margin cases should be selected, as well as patient populations reimbursed on an episodic basis, for which length-of-stay reduction and decreased resource utilization have a positive effect on costs.

Rates of infection, complication, errors, morbidity, mortality, and readmission; patient satisfaction and other quality data; and cases requiring an intensive level of interface between points in the continuum (such as those requiring complex discharge planning efforts) are desired quality improvement targets. Additional examples of indicators include some of those used at Beth Israel Medical Center in New York: improved product and personnel resource use; decreased absenteeism, turnover, and vacancy rates; decreased wait time for tests and procedures; and uniform treatment within physician groups.[33]

It is important to recognize that quality initiatives may be at work at many places in the organization using different tools. Departmentally, the case management program must be positioned within or closely aligned with the organization's main continuous quality improvement or total quality management initiative. At Lovelace Health Systems in Albuquerque, for example, the quality management department was restructured and renamed the department of clinical practice improvement and quality management better to reflect its purpose and mission, including support of the Lovelace Episode of Care Program, which currently includes nine disease-specific multidisciplinary teams.[34] Managing this transition from old models of quality improvement and care management to a coordinated effort can be leadership's greatest challenge, due to resistance to change, long-standing departments and traditions, and potential jockeying by different professional disciplines.

From the outset, strong leadership must focus on the creation of a conducive environment, ensuring that appropriate resources are provided for and managing key constituencies. The environment for case management should welcome and reward change and innovation, particularly if the quality/case management effort is an outgrowth of old departments and functions such as utilization review, discharge planning, or quality assurance. Resource availability includes human resource needs as well as information systems: personal computer based and/or linked to the organization's main information infrastructure. If information systems are a significant constraint, leadership must educate and inform appropriate executives so that these needs can be met, and expectations for demonstrated outcomes aligned with the temporarily limited information. Obtaining resources by partnering with vendors, pharmaceutical firms, payers, or foundations for funding research on management of specific patient types is also within the role of nursing leadership.

Managing key constituencies is perhaps the most critical role leadership plays in ensuring success in delivering quality in the case management initiative. Line management should be required to continually inform and involve the internal stakeholders including other nurses and care givers within the system such as physicians, pharmacists, social workers, and dietitians. Senior management must routinely incorporate case management plans, their development, and successes in communications with the board and all physicians. Regular communication with the board is paramount, so that program results can be demonstrated, and board members can hear evidence that is more than anecdotal about delivering quality patient care in an environment of fiscal and other resource constraints.

Physician buy-in and involvement are critical to the program's success. Commitment, as well as understanding, increases when physicians are educated, in a data-intensive fashion, to quality improvement and resource management objectives. In addition, suspicions can be allayed when physicians are involved in leading the effort, selecting target disease groups, and designing guidelines and indicators. At Mercy Hospital Anderson in Cincinnati, physicians embraced their internal and external case management model because it was designed as a partnership with the medical staff and provided effective alternatives to current care delivery systems for the chronically ill.[31] A physician leader with business acumen, data management skills, and an interest in quality improvement, as well as clinical expertise and respect among his or her peers, should be in place.

The importance of including external constituencies in communications cannot be overemphasized. Upon entry to the system, patients and family members should receive information describing case management services and patient benefits, in addition to customer satisfaction assessment surveys. Payers will welcome involvement at some level: from routine communications on quality outcomes achieved to integral membership in development by setting target diagnoses or treatments for intervention. Despite sometimes differing priorities, well-managed involvement builds stronger relationships with these important external customers. For example, Prudential Insurance Company of America's partnership with the Minnesota Employers Association Health Care Purchaser's Coalition has resulted in a 10 percent benefit differential for coalition members at any of 13 area hospitals when clinical pathways are used.[35]

Nursing leadership must bring the appropriate resources to bear and manage many different stakeholders to ensure the delivery of, and demonstrate, quality in a case management initiative. This is a difficult challenge given the high degree of change and varied constituents, but one that will be at the center of any successful organization's quality improvement efforts.

CONCLUSION

Although case management takes place in a variety of settings and is often delivered through different models, it is clear that this activity can achieve both cost-directed and quality-focused outcomes. In addition, the paradigm can be customized to the individual institution's needs, while at all times providing cost-effective, appropriate care in a means protective of, or beneficial to, the quality of care ultimately provided. It is important to emphasize what is somewhat obvious: The delivery of case management services has been, and continues to be, an activity primarily conducted and driven by nursing. This fundamental role of professional nursing is important for nursing leadership as well as other health care leaders to recognize: Working in concert with other professional disciplines, professional nurses can have a significant effect on the ways and means by which health care services are delivered now and in the future. Continued development of case management tools and systems can only benefit the ability of providers and health systems to provide excellent care in an intensely competitive environment of limited fiscal resources.

REFERENCES

1. Donabedian A. Quality of care: past achievements and future challenges. In Wyszewianski L, ed. *Inquiry.* 1988;25:13–22.
2. Jones K. Maintaining quality in a changing environment. *Nurs Econ.* 1991;9:159–164.
3. Lohr K, Yordy K, Their S. Current issues on quality of care. *Health Aff.* 1988;7(1):5–18.
4. Joint Commission on Accreditation of Healthcare Organizations. *LEXICON: Dictionary of Healthcare Terms, Organizations, and Acronyms for the Era of Reform.* Oakbrook Terrace, Ill: Joint Commission on Accreditation of Healthcare Organizations; 1995.
5. Donabedian A. The seven pillars of quality. *Arch Pathol Lab Med.* 1990;114:1115–1118.
6. Larrabee J. The changing role of the consumer in health care quality. *J Nurs Care Qual.* 1995;9(2):8–15.
7. Rudolph B, Hill C. The components of hospital quality: a nursing perspective. *J Nurs Care Qual.* 1994;9(1):57–65
8. Nelson E, Batalden P. Patient-based quality measurement systems. *Qual Manage Health Care.* 1993; Fall:18–29.

9. Donabedian A. The quality of care: how can it be assessed? *JAMA*. 1988;260:1743–1748.

10. Wilde B, Starrin B, Larsson G, Larsson M. Quality of care from a patient perspective: a grounded theory. *Scand J Caring Sci*. 1993;7:113–120.

11. Davis S, Adams-Greenly M. Integrating patient satisfaction with a quality improvement program. *J Nurs Adm*. 1994;24(1):28–31.

12. Ware J, Jr., Davies-Avery P, Snyder M. A taxonomy of patient satisfaction. *Health Med Care Services Rev*. 1978;1(1):1–15.

13. Nelson C, Larson C. Patients' good and bad surprises: how do they relate to overall patient satisfaction? *QRB*. 1993;March:89–94.

14. Donabedian A. Quality, cost, and cost containment. *Nurs Outlook*. 1984;32:142–145.

15. Aiken L. Charting the future of hospital nursing. *Image: J Nurs Scholarship*. 1990;22:72–78.

16. American Nurses Association Task Force on Case Management in Nursing. *Nursing Case Management*. Kansas City, Mo: American Nurses Association; 1988.

17. Zander K. Nursing case management: strategic management of cost and quality outcomes. *J Nurs Adm*. 1988;18(5):23–30.

18. Cesta T. The link between continuous quality improvement and case management. *J Nurs Adm*. 1993;23(6):55–61.

19. Zander K. Hospitals find case management can bridge the gap between total quality and patients. In Bean B, ed. *Hosp Case Manage*. 1993;1(1):16–17.

20. Juran JM. *Juran on Leadership for Quality*. New York, NY: The Free Press; 1989.

21. Gibson S, Martin S, Johnson M, Blue R, Miller D. CNS-directed case management: cost and quality in harmony. *J Nurs Adm*. 1994;24(6):45–47.

22. Tahan H, Cesta T. Developing case mangement plans using a quality improvement model. *J Nurs Adm*. 1994;24(12):49–58.

23. Wimpsett J. Nursing case management: outcomes in a rural environment. *Nurs Manage*. 1994;25(11):41–43.

24. Smith J. Changing traditional nursing home roles to nursing case management. *J Gerontol Nurs*. 1991;17(5):32–39.

25. Flynn A, Kilgallen M. Case management: a multidisciplinary approach to the evaluation of cost and quality standards. *J Nurs Care Qual*. 1993;8(1):58–66.

26. Vautier A, Carey S. A collaborative case managment program: the Crawford Long Hospital of Emory University model. *Nurs Adm Q*. 1994;18(4):1–9.

27. Sinnen M, Schifalacqua M. Coordinated care in a community hospital. *Nurs Manage*. 1991;22(3):38–42.

28. Rogers M, Riordan J, Swindle D. Community-based nursing case management pays off. *Nurs Manage*. 1991;22(3):30–34.

29. Erkel E. The impact of case management in preventive services. *J Nurs Adm*. 1993;23(1):27–32.

30. Winslow R. Health care providers try industrial tactics to reduce their costs. *Wall Street Journal*. November 3, 1993.

31. Morningstar L, ed. Quality management: a job for hospital case managers? *Hosp Case Manage*. 1994;2:53–72.

32. Green SL, Malkemes LC. Concepts of designing new delivery models. In Nackel JG, Vestal KW, eds. *J Soc Health Systems.* 1991;2:22.

33. Bean B, ed. How to measure and assess the quality of your case management efforts. *Hosp Case Manage.* 1993;1:81–100.

34. Lucas J, Gunter MJ, Byrnes J, Coyle M, Friedman N. Integrating outcomes measurement into clinical practice improvement across the continuum of care: a disease-specific episode of care model. *Managed Care Q.* 1995;3(2):14–22.

35. Bean B, ed. Employers, hospitals, and insurance company team up to offer pathways. *Hosp Case Manage.* 1993;1:61–80.

■ 9 ■

Evaluating the Effectiveness of Case Management Plans

Hussein A. Tahan, MS, RN, CNA
Toni G. Cesta, PhD, RN

The current health care environment has shifted its emphasis to high quality at low cost.[1-13] Case management models of patient care have been implemented to meet these demands. Among the goals of case management are (1) providing patients with the highest quality care at the lowest possible cost and (2) improving patient care outcomes.[4,6-8,10-20]

To meet these goals, contemporary case management models use specific tools called case management plans. This chapter provides the methods for evaluating the effectiveness of such plans and their impact on the quality of care. It also presents one approach to managing outcomes as they relate to case management.

Evaluating the effectiveness of case management plans is as important as their development and implementation. Perhaps the best way to evaluate them is through the use of data. Data collection and analysis are imperative in any process used to demonstrate the effectiveness of case management plans. One data element that can be gathered from case management plans is variations from the plan. Variance data can then be analyzed and decisions to improve the systems and processes around patient care will be made.

Variance data are of two types. The first type includes deviations from the case management plan. This kind of variance occurs when a patient care activity is not performed by the health care provider, as specified on the case management plan. To be considered a variance (deviation), the activity is either purposely (intentionally) cancelled, omitted, or delayed. The second type of variance data involves issues associated with achieving the expected

Source: Reprinted with permission from *Journal of Nursing Administration,* Vol. 25, No. 9, September 1995, pp. 58–63.

outcomes of care. This kind of variance occurs when an expected outcome of care is not met for whatever reason. This variance usually results in altering the sequence of patient care activities on the case management plan to meet the expected outcome.

VARIANCE ANALYSIS

A variance is defined as anything that is not achieved within the predetermined time frame on the case management plan (e.g., any patient care activity or outcome that is not performed or achieved as preplanned or expected).[9,12] Variances can be identified either on admission or during the hospital stay.

A variance on admission is defined as a patient's pre-existing condition (comorbidity, secondary diagnosis, allergy) that demands a change in the case management plan. For example, a patient who is admitted for management of asthma also is diabetic. In this case, antihyperglycemic agents are prescribed, which are not usually part of the standard asthma case management plan. Another example is patient allergies. In this case, the antibiotic of choice to treat a certain infection cannot be ordered because of a pre-existing allergy to that antibiotic. The case management plan is altered, and a different antibiotic is ordered.

Deviations from the case management plans during the hospital stay also are considered variances. They are related to delays in performing patient care activities, deletions, or additions of tests, procedures, treatments, and medications.[2,3,12,21-23] Deviations from the case management plans can be classified into operational-, community-, practitioner-, or patient-caused variances (Exhibit 9-1).

Operational variances also are called system variances because they are related to the functioning of the organization and the way in which activities are carried out. For example, a computerized axial tomography scan is not done because the machine is broken.

Whereas operational variances are within the hospital walls, community variances are related to systems beyond the hospital walls. Community variances are more difficult to solve and control because they are multisystem in nature. An example of a community variance is the inability to discharge a patient because a long-term care bed or home care service is not available.

Practitioner variances also are called health care provider variances. They are related to situations in which the health care provider is the reason for a delay in care or why an expected outcome is not achieved. Examples are medication errors (e.g., a nurse giving the wrong drug) or incorrect tests or procedures being ordered by the physician.

Exhibit 9-1 Examples of Variances

A. Operational Variance
  1. Machine breakdown
  2. Delay in test or procedure
  3. Lost laboratory requisition or specimen
  4. No rehabilitation technician on weekends
B. Community Variance
  1. No nursing home bed available
  2. No visiting nurse service available
  3. No family available to accompany the patient on discharge
  4. Wheelchair cannot be delivered home until four days after discharge
C. Practitioner Variance
  1. Ordering unnecessary test or procedure
  2. Medication error
  3. No consent obtained
  4. Omission of a test or procedure
D. Patient Variance
  1. Test refusal
  2. Change in condition
  3. Patient allergy
  4. Sign out against medical advice

Patient variances usually are caused by the patient. A typical example is refusal of a test or procedure or noncompliance with medical regimen.

Variances in care are evaluated based on the time frames used in the case management plan. These time frames are studied closely while developing a case management plan and are based on the clinical area or service.[19–21,23] For example, an emergency department case management plan is developed based on time frames of minutes, which means that treatments or activities are rendered within time intervals of minutes. If a treatment is not provided within the time frame specified on the plan, it is considered a variance.

Variances also are classified as negative or positive.[24] A negative variance is an action that results in an undesired outcome. Every time an activity is not accomplished during the time frame specified on the case management plan, it is considered a negative variance. Examples are echocardiography done on day 3 instead of day 2, a delay in treatment because of broken equipment, or the complete omission of a treatment. Most of the time, negative variances result in a delay in the care and an increase in length of stay. They are best prevented through better management of care.

A positive variance, on the other hand, is an action that is justified or explained. A variance on admission usually is classified as a positive variance. If a patient's recovery progresses faster than the plan specifies or if a desired outcome is achieved before it is expected to happen, it is considered positive variance.

EXPECTED OUTCOMES OF CARE

Clinical quality indicators usually identify the expected outcomes of care. By indicating these prospectively, quality is identified and maintained. Clinical quality indicators should be interdisciplinary in nature. They should be developed in conjunction with the case management plans by the same members of the interdisciplinary team who originally developed the plan.

Clinical quality indicators are the projected outcomes of care that each service or discipline involved in the provision of care for a particular patient is expected to accomplish before the patient's discharge. They are developed prospectively by representatives from these disciplines, who are a part of the interdisciplinary team charged with developing a certain plan. Then, these indicators are applied to the patient at the time of admission. They represent the "gold standard" for that diagnosis or surgical procedure.

Clinical quality indicators are also called clinical outcomes or outcome indicators. They are the result of health care processes and are best described as milestones to recovery. These outcomes are either intermediate or discharge indicators (Exhibit 9-2).

Intermediate patient outcomes are triggerpoints or milestones established on the case management plan to alert the health care provider to implement certain actions. They are intended to denote a needed change in the course

---

Exhibit 9-2 Asthma Quality Indicators

A. Intermediate Indicators
  1. Intravenous corticosteroid discontinued when peak flow is ≥200-250L/s
  2. Intravenous corticosteroids are changed into prednisone, by mouth, when peak flow is ≥ 200–250 L/s
  3. Able to demonstrate the use of metered dose inhaler with spacer
B. Discharge Indicators
  1. Peak flow is ≥ 200–250 L/s
  2. Minimal/free of shortness of breath or chest tightness
  3. Follow-up appointment is arranged
  4. Minimal/free of wheezing
  5. Able to use the metered dose inhaler with spacer
  6. Verbalize understanding of disease process, risk factors, medications, and allergens that cause asthma attack

of care or therapy. These outcomes are to be achieved during the patient's hospital stay. "Change intravenous antibiotics to oral if patient is afebrile for 24 hours," would be an example of an intermediate patient outcome.

Discharge patient outcomes, on the other hand, are the pre-established criteria for discharge. These outcomes should always be met before or at the time of discharge. They are developed based on the patient's diagnosis or reason for admission to the hospital. One example of a discharge outcome is a patient who is free of shortness of breath.

Clinical quality indicators or expected patient outcomes are always diagnosis or surgical procedure specific. They should be included and highlighted in the case management plan and developed concurrently with it. Usually, each member on the team responsible for developing a case management plan is asked to develop quality indicators related to his or her discipline's portion of the plan. These indicators reflect the standards of care and the best practice for that diagnosis or procedure. They also serve as a monitoring mechanism to ensure the provision of quality care.

Variances are documented daily as they occur. Variances related to outcome indicators are classified as unmet clinical indicators or outcomes. Variance analysis and trending of the data collected are invaluable in determining the reason(s) an expected patient outcome or clinical quality indicator has not been met.

A critical task of the nurse case manager is a daily review of the case management plan, with an analysis as to the degree to which the expected outcomes were achieved. Evaluation of the intermediate indicators and instituting the necessary changes to meet these indicators help ensure that the patient is progressing toward the desired outcomes in a timely fashion. Whenever a problem or a variance is identified (i.e., a desired outcome is not met), the nurse case manager will determine why the problem arose and try to correct it. He or she may institute some changes in the case management plan that are thought to have a positive effect on the patient's condition and correct the problem.

OUTCOMES MANAGEMENT

Currently, health care organizations are being pressured by customers, third-party payers, insurance companies, and regulatory agencies such as the Joint Commission on Accreditation of Health Care Organizations, peer review programs through Medicare, and the state health departments to develop strategies to help improve the quality of care. Outcomes management is one such strategy. Although outcomes management systems are one means by which to demonstrate the effectiveness of care, they remain relatively costly and difficult to implement. We chose to present one approach to outcomes management that is used at Beth Israel Medical Center in New York City to evaluate the effectiveness of case management plans in the provision of care (Figure 9-1).

Before the implementation of any outcomes management system, it is important to define the goals. Some of these goals as they relate to case management are (1) to determine if health care providers follow the case management plans consistently; (2) to determine if the planned results (expected outcomes) are met; (3) to identify the problems in the processes that need to be changed or revised if planned results are not met; and (4) to analyze and trend the data and design a mechanism for feedback and corrective actions.

This approach to outcomes management system consists of four core components: (1) data collection tools development; (2) outcomes measurement; (3) outcomes monitoring; and (4) outcomes management. This approach was developed based on a selective literature review related to outcomes management.[2,3,8,9,23,25-28] An outcome is defined as the result of a health care process or patient care activity. Some examples of outcomes are in-hospital complications, deaths, length of stay, patient functional status on discharge, readmissions, and patient satisfaction with care. The following discussion refers to outcomes that are related to the use of case management plans (i.e., variances of care and quality indicators).

Tool Development

Data collection tools should be developed before starting the data collection process. Tools help one focus on the type of data to be collected, streamline the process, and should be designed in a way that meets the goals of the outcomes

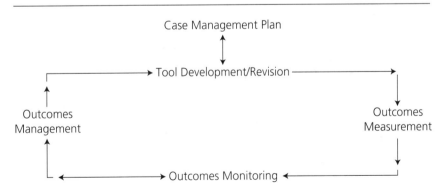

Figure 9-1 Outcomes Management Associated with the Case Management Plan

management system. Because variance analysis and expected outcomes are the indicators used to evaluate the effectiveness of case management plans, the data collection tools should be developed to be used for that purpose.

The variance data collection tool should include the type of variances, the date each variance is identified, and whether it is justified as positive or negative.

The expected patient outcomes data collection tool should be diagnosis specific and coincide with the expected outcomes identified on the case management plan. Data collected should reflect whether each expected outcome is met. In case the expected outcome is not met, the reason should be stated if known.

Outcomes Measurement

Outcomes measurement is defined as the systematic quantitative observation of variances and outcome indicators, at one point in time, using the data collection tools that are developed based on the case management plan. This approach provides a one-time assessment of the provision and outcome of patient care. It also provides nursing administrators with a mechanism for identifying any gaps in patient care and deficient areas or areas of nonconformity with the standards of care that are established by regulatory agencies. Outcomes measurement also may serve as a baseline assessment of patient care that is an essential step when developing action plans for improving patient care processes and care outcomes.

Outcomes Monitoring

Outcomes monitoring is the ongoing/repeated measurement of variances and outcome indicators, with close attention to what might have caused the observed outcomes. The care processes should be studied very carefully so that inferential causes can be determined. Assessment, reassessment, and evaluation of patient care processes are necessary every time the action plans for improving patient care delivery are constructed. Outcomes monitoring usually provides nursing and health care administrators with the data needed to examine what is working of the recommended action plans. It also helps administrators make better decisions when evaluating the impact of these action plans on patient care activities and processes.

Outcomes Management

Outcomes management is the analysis and trending of the information collected through outcomes measurement and monitoring. Decision making is done, based on the analysis, to improve the effectiveness of the case management plans and the quality of care. Data obtained can be used in a quality improvement frame work. Quality improvement teams can be established, based on the data collected, to examine the patient care processes and systems. Such teams usually are charged with examining the quality barriers and improving the efficiency of patient care. Data can be brought back to administration for administrative intervention or to the attention of the multidisciplinary team who developed the case management plan. Providing feedback to all the key personnel involved in the provision of care is an important factor in the success of outcomes management.

Sometimes, the data collected might not be exactly what was planned when the tools were designed. In such cases, the data collection tools must be revisited and the adjustments needed made. The revised tools must be used in the same fashion as the old ones (i.e., following the same process).

Nurse case managers are the best persons to collect data because of their optimal involvement in the management of care. Other health care providers who can help in data collection are utilization review nurses and quality care coordinators.

The best time to collect variance data is at the time the variance occurs. Concurrent reviews are more likely to yield accurate results. Intermediate indicators are best evaluated during the hospital stay within the time frames specified in the case management plan. However, the discharge indicators are best evaluated at the time of the patient's discharge. This evaluation is important because it focuses on the overall expected outcomes of care, in which the various members of the health care team have participated.

Reviewing the plan in relation to the patient's condition, the actual versus the projected interventions, and the actual versus the expected outcomes of care provide a strong mechanism for evaluating the effectiveness of case management plans.

CONCLUSION

Over the past decade, case management models of patient care delivery have become more popular. Case management plans have been used as the main strategy for quality improvement and cost containment. However, improving the quality of care does not end at developing and implementing case management plans. Evaluating these plans is just as important. This chapter presented health care administrators with some methods of evaluating the effectiveness of case management plans on the provision of care (i.e., variance analysis, outcomes measurement, and outcomes management). It serves as an example for hospital and nursing administrators to adapt into their organizations. It also helps them survive their struggles in the world of outcomes management.

REFERENCES

1. Barnes RV, Lawton L, Briggs D. Clinical benchmarking improves clinical paths: experience with coronary artery by-pass grafting. *Joint Commission J Qual Improvement.* 1994;20:267–276.

2. McGinnity ES, Pluth TE. Managing orthopedics and neurosciences costs through standard treatment protocols. *Hospital Technology Special Report, American Hospital Association.* 1994;13:1–25.

3. Meyer JW, Feingold MG. Using standard treatment protocols to manage costs and quality of hospital services. *Hospital Technology Special Report, American Hospital Association.* 1993;12:1–23.

4. Ling K. Initiation and evaluation of managed care at the Johns Hopkins Hospital. *Nurs Adm Q.* 1993;17(3):54–58.

5. Smith GB. Hospital case management for psychiatric diagnoses: focusing on quality and cost outcomes. *J Psychosoc Nurs.* 1994;32(2):3–4.

6. McKenzie CB, Torkelson NG, Holt MA. Care and cost: nursing case management improves both. *Nurs Manage.* 1989;20(10):30–34.

7. Green SL, Malkemes LC. Concepts of designing new delivery models. *J Soc Health Syst.* 1991;2(3):14–24.

8. Sowell RL, Meadows TM. An integrated case management model: developing standards, evaluation, and outcome criteria. *Nurs Adm Q.* 1994;18(2):53–64.

9. Weillitz PB, Potter PA. A managed care system: financial and clinical evaluation. *J Nurs Admin.* 1993;23(11):51–56.

10. Vautier AF, Carey SJ. A collaborative case management program: the Crawford Long Hospital of Emory University model. *Nurs Adm Q.* 1994;18(4):1–9.

11. Ethridge P, Lamb G. Professional nursing case management improves quality, access and costs. *Nurs Manage.* 1989;20(3):30–35.

12. Cohen EL, Cesta TG. *Nursing Case Management: From Concept to Evaluation.* St. Louis, Mo: Mosby-Year Book Inc; 1993.

13. Cunningham LG, Koen MJ. Acute care case management: integration for providers and payors. *Case Manager Advisor.* 1994;5(5):53–60.

14. Ethridge P. A nursing HMO: Carondelet St. Mary's experience. *Nurs Manage.* 1991;22(7):22–27.

15. Zander K. Managed care within acute care setting: design and implementation via nursing case management. *Health Care Superv.* 1988;6(2):27–43.

16. Tahan HT. The nurse case manager in acute care settings. *J Nurs Adm.* 1993;23(10):53–61.

17. Olivas GS, Armanasco DT, Erickson JR, Hanger S. Case management: a bottom line care delivery model: part I, the concept. *J Nurs Adm.* 1989;19(11):16–20.

18. Crummette BD, Boatwright DN. Case management region wide. *Nurs Manage.* 1991;22(3):62–64.

19. Guiliano KK, Poirier CE. Nursing case management: critical pathways to describe outcomes. *Nurs Manage.* 1991;22(3):52–55.

20. Tahan HT, Cesta TG. Developing case management plans using a quality improvement model. *J Nurs Adm.* 1994;24(12):49–58.

21. Ferguson LE. Steps to developing a critical pathway. *Nurs Adm Q.* 1993;17(3):58–62.

22. Nyberg D, Marschke P. Critical pathways: tools for continuous quality improvement. *Nurs Adm Q.* 1993;17(3):62–69.

23. Katterhagen JG, Patton M. Critical pathways in oncology: balancing the interests of hospitals and the physician. *J Oncol Manage.* 1993;2(4):20–26.

24. Hampton DC. Implementing a managed care framework through care maps. *J Nurs Adm.* 1993;23(5):21–27.

25. Davies AR, Doyle AT, Lansky D, et al. Outcomes assessment in clinical settings. *Joint Commission J Qual Improvement.* 1994;20(1):6–15.

26. Wimpsett J. Nursing case management: outcomes in a rural environment. *Nurs Manage.* 1994;25(11):41–43.

27. Kelly KC, Huber DG, Johnson M, et al. The medical outcomes study: a nursing perspective. *J Prof Nurs.* 1994;10:209–216.

28. Cleary PD, Greenfield S, Mulley AG, et al. Variations in length of stay and outcomes for six medical and surgical conditions in Massachusetts hospitals. *JAMA.* 1991;266:73–79.

■ 10 ■

Variance Analysis

Barbara Barth Frink, PhD, RN, FAAN
Larry Strassner, MS, RN, CNA

This chapter provides conceptual and programmatic guidance on variance analysis in the context of case management and critical paths. The chapter is divided into four areas of discussion: The first section is focused on contextual and strategic factors influencing the development of case management/critical path programs; the second section is focused on variance analysis as a concept, classification schema, and planning the variance indicators for a critical path; the third section presents issues of information management of critical path variance data, including supporting technology; and the fourth section concludes the chapter, summarizing factors to consider in analysis, interpretation, reporting, and presentation of the variance data.

First, it is important to understand the conceptual placement of the case management/critical path system. The case management model (in whatever form it is structured) exists within the policy umbrella of clinical quality improvement, effectiveness, and outcomes. Critical paths are an extension of practice guidelines concepts; they are a set of interdisciplinary recommendations for care of a specific condition in a temporal model. They are designed operational environments as opposed to evidence-based practice guidelines. They are designed to reduce variation and establish guidelines for care within an individual institution. Careful evaluation of critical path outcomes provides data on the strengths and limitations of clinical processes and the link to outcomes; the path itself does not improve clinical performance. The critical path provides the structure, process, and outcome elements for use in variance analysis, which yields the data to inform decisions about clinical performance improvement.

Acknowledgment: The authors acknowledge Mark Bruder, BS, for graphic design of figures.

STRATEGIC INITIATIVES OF THE ORGANIZATION: MANAGED CARE

The revolution in health care is changing the once "hospital-centric" health care environment to a community-based model of health promotion and disease prevention. This profound change is reflected in managed care initiatives, which range from first-stage price discounts to third-stage capitated payments in which providers assume the risk for enrolled populations.[1] Health care providers are facing significant challenges to demonstrate that care delivery is appropriate, comprehensive, cost efficient, and of high quality.[2] Changes in financial risk, increasing accountability, performance documentation, and outcome measurements are shifting health care providers' focus from planned care to managed care. Hospitals, once known as "revenue generators," are now viewed as cost centers providing an event or an episode of care.[1,3] Managed care, once applied only to high-cost chronically ill and disabled patients, is now being expanded to include all patients. Consumers and payers are demanding an integrated interdisciplinary health care system that provides comprehensive care from birth to death, not just events or episodes of care during hospitalization. Consumers are also becoming more emphatic about the need to maintain and sometimes improve the quality of care that is provided while simultaneously expecting access and affordability of care.[4] In an effort to respond to these challenges, many hospitals across the country have established formal initiatives for monitoring, measuring, and managing clinical processes. The initiatives often include hospital case management programs and the design and implementation of critical pathways.

Case management models and the use of critical paths have been powerful strategies in demonstrating decreases in length of stay and cost savings relating to the hospital episode of care.[5-9] However, the need to move case management efforts beyond the walls of the hospital toward fully integrated case management systems is becoming increasingly apparent as multihospital systems and managed care organizations begin to adapt to disease management models. Organizations must strategically prepare and respond to managing patients as identified by Handy et al,[10] in Figure 10-1.

A fully integrated case management system that is flexible and responsive is essential to meet the challenges of health care. The requirements of an integrated case management/critical path system may be found in Exhibit 10-1. This exhibit provides a checklist of structure and process elements used in assessment and implementation of a case management/critical path program.

Lumsdon and Hagland[11] identified that some hospitals are implementing patient-centered care and using critical pathways as the clinical tools that accompany environmental and work redesign. Patterson[12] at Baptist Memo-

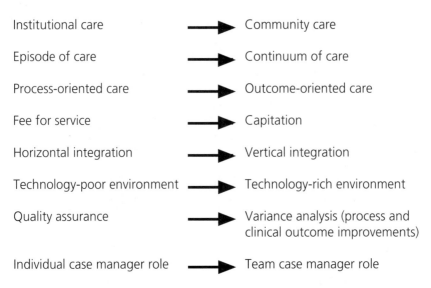

Institutional care ➤ Community care

Episode of care ➤ Continuum of care

Process-oriented care ➤ Outcome-oriented care

Fee for service ➤ Capitation

Horizontal integration ➤ Vertical integration

Technology-poor environment ➤ Technology-rich environment

Quality assurance ➤ Variance analysis (process and clinical outcome improvements)

Individual case manager role ➤ Team case manager role

Figure 10-1 Strategic Changes in Health Care Delivery. *Source:* Information from *Nurse Case Managers: A Snapshot of Roles and Settings* by J. Handy, S. Kedrowski, E. Lynette, and J. Quinn, Case Management Across the Continuum Conference, Contemporary Forums, May 1995.

rial Hospital in Memphis, Tennessee, one of the largest hospitals in the country, identified that nursing case management has increased patient/family satisfaction and improved both operational effectiveness and efficiency. Case management has grown in this organization to include 45 case managers and 20 interdisciplinary teams. Case management at The Johns Hopkins Hospital, a 1,000-bed tertiary/quaternary academic health center in Maryland, is based on a multidisciplinary clinical care system. A master's prepared registered nurse case manager is designated to coordinate care for a select group of patients across the continuum of hospitalization. The critical path is the patient's multidisciplinary plan of care; it is used to plan, deliver, monitor, and concurrently review care provided to patients. Currently, case managers coordinate episodic acute care for select surgical, pediatric, medical, and oncology patients.

Case Management

Various definitions of case management exist in the literature. The specific model definition is dependent on the discipline that uses it, the setting in which it is implemented, and the personnel and staff mix used in its imple-

Exhibit 10-1 Assessment of Case Management/Critical Path Program

	In Place	Working On	Not Begun
1. Program Structure			
Case management and critical paths are identified in the institution's annual goals and objectives and/or mission statement			
Goals and objectives of the program have been identified and approved by executive management			
A reporting mechanism has been established whereby executive management receives progress reports of the program			
Institution specific definitions have been defined and approved by the executive management			
Organizational infrastructure supports the program:			
Multidisciplinary steering committee			
Full-time project director			
Interdependencies of other departments (QA/UR, Social Work, Information Services, Finance, clinicians)			
Graphic design support			
Secretarial support			
2. Case Managers			
Job description			
Performance evaluation			
Orientation program			
Defined relationships with Social Work, QA, primary nurse, MD clarified			
Direct report to whom			
3. Critical Paths			
Multidisciplinary teams develop, evaluate, revise, and approve critical path			
Care across the continuum (ER, OR, PACU, Inpatient, Outpatient, Home Health)			
Consistent format defined			
Part of the medical record			
Multidisciplinary content			
Multidisciplinary documentation tool			
Order sets support path interventions			
Preprinted discharge instructions (optional)			
Patient/family critical path			

continues

Exhibit 10-1 continued

	In Place	Working On	Not Begun
4. Education			
Initial education included all departments, MDs, and RNs			
Ongoing education (orientation, hospital newsletter, MD newsletters)			
Institution-specific resources ("how to" manuals, reference guides)			
5. Program Evaluation			
Defined what data elements to collect for each path			
Fiscal			
Quality			
Clinical outcomes (intermediate, discharge, and postdischarge)			
Variance analysis			
Patient/family satisfaction			
Defined who will collect data			
Define what data bases are to be used			
Defined criteria for performances according to managed care contracts			
Defined mechanisms for reporting data to the executive management, critical path teams, and hospital CQI structure			
Define how and what data to use for marketing to managed care organizations			
6. Variance Analysis			
Institution-defined variance			
Multidisciplinary teams define critical path-specific interventions and outcomes variances they wish to track			
Who will collect variance data?			
Technologies to collect variance data			
Will it be part of medical record?			
How is it integrated with CQI efforts?			
7. Automation			
Used to develop critical paths			
Documenting on line to critical paths			
Documenting multidisciplinary variance on line			
MD order sets on line that support critical path			
Decision support system used concurrently or retrospectively to analyze clinical data			

Source: Courtesy of Larry Strassner, The Johns Hopkins Hospital, Baltimore, Maryland.

mentation.[13] Industry in the 1950s used two tools, critical path method and program evaluation and review technique to plan, organize, coordinate, and manage its processes that were often complex, included long periods of time, and were spread across large geographic areas. The recent prominence of clinical pathways in health care is based in part on the work of Zander and associates at The New England Medical Center.[14] Luttman et al.[15] identify that a popular approach to plan and manage care has been the development and implementation of clinical pathways. They make an important distinction between the terms *critical pathway* as applied in industry and the *clinical pathway* development in health care. They identify that the health care industry has not taken full advantage of the critical path methodologies used in industry and that there is some confusion in health care organizations over the term *critical path* due to multiple interpretations of the term *critical*. Lumsdon and Hagland[11] reported results of a survey of 581 U.S. hospitals conducted by *Hospitals and Health Networks* in regard to methods used to manage clinical processes. When queried as to what tools they used to manage care, 42 percent or 244 of the hospitals used critical paths, 13 percent or 75 used practice guidelines/parameters, 12 percent or 70 used clinical guidelines, and 8 percent or 46 used clinical protocols/algorithms. The hospitals identified 34 distinctive names used to manage the care process in addition to critical path, clinical, or practice guideline. This reflects both differences in methods of care management practice, lack of standardized approach and use of common language, and diverse views on the definition and scope of critical paths.

Case management research has been conducted by nursing and other disciplines. Lamb,[16] in a recent research review of case management, reports that the state of the science does not meet the current demand for answers to complex health care restructuring questions. She recommends a strategic effort by the nursing community that would focus an interdisciplinary research team on linking case management process to outcomes and standardizing outcome indicators across studies. Lamb's integrative research review provides a framework for the critical next steps in evaluating case management programs.

For the purposes of this chapter, *case management* is defined as a multidisciplinary clinical system that uses registered nurse case managers to coordinate the care for select patients across the continuum of a health care episode. The continuum is defined as a customer-oriented seamless system providing a comprehensive array of health, mental health, and social services across all levels and sites of care to improve the health and status of a defined population over time. The technologies of case management are health screening tools, risk assessment instruments, critical paths (episodic and continuum), care plans, clinical algorithms, and variance analysis. The *critical path* is the tool used within the case management system to plan, deliver, monitor, document, and concurrently review the care provided by multiple disciplines. It is the patient's plan of care and includes multidisciplinary interventions and expected intermediate and discharge clinical patient outcomes plotted against a time line (episodic or continuum) for a homogeneous population or case type.

VARIANCE ANALYSIS

Compared to the volume of literature on critical path development, the subject of critical pathway variance analysis is relatively undeveloped. Yet, critical pathway analysis is essential in achieving expected patient outcomes, improving processes of care, and attaining organizational financial goals. The development and implementation of the critical pathway are only the first steps toward improving fiscal clinical processes and patient outcomes. Usually the path is customized for each institution and represents a consensus of the clinicians caring for this population based on research literature, professional experience, and unique system issues. Consensus reflects the clinicians' conception of the "best practice" for this group of patients. Within the framework of quality improvement, the design and implementation of the critical path model is only the beginning. The true value of such a model is proved over time as deviations from the expected outcomes are measured and analyzed in light of their relationship to the structures and processes of care and then used to improve outcomes for the cohort of patients. This monitoring is often referred to as variance analysis.[17]

Source of Patient Outcomes

The patient outcomes defined in a critical path model represent a junction of two very different philosophic and academic models in health care: the clinician/basic science model and the social scientist/health economist model. Understanding these differences is fundamental to understanding the complexity of variance data. Critical paths are designed for cohorts of patients who meet predetermined eligibility criteria, experience specified care processes within specified time periods, and are expected to achieve certain outcomes. That definition could also be applied to research protocols in randomized clinical trials. However, critical paths are designed for operational day-to-day use; they are not a research process superimposed on clinical operations.[18] One clinical area in which critical paths and research protocols are closely aligned is clinical oncology in cancer research centers. A high percentage of clinical oncology care in these centers is driven by research protocols that guide specific care processes for patients over a time and treatment continuum. In these cases, the critical path provides the coordination of the randomized clinical trial protocol components.

Randomized clinical trials are the primary research methodology of the biomedical model of health care, with intellectual roots in biology, biochemistry, and physiology. Thus, patient outcomes resulting from the biomedical model are "biological, physiological, and clinical."[18] By contrast, the social science model, sometimes called *quality of life model* of health care has its intellectual roots in sociology, psychology, and economics. The primary research methodology of this tradition is focused on measurement of complex behavior, feelings, attitudes, dimensions of functioning, and well-being. Patient outcomes resulting from the quality of life model are measures of health status, functional status, or mental status. For those who are interested, Wilson and Cleary[18] present a conceptual model for patient outcomes in an attempt to link clinical outcomes with quality of life outcomes. This fundamental difference in the scientific roots of patient outcomes adds to the complexity of using outcome data to improve clinical performance and to conduct *outcomes research*. Differing interpretations of variance data among groups and individuals may be influenced by these different scientific traditions, which in turn may influence performance improvement activities.[19] The fundamental assumption of the value of critical paths is that both patient quality and costs (patient and institutional) can be improved through their implementation, analysis, and feedback. This assumption is based on the use of statistical inference to identify and control clinical process variation. Understanding process variation is fundamental to both the design of the variance measurement system and to interpretation of the resulting data. The design of critical paths is targeted to control both inputs and processes and then to measure variation in the outcomes systematically. Interpretation of the variation patterns provides feedback to adjust the processes of care continuously to yield improved patient outcomes.

Definitions of Critical Path Variance

Variance is commonly defined as "the state of being variable or variant" or "the state of being in disagreement."[20] In the context of critical path analysis, the most elemental definition of variance is the deviation of actual outcomes from a predetermined norm, standard, rate, goal, threshold, or expected outcome. Analysis, of course, is the process of assigning meaning and interpretation to data and converting the data into information. Luttman et al.[15(p.9)] define variance as "any activity (treatment, procedure, test or clinical outcome) that does not occur at all, or does not occur in the scheduled time period." Bowers[21] defines variance as "a deviation from the patient care activities outlined on the critical path/CareMap® tool which may alter the anticipated discharge date, the expected cost, or the expected outcomes." Another definition of critical path variance is the difference between the planned interventions and patient outcomes as stated on the critical path and in the allotted time frame, as compared with the actual interventions, outcomes, and time frame.[22] Although various definitions exist for variance, the concept of deviation from some predetermined standard is the common theme.

Variance analysis implies a single activity that provides feedback on the actual versus the expected achievement of goals specified on a critical path. It is, however, a much more complex activity involving statistical inference on data sets, documentation of process control variation, identification of causal relationships, feedback, and use of clinical practice data to inform policy.

It is unfortunate that the terms *variance* and *variance analysis* have become so widely used in the context of critical path analysis, as they have very different meanings from the statistical terms *variance* and *analysis of variance*. *Variance* is one measure of variability of a sample. In statistical terms, it is the standard deviation, which is computed from the sum of the squared deviations divided by $(N - 1)$. For clarity of discussion and clinically relevant examples, see reference 23. *Analysis of variance* is a statistical test used to determine if all groups in a sample are equal and drawn from the same population. It requires that the dependent variable be interval- or ratio-level data and that the independent variable(s) are nominal-level data. It is computed by measuring the variance of each group separately and the variance of the total group (each computed by finding the sum of squares). The variances within each group and among the groups are summed to give the total variation. For clarity of discussion and clinically relevant examples, see reference 24. For further discussion, see any basic statistics text.

Classification of Causes of Variance

Several authors have identified four standard categories for classifying the causes of variances. Cesta and Cohen[13] identify the four variance categories as operational, health care provider, patient, and unmet clinical outcomes. Examples of operational variances are broken equipment, unavailability of bed for patient transfer or discharge, and inefficient or unavailable scheduling for service such as physical therapy or radiographic studies. Health care provider variance includes any situation in which the health care provider is the cause of the delay in achieving an expected outcome. Examples are delays in provider-initiated diagnostics, treatment, medications, discharge planning, or lack of coordination of care among disciplines. Patient variances include any patient-related delays such as refusal of treatment or change in physiologic status. Unmet clinical outcomes are the intermediate and discharge patient outcomes developed in conjunction with the critical path, such as the patient has not as yet experienced normal cardiac output or specific normative laboratory values.

Zander[25] also identified four categories for the causes of variances such as patient/family, care giver/clinician, hospital/system, and community. The Cesta and Cohen schema integrates Zander's hospital/system and community categories into the one category of operational variance. Zander also uses the same categories for defining variances related to patients' intermediate and discharge outcomes and does not use a separate unmet clinical outcomes category. Coffey and colleagues[26] use the same definitions as Zander for each variance category. Bueno and Hwang[27] from the Robert Wood Johnson University Hospital identified four variance categories used by their case managers to identify variances: patient, health, care giver, and environment. Although these four-element classification schemes are similar in that they share some common elements, the lack of standardization and lack of common language prevent comparison of data across institutions or sites.

By contrast, Robinson and colleagues[28] identified only two variance classification categories: patient and system. However, within these categories is a variance identification decision tree that includes items such as comorbid factors, delays in testing, and resource consumption. Hoffman[6] applied a different method for identifying variance categories. He used the content categories of the critical path as the variance categories. That is, he tabulated the frequency of variances in categories such as laboratory tests, medications, activity level, diet, and discharge goals. Mikulaninec[29] recommends the approach of individualizing a path first based on patients' comorbidities and socioeconomic factors. Thereafter, any deviations from the individualized path is defined as a variance. In summary, categories of variance have been defined in direct response to the content on critical paths, rather than to standardized expected outcome categories.

Many organizations have selected categories of variance as defined above for consistency in reporting at the institutional level. The critical path development teams are responsible for defining the types of variances within each category. Clinician teams are the most knowledgeable group to specify the types of variances that are meaningful in managing care for their patient population. The *types* of specific patient variances may differ depending on the population. For example, the type of patient variance for a post-abdominal surgical patient who is unable to tolerate a regular diet may be bowel obstruction or hypoactive bowel motility. A type of patient variance for a post-myocardial infarction patient who is unable to tolerate a regular diet may be continued chest pain. Another example of types of variances comes from the work of Bueno and Hwang.[27] They identify specific variances within the health category such as circulatory, embolism/thrombosis, diarrhea, infection, pain, and arrest. Specific variances that may be within the care giver/clinician category are no physician order, health care provider decision/preference, health care provider response time, or health care provider unavailable.

It is important to apply some standard categories to variance identification but allow the flexibility of the clinicians to define the types of variances. An advantage to clinician control of specific variance identification is the likelihood of clinician investment in the process with consequent support for variance data collection and analysis. Requiring a rigid structure for categories and types of variances may not provide clinicians with enough specific data appropriate to their patient population to identify opportunities for improvement. This runs the risk of variance collection being viewed solely as an administrative requirement, with the subsequent loss of these data in managing patient care.

In all these classification schemes, variances are stated as positive or negative. A positive variance occurs when the patient meets the expected clinical outcomes or receives the defined clinical processes before the established time line. For example, a positive variance is recorded for a coronary artery bypass patient who tolerates a regular diet on postoperative day 3 as opposed to the stated goal of regular diet on day 4 or who has the chest tube discontinued on day 2 as opposed to day 3 as stated on the critical path. An example of a negative variance is the patient not discharged by the day stated on the critical path.

Although classification of variance data by categories and types assists in describing and codifying the data, this may lead to a simplistic analysis of outcomes based on the assumption that categories are mutually exclusive and that specific types of variance are independent. One of the challenges of variance and outcomes analysis is to explore the relationships among care processes and outcomes continually to identify the root causes of outcomes and dependencies among critical variables. The performance improvement cycle generated by critical path data requires specification for collection, analysis, use, storage, and reporting of the data.[30,31]

Relevance and Quantity of Variance Data

Just as there is no one right way to develop critical paths or case management programs, there is also no one right way to define what variance data to collect. The initial work of defining how much and what kind of variance data should be collected centers around the definition of variance. For example, Schriefer[32] reported that often variance data were collected for all interventions and/or patient outcomes that were identified on the critical path that did not occur at all or did not occur within the scheduled time period. Although all these variances may have had some importance for documentation, regulatory, or medical/legal reasons, it soon became evident that all these variances did not significantly affect the patient's length of stay or have a negative effect on the care processes.[15] Often, this level of capturing all items as variance is used during the pilot phases of the critical pathways to validate the sequence of practice patterns as defined by the critical path development team. Organizations quickly learned that although this provided them with patient and system performance data, they were now drowning in data. Clinicians found the data difficult to interpret, hospitals found data systems difficult to maintain, individuals responsible for collecting the data were overwhelmed, and data integrity was an ongoing issue.

Identifying the quantity of variance data to collect is related to the complexity of the care processes, the resources available, the frequency of collection, and the desired outcomes. Zander[25] relates the amount of variance data desired to the CareMap® structure and processes. She identifies that reviewing the CareMap® tool once a day will provide low to moderate amounts of variance data. Frequent data collection and total standardization of outcomes and tasks, with no patient individualization, will yield high amounts of variance data of questionable value. The complexity of the path that produced the outcome will be inversely proportional to the value of the outcome.[33] Pilot testing the content and process of variance measures is recommended.

Another method of identifying what data to collect is to have the critical path team define the critical variances for collection. Critical variances are identified as activities that affect the flow of patients through the system. To accomplish this, the team may develop a specialized flowchart that shows sequential relationships among the activities and the clinical outcomes in the care process. Using this approach to monitor critical pathway activities greatly reduces data collection and analysis. Within this approach, the team may also decide to collect additional variance related to high-cost tests, procedures, or specific quality improvement indicators. For example, the team may want to capture frequency of and indications for MRI or CAT testing for a particular neurosurgical patient pathway.

Luttman et al.[15] identified from this experience that the critical variance approach had two problems: Few of the variances correlated with length of stay, and many of the supposedly independent variances correlated with each other. They used the term *gateways* as a measure of patient progress through the system. When a patient approaches a gateway, there are three possible directions: progression to the next phase, falling off the path/discontinuing, or extra days of stay. At each gateway, a team constructs a cause-and-effect diagram for failure to progress. Variance data are collected for only this gateway variance, along with the coded reason from the cause-and-effect diagram. The cause-and-effect diagram has assisted in identification of root causes and decreased the tendency to select several causes for path variance.

In summary, whatever method one uses to define what and how much variance data to collect, it is essential that (1) clinical patient outcomes be part of the analysis, (2) multidisciplinary clinician teams identify and define the variances to be collected, (3) interventions and outcomes are specified for all appropriate clinician groups, and (4) an infrastructure to support data collection, analysis, storage, and reporting is established and funded.

INFORMATION MANAGEMENT OF CRITICAL PATH DATA

Collecting Variance Data

Just as there are several classifications for variances and various methodologies to identify what specific variances are collected, there are many practical ways to collect critical path variance data. The one universally agreed-on concept is that variance data must be collected concurrently for individual patients and aggregated for trends and analysis for patient populations if we are to improve care and ultimately improve health care outcomes. It must be emphasized that there is a paucity of literature devoted to information management of critical path data, variance analysis, and improvement of patient outcomes in contrast to the literature devoted to case management/critical path development and implementation. The infrastructure required for information management of variance data requires financial and human resources. Investment in these resources should be carefully considered in the planning and implementation of a critical path program.

Resources for Data Collection

Just as there are many technologies to collect variance data, there are also various schools of thought on who should collect or document variance data. With the recent changes in health care and the demand for more efficient data-driven care, organizations are experimenting with various methods and personnel to collect clinical data. One clear trend is that organizations are assigning data collection to already established roles in the organization and not adding personnel. To date, no one single recommendation has evolved in the literature defining who should collect variance data. Cesta and Cohen[13] identify the case manager as the individual responsible to identify, document, and intervene to correct the variance. Etheredge[34] identified that primary nurses at the point of care identify, document, and report variances in the intershift report. Schriefer[32] identified that all care givers (nurses, therapists, dietitians) manually document variances on the critical path and in the progress notes but that utilization review staff are responsible for collecting and aggregating select variances that have an effect on length of stay, cost per case, patient satisfaction, and readmissions, to name a few. Gentile,[35] in a recent interview for *Hospital Case Management*, reports that she employs two registered nurses to perform retrospective chart reviews and collect daily critical path variances.

The concept of concurrently collecting variance data as part of the normal process of providing patient care is a relatively new concept for many disciplines. More recently, this task has been assigned to the nurse case manager or nurse caring for the patient on a daily basis. A word of caution to organizations endorsing this approach is that it places nurses in the role of categorizing and defining variances for other disciplines. For instance, if one of the outcomes for a post-coronary artery bypass graft patient is walking 100 feet on day 3 and the discipline responsible for assisting the patient to achieve this outcome is physical therapy, then it should be physical therapy that identifies if the outcome was achieved or not achieved and thus defines the variance. This concept supports the multidisciplinary approach to developing, implementing, and evaluating care according to the critical path. Regardless of the method used to collect the data, the following questions must be considered when selecting individual data collectors:

- Who is responsible for documenting variance?
  1. All disciplines involved in providing the care
  2. Case manager only
  3. All nursing staff
  3. Non-care givers
- How is variance documentation integrated?
  1. As part of the clinicians' documentation
  2. An addition to the current work and documentation requirements
- How are individual patient variance data aggregated?
- How is data integrity ensured?
  1. Missing data
  2. Incorrect coding of variance

- How often and who will analyze the data?
- Does the system provide standard/customized reports that are clinician friendly, easily understood, and able to be applied to make improvements?

It is essential that whoever collects variance data be thoroughly trained in both the method of collection and the definition of the variance categories and types. Standard methods for ensuring interrater reliability should be used.

How Are Variance Data Collected?

There are several approaches for collecting variance data: manually, fully integrated clinical information system, and intermediate or semiautomated approaches.

Manually

Most organizations initially track variances manually.[11] Experiences and anecdotal reports from other organizations have indicated that this is the most common approach today. Most organizations are evaluating technologies to support the automation of this process, yet in balancing the need for availability of data with timeliness and cost of automation, many initially began with manual chart documentation. Some pathways have a variance section at the bottom of the path where the care provider, often the nurse, documents the type of variance;[32] some use perforated forms attached to the path that are completed and removed at time of patient discharge and sent to a central office for data aggregation and reporting,[36] and some have placed boxes beside each intervention or outcome on the critical path requiring a checkmark in the appropriate box (met, unmet, yes, or no) by the discipline.[8] In documenting variance directly on the critical path, it is often a requirement that for each variance a note is written in the progress note section or on the nursing flowsheet describing how the care giver is addressing that variance and, if needed, providing more detail about the variance. For example, a nurse identified that the patient did not achieve a pain relief goal in less than 3 days as defined on the critical path. The progress note may read, "Ineffective pain relief, patient continues to identify pain rating of 5 to 6 after PO demerol and IM morphine. Pain service notified, will begin intravenous patient-controlled analgesia." Often these individual variances are addressed concurrently by the multidisciplinary team providing the patient care.

The aggregation of these data to review trends is somewhat complex and cumbersome. Data collected by the health care provider must be transported from the document into a software program to aggregate the data in a way that is meaningful to the clinicians. Often this requires retrospective chart reviews or the batch processing of individual variance forms. Relevant information that may assist clinicians in understanding the variances is often located in the patient progress notes. Progress notes are recorded in narrative format and may be difficult to codify. Consistency in coding may be a problem if the individual doing the coding from the progress notes is not the clinician caring for the patient. Retrospective chart reviews, although used for many purposes in patient care, may not always provide the clinicians with the most accurate or appropriate data. Manual collection of data and retrospective chart reviews by individuals not providing care to the patient or not having knowledge and expertise in care of that patient population create data integrity concerns and issues.

Batch processing of individual variance forms, although completed by the clinicians caring for the patient, may have missing or inaccurate data elements. Often these forms are entered into a data base by central office staff who are often unfamiliar with the data. Thus, missing data elements and unclear or inaccurate data may need to be returned to the clinicians for concurrent review or additional chart review. This process has an effect on data timeliness as well as data integrity.

Integrated Computer Systems

Computer-based systems are rapidly growing to meet the challenge of integrating critical path development, documentation, collection, and analysis of variance data on line. Di Jerome[37] describes a computerized critical pathway and variance system in use at Summa Health System in Akron, Ohio. This system has the ability to alter the path on line to meet the individualized needs of the patient. It also collects variance and provides trends for analysis. Currently, Nolten,[38] at Scripps Health Care System, LaJolla, California, is beta testing the SMS (Shared Medical Systems) CareCenter system in the maternal child health division for normal newborn, normal vaginal delivery, and Caesarean section CareMaps®. In a recent supplement in *Hospital Case Management*,[39] 26 large vendor companies were identified throughout the United States offering critical pathway systems or modules to help in the development and management of critical paths. A key criterion for an integrated critical path management system is that automated physician order entry should be fully implemented. In anecdotal reports from various hospitals across the United States, few hospitals to date have achieved a fully integrated clinical information system that supports critical path development, clinical documentation, and variance collection and analysis.

Intermediate Semiautomated Methods

Intermediate technologies exist to support variance data collection and analysis as a part of an integrated clinical information system. Many of these technologies, although they can stand alone, may be integrated with a hospital clinical information system. Nolten and Zawadski[40] identified the need to develop open architecture systems that support multiple information sets, various software applications that talk to one another, linked together in an organized way within a single service, across multiple services, and across multiple agencies. Grobe[41] describes information systems as the anchor of the entire clinical performance improvement, effectiveness, and outcomes cycle. The information infrastructure required to support an organization-wide critical path/outcomes management program should be included in the initial development and program planning. The demand for quality and outcomes data requires a different design than traditional transactional hospital information systems.[42] Industry migration from mainframe environments to client/server network environments also affects the management of quality and outcomes data. Estimates are that some health care organizations have invested approximately $100 million over three years to develop effective outcome information based on clinical and management information systems.[1]

Three stand-alone technologies (the laptop computer, the Newton™, and an optical scanner) are presented as intermediate or semiautomated methods for conducting variance analysis. Each method meets the criteria for timely input at the point of care and potential to link with other hospital data systems. This discussion is based on anecdotal experience with these technologies at The Johns Hopkins Hospital during implementation of a critical path program (1993–1995).

Laptop Computer. The laptop computer is one technology that supports variance data collection and analysis. A proprietary DOS™-based software program was customized by a vendor for several surgical critical paths. The program required 12 megabytes to run, and the data base required 2 megabytes of storage per 100 patients. Data were captured directly to the laptop and downloaded to a data base on a personal computer. User input was included at the beginning of the software customization.

User procedure: The patient's name and user-specific demographics are entered into the system. The appropriate path is selected from the listing, and the patient is then entered onto a path. The path may now be individualized to meet the unique needs of the patient by deleting or adding any specific interventions or outcomes. A screen describing management of patient care activities lists all the standard and individualized patient interventions planned for a particular day according to the critical path. For each intervention that does not occur, a standard variance category is selected. Additional comments may also be entered to explain the variance further. As discussed earlier, the selection of a standard variance category alone may not give the clinicians the added detail necessary to analyze the aggregate data; therefore, the comment field provides the clinician with more detail. This software has the capability to collect variance data on all interventions or select critical variances as defined by the clinicians. Reports may be generated directly from the software package or the data may be downloaded into a relational data base residing on a server or stand-alone personal computer for additional reporting and format designs in other software programs.

Although the laptop is relatively inexpensive, there are both hardware and software issues to consider before implementing this technology in the acute care setting. Hardware issues are: (1) the laptop is somewhat heavy and cumbersome to carry; (2) it has a short battery life of a few hours; and (3) availability of the devices for clinicians needs to be balanced with security of the devices on a clinical unit. Software issues include: (1) response time of the program is not adequate to collect data concurrently during physician rounds, thus retrospective chart review is required; (2) the program output is not integrated in any way with current documentation, and thus it may be viewed as an added work requirement; (3) there is redundancy of collecting patient demographics that are also captured on the hospital registration system; and (4) it does not easily lend itself to point-of-care data collection by all providers of care to the patient on a critical path.

Laptop technology may have greater applicability in a setting where episodic care, such as a clinic visit, is provided by one or two individuals who collect data concurrently as part of the clinic visit. This technology is currently used in some settings by utilization review nurses during retrospective chart reviews and is beginning to be applied to the collection of critical path variance.[35]

Newton™ Hand-Held Computer. A small (approximately the size of a calculator) hand-held pen-based laptop computer (Newton™) is another intermediate technology that may assist in variance data collection and analysis. The difference in this technology from the laptop is its size, the use of a stylus that recognizes handwriting to enter and retrieve data, and the ability to download the data to any desktop workstation simply by connecting a cable to the Newton™. The software functions are similar to the previously described laptop software functions, with the added capability of storing patient resource information such as primary physician telephone numbers, beeper numbers, insurance information, and home health nurse details. The technology is designed to function as an individual's notebook and as such is not as conducive to multiple users or collection of data concurrently in the acute care setting. Thus, often a case manager or utilization review nurse is assigned to one device. The same issue of redundancy of adding patient information to the system and security of the devices exists as in the laptop. The current software does not create reports. It is used primarily as a repository for data, which is transferred to a desktop workstation. Reports are developed and printed from other software products. Software maintenance and upgrading is somewhat time consuming.

Card Scanner. Although this technology has been applied in many settings, such as education, its use in health care as a method to capture point-of-care variance data is relatively new. Bueno and Hwang[27] discuss the use of the optical scanner where nurse case managers at the time of patient discharge finalize variance identification. The data are collected through the scanning device. Reports are then generated using a statistical package to determine frequencies, averages, and ratios.

At The Johns Hopkins Hospital, the use of scanner technology has been piloted on one unit at the point of care and is part of the normal documentation requirements of all disciplines. We are currently evaluating the use of the optical scanning device and software in a network environment. The system requirements are a Windows™-based 486 clinical workstation, software, scanning device, and printer. Issues of feasibility and scalability with multiple critical paths and multiple clinical units are being evaluated.

User procedure: As part of their normal patient documentation, nurses and other health care professionals collect daily variance data and record them directly onto a scanner form (card). This card includes critical path-specific patient information such as patient comorbidities or risk factors, age, attending physician, patient outcomes, and resource utilization items. All data to be collected are defined by the team responsible for developing the critical path. One card is used for the patient's entire length of stay and may be scanned by many users and multiple times a day until all items are completed relevant to the critical path. For example, the nurse completes item 1 on postoperative day 1 "achieved a pain relief goal 3/10" and scans the card. Later that day, the physical therapist completes item 4 "OOB with assistance QID" and scans the card. A sample of a card scanner form is displayed in Exhibit 10-2. The scanning literally takes seconds to complete. If there is an error in completing the form such as incomplete data, missed data, duplicate selections in a single category, or data recorded on the wrong path day, the system will refuse the data. The computer screen prompts the user to the exact place on the scan form where the error was detected. This assists in ensuring data integrity and avoiding missing data.

An important point to reiterate here is that to apply point-of-care variance collection, one must integrate data collection as a normal part of documentation and not add it to the current documentation requirements. Therefore, it is very important to assess and make appropriate changes to patient care documentation that include all relevant disciplines. Charting by exception has

Exhibit 10-2 Sample Card Scanner Form

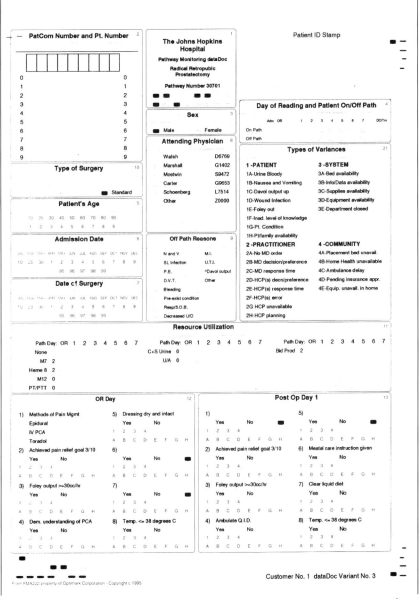

continues

Exhibit 10-2 continued

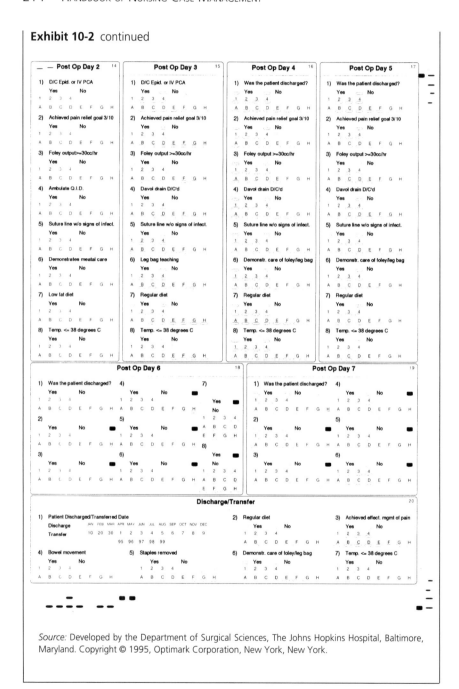

Source: Developed by the Department of Surgical Sciences, The Johns Hopkins Hospital, Baltimore, Maryland. Copyright © 1995, Optimark Corporation, New York, New York.

been one method that has enhanced critical path and variance documentation without increasing documentation requirements.

An example of charting by exception that correlates with a report available through the card scanner technology is the daily summary of patient progress toward outcomes. This report may replace the nursing daily patient narrative note, the physician progress note, and other disciplines' progress notes. If the patient achieves the expected outcomes as indicated by "yes," then no additional documentation is necessary other than a signature. If the patient does not achieve the expected outcomes as indicated by "no," then a narrative note by the specific responsible health care professional is written regarding how this variance is being addressed.

The software associated with the scanner technology concurrently provides data to the users at the point of care. The user in a Windows™ environment selects an administrative report icon that displays a selection of available reports. The user then selects the time frame and the particular critical path for report generation. Examples of some reports available on the nursing units are previous 24-hour patient variances for all patients or a particular patient on the unit, laboratory study trends by test (e.g., complete blood count) and by physician, and length of stay by critical path and by physician. Some of the reports such as length of stay have critical path benchmarks built into the format (Exhibit 10-2). Another report used to assist the critical path develop teams in identifying opportunities for improvement is the aggregate report of the most frequently occurring variances for all patients on a particular path and patient outcome data aggregated per day and on discharge.

The power behind this technology lies in the accessibility of concurrent data at the point of care where patient care decisions are made. It focuses nursing and other disciplines on patients' accomplishments toward outcomes and, as such, provides clinicians with real-time data to manage patients while supporting the assessment of aggregate outcomes. It also places codification of variances directly in the hands of the clinicians caring for the patient and integrates variance collection with patient care documentation. Because a variance data base is generated by the software, concurrent and aggregate data can be communicated easily to groups or departments that analyze aggregate data for trends and financial outcomes. Figure 10-2 depicts the interaction of scanner technology with clinical and other departments.

Results of Variance Analysis

Variance analysis is only one element of the performance improvement process. It provides guidance for the next step both at the individual patient level and the aggregate level. Several factors are critical to the validity of the

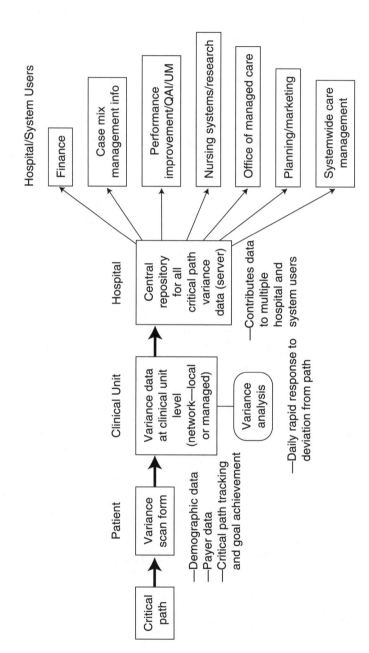

Figure 10-2 Relationship of Critical Path Scanning Technology to Other Organizational Initiatives. *Source:* Courtesy of Barbara Frink and Larry Strassner, The Johns Hopkins Hospital, Baltimore, Maryland.

process. First is the validity and relevance of the indicator that is measured. The second is the issue of risk stratification of the critical path population, and the third is context of the interpretation of the data. The familiar phrase "garbage in, garbage out" is sometimes used to describe automation of useless or incorrect data or processes. In the case of critical paths and variance analysis, there is a danger of "garbage in, gospel out." The analysis of critical path outcome data is at an early stage of development. Little is known about clinical processes in regard to variation and control.

Risk adjustment of patients on paths, using a standardized methodology, is vital to interpreting clinical variance data and to comparing data across settings and institutions. Risk adjustment, including measures of severity, is a complex area of research that is critical to developing valid outcomes management systems.[43,44] At the least, institutional standards, such as a case mix adjustment, should be applied to all patients on a critical path before aggregating the outcome data. The risk stratification provides the context for data interpretation, including patterns of variation and identification of data significantly outside of a normative range, commonly referred to as outlier data. Failure to adjust for risk can lead to the overestimation of variation in a clinical process and incorrect identification of outlier data.[17,45,46] The context of the measurement and the level of analysis of variance data are also important in interpretation. Variance data at the individual patient level, used for patient management, have one meaning. Variance frequencies at the aggregate level for a cohort of patients may present a different interpretation. Variance frequencies across cohorts, such as aggregating system variation data across five critical paths, will present a system quality interpretation.[47,48]

Descriptive data about categories, types, and specific variances in expected patient outcomes provide valuable input for making changes to manage individual patients at the point of care. Frequency distributions of categories of variance provide direction for managing groups of patients and may point to particular areas for further study or improvement. For example, if 20 percent of all patients on a coronary artery bypass graft critical path experience a negative variance in the timely discharge from the intensive care unit, a system variance has been identified that can easily be quantified in both the cost to the individual patient and the institution. Solving the system problem may entail a process analysis of intensive care unit patient flow, bed utilization, general care unit bed availability, or other relevant system processes. It is in examination of the clinical and system processes that the root cause is discovered. Aggregate data across critical paths may give further indication of system performance. For example, variance data across all pediatric critical paths on expected pain management outcomes may demonstrate that pediatric pain management processes are widely variant or generally a process in control. Such data provide direction for policy evaluation and effectiveness as well as serving as indicators of quality for an external audience, such as consumer groups or payers. Figure 10-3 depicts relationships of variance analysis to clinical, operational, and system performance improvement as well as research. Through systematic evaluation and research on the relationships between clinical processes and outcomes, knowledge of processes that affect results can be used to improve clinical performance.[49,50]

The interpretation of data can be greatly influenced by the visual presentation. Variance data from critical paths should be used to make substantive changes in clinical and financial performance for both patients and organizations. Presentation of meaningful data to appropriate audiences can have a powerful effect on institutional and individual performance. Some understanding of principles of design, publishing, and graphics will enhance the presentation of variance data and contribute to its potential usefulness in improving quality. Software and hardware that enable the visualization of quantitative data are increasingly affordable and available. Development of visual cues that enhance the depiction and meaning of data is one of the challenges of communicating credible variance data to multiple audiences.[51]

Transformation of Data into Information

The display of data using control charts can provide a tool for increasing understanding of variation in care processes. Finison et al.[52] and Kritchevsky and Simmons[53] provide reviews of this method as applied in the health care environment. Tufte,[54-57] well-known author and publisher of methods for the display of quantitative and symbolic data, provides the following principles of data display:

- Show causality mechanisms or dynamics wherever possible.
  1. The display of the data should match the analytic goal.
  2. Data displays should always note the data source, any problems in the data, and the methodology.
  3. Whenever appropriate, show both the mean and variation of the data.
  4. Order data displays by meaningful content such as in ascending or descending order, not alphabetically.
- In displaying financial data:
  1. Show an assessment of change.
  2. Show both the mean and standard deviation.

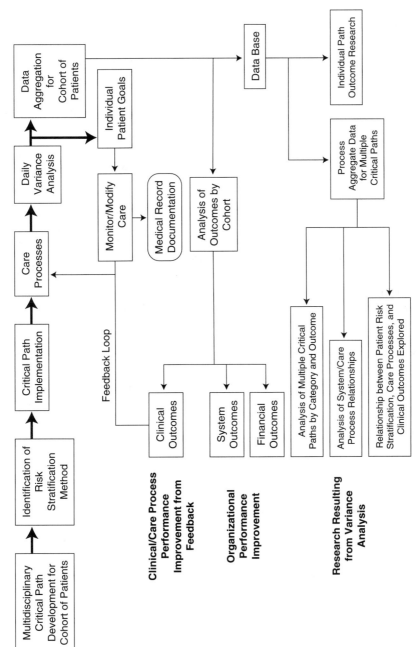

Figure 10-3 Variance Analysis in Critical Paths. *Source:* Courtesy of Barbara Frink, The Johns Hopkins Hospital, Baltimore, Maryland.

3. When showing financial data against time, always adjust for inflation and report standardization.

4. Show cause and effect relationships whenever possible. Most financial displays are often descriptive.

5. Use the *New York Times* and *Wall Street Journal* data tables as models of well-designed, high-resolution financial tables.[57]

- For dynamic process data, show the process on many variables within the eye span.[56]

CONCLUSION

This chapter focused on the concept of variance analysis in the context of case management/critical path programs. Variance analysis was defined and issues related to variance classification, infrastructure, data collection, data analysis, and interpretation were discussed. Both content and process areas of critical path program development were included to provide context for the variance analysis. The analytic process was defined as one element in a cycle of performance improvement targeted at both improvement of individual patient clinical outcomes and operational system outcomes. Properly constructed, well-managed paths and outcome data lead not only to performance improvement but also to outcomes research at the patient cohort and systems level. It should be emphasized that the use of variance analysis with well-defined data infrastructures and comprehensive critical path programs is at an early stage of development in U.S. hospitals. It is expected that continued enhancement of the analytical and performance improvement aspects of such programs will assist hospitals in effective management of patients in the new health care environment.

REFERENCES

1. Shortell SM, Gillies RR, Devers KJ. Reinventing the American hospital. *Milbank Q.* 1995;73:131-160.

2. Epstein A. Performance reports on quality–prototypes, problems and prospects. *N Engl J Med.* 1995;333:57-61.

3. Keegan AJ. Hospitals become cost centers in managed care scenario. *Healthcare Financial Manage.* August 1994:36-39.

4. Krivenko CA, Chodroff C. The analysis of clinical outcomes: getting started in benchmarking. *Joint Commission J Quality Improvement.* 1994;20:260-266.

5. Barnes RV, Lawton L, Briggs D. Clinical benchmarking improves clinical paths: experience with coronary artery bypass grafting. *Joint Commission J Quality Improvement.* 1994;20: 267-274.

6. Hoffman PA. Critical path method. An important tool for coordinating clinical care. *Joint Commission J Quality Improvement.* 1993;19:235-246.

7. Southwick K. Memphis' huge Baptist Memorial—fast-track institution wide case management for quality and efficiency gains. *Strategies Health Care Excellence.* 1993;6(11):1-8.

8. Vandenbusche P. Medication profile key to surpassing LOS reduction goal. *Hosp Case Manage.* 1995;3:59-62.

9. Verona DM. Case management guidelines. In: Ball M, Simborg D, Albright J, Douglas J, eds. *Healthcare Information Management Systems, A Practical Guide.* New York, NY: Springer-Verlag; 1995:97–107.

10. Handy J, Kedrowski S, Lynette E, Quinn J. Nurse case managers: a snapshot of roles and settings. Lecture at Case Management across the Continuum, sponsored by Contemporary Forums: May 7–9, 1995; San Francisco, Calif. Abstract.

11. Lumsdon K, Hagland M. Mapping care. *Hosp Health Networks.* October 1993;20:34-40.

12. Patterson J. Baptist Memorial Hospital. *Patient Focused Healthcare J.* 1994;2:6.

13. Cesta T, Cohen E. *Nursing Case Management from Concept to Evaluation.* St. Louis, Mo: CV Mosby; 1993.

14. Zander K. Nursing case management: strategic management of cost and quality outcomes. *J Nurs Adm.* 1988;18(5):23–30.

15. Luttman HR, Laffel G, Pearson S. Using PERT/CPM to design and improve clinical processes. *Quality Manage Health Care.* 1995;3:1–13.

16. Lamb GS. Case management. In: Fitzpatrick JJ, Simmons JS, eds. *Ann Rev Nurs.* 1995;13:117–136.

17. Rosenthal GE. Potential for bias in severity adjusted hospital outcomes data: analysis of patients with rheumatic disease. *J Rhematol.* 1994;21:721–727.

18. Wilson IB, Cleary PD. Linking clinical variables with health-related quality of life. *JAMA.* 1995;273:59–65.

19. Brooten D, Naylor MD. Nurses' effect on changing patient outcomes. *J Nurs Scholarship.* 1995;27:95–99.

20. *Webster's Ninth New Collegiate Dictionary.* Boston, Mass: Riverside Publishing Company, 1995.

21. Bowers K. Case management along the continuum. Lecture sponsored by Contemporary Forums: May 7–9, 1995; San Francisco, Calif. Abstract.

22. Strassner L. *How To Develop and Evaluate Critical Paths.* Baltimore, Md: The Johns Hopkins Hospital; 1994.

23. Jacobsen BS. Univariate descriptive statistics. In: Munro BH, Page EB, eds. *Statistical Methods for Health Care Research.* Philadelphia, Pa: JB Lippincott; 1993:19–37.

24. Munro BH. Differences among group means: one-way analysis of variance. In: Munro BH, Page EB, eds. *Statistical Methods for Health Care Research.* Philadelphia, Pa: JB Lippincott; 1993: 109–127.

25. Zander K. Care map tools and case management across the continuum. Lecture sponsored by the Maryland League for Nursing: September 30, 1993; Baltimore, Md.

26. Coffey RJ, Richards JS, Remmert CS, LeRoy SS, Schoville RR, Baldwin PJ. An introduction to critical paths. *Quality Manage Health Care.* 1992;1:45–54.

27. Bueno MM, Hwang RF. Understanding variances in hospital stay. *Nurs Manage.* 1993;24:51–57.

28. Robinson JA, Robinson KJ, Lewis DJ. Balancing quality of care and cost-effectiveness through case management. *ANNA J.* 1992;19:182–188.

29. Mikulaninec CE. An amputee critical path. *J Vasc Nurs.* 1992;10:6–9.

30. Spath PL. The quality-cost connection: clinical path development should be a team effort. *Hosp Peer Rev.* December 1993:196–199.

31. Steinwachs DM. Patient outcomes of health care: integrating outcomes into management information systems. In: Ball M, Sinborgs D, Albright J, Douglas J, eds. *Healthcare Information Management Systems, A Practical Guide.* New York, NY: Springer-Verlag; 1995:108–118.

32. Schriefer J. Managing critical pathway variances. *Quality Manage Health Care.* 1995;3:30–42. Abstract.

33. Sterman JD. Misperceptions of feedback in dynamic decision making. *Organizational Behavior Hum Decision Processes.* 1989;43:301–335.

34. Etheredge ML. *Collaborative Care Nursing Case Management.* Chicago, Ill: American Hospital Publishing, Inc; 1989.

35. Gentile C. PA hospital computerized variance analysis system aids pathway team. *Hosp Case Manage.* 1995;3:1–4.

36. Cesta T. Integrating case management plans into documentation; multidisciplinary path documentation. Lecture at Case Management along the Continuum, sponsored by Contemporary Forums: May 7–9, 1995; San Francisco, Calif.

37. Di Jerome L. The nursing case management computerized system: meeting the challenges of health care delivery through technology. *Comput Nurs.* 1992;10:250–258.

38. Nolten D. Planning for critical pathways—across the health continuum. Lecture at Case Management along the Continuum, sponsored by Contemporary Forums: May 7–9, 1995; San Francisco, Calif.

39. American Health Consultants. Vendors hot on the trail to capture pathway market. *Hosp Case Manage.* 1995;3(suppl).

40. Nolten D, Zawadski R. Information and case management; defining a new generation of support systems. Lecture at Case Management along the Continuum, sponsored by Contemporary Forums: May 7–9, 1995; San Francisco, Calif.

41. Grobe SJ. Informatics: the infrastructure for quality assessment and quality improvement. *J Am Med Informatics Assoc.* 1995;2:267–268.

42. Zielstorff RD, Hudgings CI, Grobe SJ. *Next-Generation Nursing Information Systems. Essential Characteristics for Professional Practice.* Washington, DC: American Nurses Publishing; 1993.

43. Ellis PJ, Wu AW, Ahmed F, Moore R, Rubin HR, Steinberg EP. A new comorbidity index based on hospital discharge abstracts predicts hospital mortality. Lecture at The Johns Hopkins University School of Medicine and School of Hygiene and Public Health and Program for Medical Technology and Practice Assessment and The Johns Hopkins Hospital, 1994; Baltimore, Md.

44. Iezzoni LI, Greenberg LG. Widespread assessment risk-adjusted outcomes: lessons from local initiatives. *J Quality Improvement.* 1994;20:305–316.

45. Petryshen P, Pallas LL, Shamian J. Outcomes monitoring: adjusting for risk factors, severity of illness, and complexity of care. *J Am Med Informatics Assoc.* 1995;2:243–249.

46. Salem-Schatz S, Moore G, Rucker M, Pearson SD. The case for case-mix adjustment in practice profiling: when good apples look bad. *JAMA.* 1994;272:871–874.

47. Hegyvary S. Issues in outcomes research. *J Nurs Quality Assurance.* 1991;5:1–6.

48. Verran J, Mark B. Contextual factors influencing patient outcomes: individual/group/environment: interactions and clinical practice interface. Patient outcomes research: examining the effectiveness of nursing practice. 1992. NIH 93-3411. Abstract.

49. Phelps CE. The methodologic foundations of studies of the appropriateness of medical care. *N Engl J Med.* 1993;329:1241-1245.

50. Batalden PB, Nelson EC, Roberts JS. Linking outcomes measurement to continual improvement: the serial "V" way of thinking about improving clinical care. *J Quality Improvement.* 1994;20:167–180.

51. Keller PR, Keller MM. *Visual Cues, Practical Data Visualization.* Los Alamitos, Calif: IEEE Press; 1992.

52. Finison LJ, Finison KS, Bliersbach CM. The use of control charts to improve healthcare quality. *J Healthcare Quality: Promoting Excellence Health Care.* 1993;15:9–23.

53. Kritchevsky SB, Simmons BP. Continuous quality improvement. Concepts and applications for physician care. *JAMA.* 1991;266:1817–1823.

54. Tufte ER. *The Visual Display of Quantitative Information.* Cheshire, Conn: Graphics Press; 1983.

55. Tufte ER. *Envisioning Information.* Cheshire, Conn: Graphics Press; 1990.

56. Powsner S, Tufte ER. A graphical display of patient status. *Lancet.* 1994;344:386–389.

57. Tufte ER. Presenting data and information. Seminar: June 16, 1995; Crystal City, Va. Abstract.

■ 11 ■

Improving Accreditation Results through Case Management

Diane B. Williams, MSHA, BSN

The broad scope and diverse nature of case management, along with a quality focus, easily lend the process to achieving successful accreditation in both the hospital and managed care environment. Whether seeking accreditation from the Joint Commission on Accreditation of Healthcare Organizations (the Joint Commission) or from the National Committee for Quality Assurance (NCQA), the resources dedicated to case management can be a valuable commodity in the survey process. How do your quality programs tap this resource in case management? Which accreditation standards are addressed by case management? How does the organization integrate continuous quality improvement initiatives with those in case management? This chapter explores the answers to these questions and more. Not only can case management improve accreditation results, but it offers health care organizations the ability to blend concurrent staff activities and save resources.

Case management has gained rapidly in popularity as a process for managing cost, quality, and customer satisfaction in a variety of health care settings. One additional and often overlooked benefit of case management is the impact the process has on accreditation. Most health care organizations participate voluntarily or through state/federal mandates in some type of accreditation survey. Accreditation is sought for the marketing advantages to patients and employers, to receive reimbursement from certain payer sources, and to validate performance and process achievements internally to staff and management.

The basic tenant of accreditation is the assurance, by an independent source, that the health care facility is providing high-quality, effective services to the customers it serves. The amount of money an organization spends pursuing accreditation varies, depending on size and organizational structure, but includes both the application fees for the survey and internal costs associated with preparation. It is not unusual for an organization to spend more than $50,000 in fees and preparation activities, so any opportunity to leverage resources from other existing programs or departments would be beneficial to the organization. Case management affords this opportunity.

This chapter focuses on two voluntary accrediting agencies: the Joint Commission and NCQA. The first accredits inpatient and ambulatory facilities, such as hospitals, long-term care, skilled nursing, free-standing surgical facilities, and home care companies. The second accredits health plans or managed care organizations.

The accreditation survey is often associated with gut-wrenching preparation involving many hours of staff and management time. To avoid the last minute "fire fight" associated with pre-survey preparation, many health care organizations have invested heavily in management theories such as total quality management (TQM) and processes such as continuous quality improvement (CQI). These concepts perpetuate an environment focused on continuous improvement using systems thinking and teams consisting of cross-functional staff members. When one compares the theories in TQM and CQI to that of case management, overlapping themes are evident:

- Customer focus through patient involvement in care decisions and ongoing education
- System/process driven rather than individual performance as a means of addressing inappropriate or less than optimal patient care
- Analysis of variation in the practice of medicine and nursing with a focus on reduction in variation as a means to improve quality and cost
- Scientific use of data and measures that establish baseline performance and incremental improvements
- Teamwork as a means of leveraging human resources, harnessing ideas, and involving all key stakeholders to induce better collaboration

Organizations that practice TQM/CQI have a foundation to support successful case management because of these similar concepts. TQM sets the leadership stage for an organization by encouraging top-down commitment. CQI redesigns the work flow and processes to facilitate horizontal communication and teamwork. Case management is the next evolutionary step, as health care organizations manage patient care each step along the continuum of services, reducing fragmentation in care, both internally and externally to the health care facility.

This chapter takes a practical approach by dissecting the standards applicable to case management published by both the Joint Commission and NCQA. The discussion on the Joint Commission refers mainly to the hospital accreditation standards, but the implications for home care and ambulatory surgery facilities are similar for standards relating to patient care. By using this approach, the reader can evaluate past performance in accreditation surveys and use the concepts in case management to improve the substance and results in focused areas of the organization.

THE JOINT COMMISSION ON ACCREDITATION OF HEALTHCARE ORGANIZATIONS

The Joint Commission's organizational mission is to improve the quality of health care provided to the general public.[1] The 700-plus hospital standards are revisited annually by the Joint Commission to challenge health care facilities continually to enhance services. In 1987, the Joint Commission introduced the Agenda for Change, an initiative to drive health care organizations toward performance-based analysis of the processes that support patient care. Although the Joint Commission does not prescribe any one particular management theory, the Agenda for Change moved the survey process away from strictly looking at an organization's capabilities to one focused on process improvements, outcome measurements, and performance-based expectations. It was during this time that many hospitals adopted the management concepts of TQM and CQI.

Since the early 1990s, the Joint Commission has placed more emphasis in the standards on the process of patient care and key functions that support the process. No longer does the Joint Commission focus the standards around individual departments in the hospital such as nursing or laboratory. Instead, the standards have come to reflect the idea that patient care requires a multidisciplinary approach, highlighting collaboration among departments and staff members as a means to maximize quality and resources. Integration of nursing, medical staff, and other allied health care professionals is necessary to meet the intent of the standards. This framework of integration on which the Joint Commission developed its standards is fundamental to case management. "Although case management may be directed toward other goals, and although the primary purpose for instituting a case management system may vary among programs, coordination of care is the basic component of all models and modalities of case management."[2] The recognition that the Joint Commission standards are steeped in the same basic theories as case management (integration, coordination, collaboration, and improvements in care) is key to the realization that the two processes (case management and accreditation preparation) are not independent activities. Organizations that pursue them as independent activities are missing the opportunity to enhance outcomes in each process and to save time and resources.

Let's look at the Joint Commission standards that are benefited by a case management program to understand better how case management can improve accreditation performance.

Patient-Focused Functions

The first group of standards related to case management are those termed patient-focused functions. The basic tenet of the patient-focused function standards is the recognition that each patient is unique in terms of health care needs and personal expectations. The health care organization is responsible for tailoring its services to meet these individual patient needs. In the current reimbursement climate, reducing variation (and subsequently expenses) in the process of patient care through the use of protocols, practice guidelines, and clinical pathways has become essential to reduce excessive resource utilization. Health care providers are expected to balance the need for individual patient care planning with that of establishing performance expectations in the form of predetermined care standards. This balancing act requires careful management, and in many hospitals, it is the case manager who is the catalyst for this process.

Case management is patient focused. The patient is the common denominator in the case management equation as case managers use the full spectrum of services provided in the delivery system, work to reduce fragmentation of care, and advocate on behalf of the patient's needs and desires. Case managers find tools such as standards of care and clinical pathways helpful in setting baseline expectations in case management but are mindful to incorporate individualized patient care issues into the management of their client's illness or disease.

The patient-focused functional standards encompass the hospital's performance in the areas of patient rights, assessment, actual care provided, education, and the care continuum. With regard to patient rights, the standards relating to mechanisms for addressing communication of patients' needs and resolution of patient complaints are particularly relevant to case management. Case managers are the link between the patient and the care givers. They clarify information for the patient, answer questions about the patient's illness or pending treatment, educate the patient on self-care and healthy life style choices, and provide a sounding board for patients to ventilate their concerns and fears. When patients have complaints about the services they have received, it is often the case manager who is the first to hear about them. In some case management programs, it is the case manager's responsibility to document and resolve these complaints. In other programs, the case manager facilitates resolution of the complaint by informing the appropriate service area of the problem.

Assessment of patients in the Joint Commission standards is dedicated to the goal of individualizing health care services to meet the needs of each patient entering the facility. It requires data collection specific to the patient and decisions for treatment based on analysis of that data. As part of any case management program, early assessment of patient needs for medical care and services, along with psychosocial issues, is characteristic of the documentation case managers acquire through a patient and family interview, review of the medical records, and discussions with providers. These assessment records demonstrate a systematic process of developing baseline data for each patient for whom the case manager is responsible.

Using the assessment information, the Joint Commission standards require care givers to make decisions about appropriate treatment and operationalize these decisions into specific treatment plans. Treatment plans are multidisciplinary and address services provided throughout the continuum of care. A primary role for the case manager is that of observer and recorder of pertinent information about the patient that allows for appropriate resource planning and coordination of services that will be required either inpatient or in the ambulatory environment. But beyond the observer role, the case manager formulates recommendations for improving the treatment plan and patient care outcomes. "All case managers must be observers, but they must be much more as well. If they never looked beyond 'what is wrong with this picture' to 'what can I do to improve this,' if they never envisioned the contributions they could make— to better the patient's condition, support the family, stretch the dollars, tighten up the treatment plan, coordinate the activities of the providers— then they would be merely a group of reporters."[3]

Patient education is constant throughout the process of patient care. Appropriateness of educational efforts is an important part of the patient-focused functions in the hospital accreditation manual. Likewise, patient education is an important role for case managers. The critical aspect here is that case managers are at the epicenter of patient care and management. Case managers are in the best position to appreciate fully the complexity of issues concerning the patient: clinical management, psychosocial dynamics, financial or insurance concerns, and discharge planning needs for each of their clients. Case management programs must clearly identify the case manager's role in patient education. This is accomplished by developing assessment tools, identifying key educational issues for populations of patients, developing mechanisms to provide this education to patients (e.g., classes, video tapes, written materials, individual or family educational sessions) and then following up with measurements that analyze the results of educational efforts on improvements in health or knowledge. These efforts demonstrate compliance with the Joint Commission standards in this area. Beyond patient education, case managers also provide education to physicians and other care providers about availability of ambulatory services, alternative health care facilities that may be appropriate for patients, and information about community services.

Finally, the care continuum is addressed by the Joint Commission as the need for the hospital organization to consider the appropriate setting and services for their patient population. Case managers well versed in discharge planning and resource management are in the perfect position to provide the organization with a documented process to support a continuum of care and meet the intent of the Joint Commission standards.

Organizational Functions

The next group of the Joint Commission standards related to case management are those termed organizational functions. The standards related to organizational functions are concerned with the processes and systems the health care organization uses to improve performance in patient care outcomes. Key to this set of standards is the use of the Joint Commission performance improvement framework (Figure 11-1). The steps in this model—to design, measure, assess, improve, and redesign—allow the health care organization both to tailor activity for specific patients and, at the same time, focus on overall improvement for the facility in health care outcomes.

A case management program can be used to implement the Joint Commission performance improvement model. Case managers have dual roles. First, case managers are concerned with the ongoing management of their individual patients. This means managing a case load on a daily basis to ensure appropriate activities are occurring. Second, case managers must concern themselves with improving the overall dynamics of the care process and outcomes achieved by the hospital. Whether the model of case management used is one dedicated to certain patient populations (i.e., the case manager is assigned to only transplant patients or to a particular unit, such as intensive care) or a program in which case managers are assigned to patients with many different diagnoses (e.g., the case manager works with all Medicare patients or any patient referred by the physician), case managers use information acquired during the assessment phase, planning, and actual patient care processes to work with other members of the delivery team to improve proactively the process and outcomes of care for the patients they serve. It is this constant use of data and expertise acquired during episodic management of patients that allows case managers to improve, longitudinally, outcomes for their clients.

A comparison of the case management process to that of the Joint Commission performance improvement model is made in Figure 11-2. The pro-

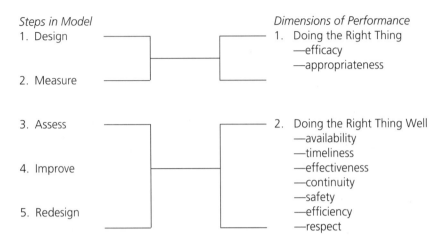

Steps in Model
1. Design
2. Measure
3. Assess
4. Improve
5. Redesign

Dimensions of Performance
1. Doing the Right Thing
   —efficacy
   —appropriateness
2. Doing the Right Thing Well
   —availability
   —timeliness
   —effectiveness
   —continuity
   —safety
   —efficiency
   —respect

Figure 11-1 Joint Commission Organizational Performance Improvement Model. *Source:* Based on the Joint Commission on Accreditation of Healthcare Organizations, *1996 Accreditation Manual for Hospitals, Vol. 1, Standards,* pp. 23–27, © 1996.

cess of case management demonstrates use of the Joint Commission's improvement model.

Other ways in which case management supports achievement of standards in the area of organizational performance include (1) a systematic process for collecting data, (2) measurement of patient care performance, and (3) resources that actually improve patient care.

Hospitals or other health care organizations that have developed case management programs should have a "plan" describing the scope, goals, objectives, accountability, and process of case management for their institutions. This case management plan would be similar in structure to a quality improvement plan; it may even be part of that document. An outline of a case management plan is presented in Exhibit 11-1. An essential component of any case management plan is that the processes of care delivery are quality driven. Key performance measures are identified, a process for data collection is described, and the role of the case manager in analyzing, reporting, and using the data to improve health care outcomes is included in this plan. This document, along with the achievements the case management program demonstrates, will aid in meeting the Joint Commission standards in the area of performance management.

The collaborative nature of case management is also important in complying with organizational performance standards. Case managers primarily act as facilitators, bringing many disciplines together to discuss and participate

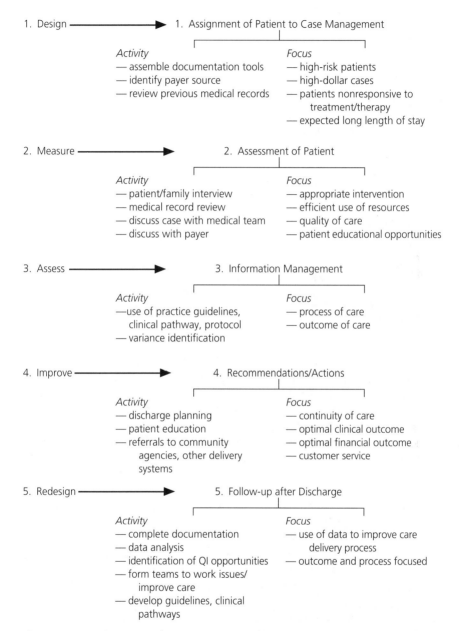

Figure 11-2 Comparison of Case Management to the Joint Commission's Performance Improvement Model. *Source:* Courtesy of T.P. Williams and Associates, Inc., Portland, Oregon.

Exhibit 11-1 Case Management Program Description

1. Executive Summary
2. Stakeholder Analysis
3. Vital Statistics and Assumptions
   —patient population
   —target diagnosis/procedure
   —linkage to outpatient services
   —organizational structure (reporting)
4. Deliverables
   —goals, expected outcomes, measures
   —financial and clinical (quality of care)
   —cost-benefit analysis
5. Data/Reporting
   —who
   —what
   —where
6. Risks
7. Implementation Strategy
   —team
   —timeliness
   —reporting

Source: Courtesy of T.P. Williams and Associates, Inc., Portland, Oregon.

actively in the management of patient care. Case managers document conversations they have had describing interaction among physicians, nursing staff, other health care service departments (respiratory therapy, physical therapy, radiology, etc), social services, patient and family, insurers, and outside agencies (home health, long-term care facilities). It is often the case manager's ideas and problem-solving activities surrounding the appropriateness of treatment and the treatment setting that prompt interaction between care providers.

Multidisciplinary collaboration with a quality focus is the hallmark of a good case management program. Such a program addresses many of the important aspects in standards compliance for the Joint Commission. Case management alone will not ensure successful accreditation. However, case management will achieve improved results in the design of tailored patient care plans, patient education, communication among members of the health care delivery team, data collection, and analysis to address systematically opportunities for improved outcomes and provisions for services at each step along the continuum of care. Used in conjunction with other quality initiatives, case management will reduce redundancy in survey preparation time and costs and result in successful Joint Commission accreditation.

THE NATIONAL COMMITTEE FOR QUALITY ASSURANCE

The NCQA was established in 1979 by the managed care industry. However, it was not until 1990, when the organization became an independent agent and after the publication of its first set of standards in 1991, that the organization came into prominence as the primary source of accreditation for managed care organizations.

The NCQA collaborated with employers, representatives from the managed care industry, and consumers of health care services to develop its standards. These standards[4] are focused on both the quality of clinical care and administrative services managed care organizations offer to the public. The standards manual is divided into six segments: quality management, utilization management, credentialing, members' rights and responsibilities, preventive health services, and medical records.

Unlike the Joint Commission, NCQA standards speak directly to case management. Although the managed care organization is not required to have a case management program, NCQA recognizes the link between utilization management and case management and evaluates the policies and procedures developed by health plans to review and approve the health care services provided to patients. Direct references to case management are seen in the utilization management standards and are addressed later in this section. But first, let's look at some of the other sections in the standards manual to identify how case management can support successful accreditation by NCQA.

Quality Management and Improvement

The standards relating to quality management and improvement address the infrastructure the managed care organization has developed to support quality improvement activities. Program description, an annual work plan, and integration of quality improvement with the rest of the managed care organization are all features in this section of the standards manual. An important fact to remember is that the quality improvement portion of the NCQA manual is weighted higher than any other group of standards in the accreditation decision.

There are standards in the quality management section that require the use of a performance improvement cycle similar to the Shewhart (plan, do, check, act) cycle of quality improvement.[5] Requirements for measurable objectives, tracking and trending of data for use in analysis, and finally, action taken as a direct result of data findings to improve the outcomes of care provided to patients, must exist. Case management should demonstrate use of this data-driven methodology. Case managers rely on benchmarking or identification of best practices to establish process and outcome measures. These measures are used to track variance. Results are recorded for discussion and study. Individual improvement actions for each patient, as well as actions for groups of patients, are conducted based on the results of analyzing variance data. Once new quality initiatives are underway, following recommendations from case managers, physicians, and other members of the health care delivery team, the case management data can assist in identification of the effectiveness of these new activities. This performance improvement cycle is documented through the case management reporting structure or quality improvement program in the managed care plan and will support achievement of NCQA standards in the quality management section of the manual.

New to the quality management standards (effective April 1, 1995) is the requirement for health management systems to demonstrate that the managed care organization has taken a proactive role in improving the health status of the population it serves. This requires that the health plan not rely solely on traditional measures of quality management, focusing on individual occurrences, but develops a program that effectively promotes identification of high-risk or chronically ill patients and then provides services to improve health status and clinical outcomes for these members.

To meet the intent of the health management systems standard, the managed care organization must aggregate population-based epidemiologic data, use this information to target high-risk members, and then develop action-oriented programs to interface with these members. Case management is one strategy used by managed care organizations that will address this standard.

"In general, case management with its concerted focus is not needed by every patient and family, nor is it usually realistic financially to provide distinct case managers to everyone. All patients need their care well-managed, but not all patients need a case manager, which requires some additional infrastructure in the organization."[6] This infrastructure for setting priorities for which patients will be identified for case management requires a well-designed triage system that targets patients for case management as soon as they enter the system or, better yet, before they seek health care services. To develop this triage system, which might distinguish patients based on diagnosis or high-risk factors (age, sex, race, family history) for certain conditions, case managers study and analyze population-based data. By using pareto, or frequency analysis, case managers identify patient population trends and focus their resources accordingly. Hence, many managed care organizations have identified female health care issues such as breast and cervical cancer, pediatric concerns such as immunization rates and asthma care, and issues for the elderly population such as accidents or falls in the home and related injuries as medical management issues for case management programs. Members with these conditions or attributes are identified and assigned to case management; educational programs developed to enhance wellness and clinical interventions, through guideline development, are established and promulgated.

Case management provides the vehicle for arriving at strategies for reaching the high-risk or chronically ill patient population. It may not be the case manager who provides all the interventions for these patients; in some instances, health care educators, managers of quality improvement, or others in the health plan may be involved in health management activities. The case management process facilitates the multidisciplinary use of talent to arrive at health management systems that are integrated into the fabric of the managed care operation. The bottom line here is, if case management is part of the managed care plans' operation, then information and activities conducted in this program are relevant to health management systems and should be incorporated into this activity. Conducting the two activities separately is a waste of resources and encourages missed opportunity to improve results.

Preventive Health Services

The preventive health services section of the NCQA standards is another area where case management activities can aid in standards compliance. This section of standards is dedicated to the use of practice guidelines for managing preventive and promotive health care services that the managed care organization offers members of the health plan. In addition, NCQA focuses on how well the managed care organization assesses its performance against preventive health guidelines. For example, are children younger than the age of 10 years appropriately immunized? How has the health plan ensured members are seeking immunization services? The answers to these questions require the managed care organization to use population-based data analysis to identify high-risk members and take appropriate action to minimize risk and improve health status.

How does the case management process enhance efforts to achieve standards compliance in preventive health services? Primarily in two ways. The first is in identification of high-risk members who would benefit from health promotion activities. Managed care organizations can readily recognize health issues germane to membership based on age or sex discriminators by analyzing enrollment or claims data. As an example, if the health plan enrolls a high number of Medicare-age members, coronary artery disease screening might be selected as a focus for study because this age group is at risk for heart attack. Other health care issues are more difficult to identify using only enrollment or claims data. If the health plan is concerned whether diabetic education has been provided to members with diabetes, claims data will not produce accurate results. Case management can be a source of information for identification of population-based health care issues not available from other sources. Either through medical record review or interviews with patients, case managers will uncover population-based health care issues that would benefit from preventive/promotive activities.

The second way case management can improve standards compliance with preventive health services is through the actual monitoring of compliance with established practice guidelines. The key to using case management for this activity is the use of a structured method for consistent data collection and analysis. This requires the case managers in the managed care organization to use variance analysis as part of their daily practice. Variance analysis is simply measuring the difference between expected results and actual results. The health plan, working together with the physician and hospital providers, establishes benchmarks for use as a "yardstick" to measure variance. These benchmarks may be guidelines, protocols, clinical pathways, or other consensus statements about medical care that members are receiving. Variance data are tracked and trended as part of the case management process to establish alternative treatment plans for individual patients and for use in aggregated data analysis to improve incrementally the process of care for a given diagnosis or treatment.

The case manager, along with other members of the health care delivery team, will use variance data to address patient care concerns. For example, the case management staff might identify a high number of pediatric patients admitted to the hospital with uncontrolled asthma. The case managers will collaborate with the involved physicians, emergency department staff, and home health agencies to establish ambulatory care guidelines and procedures for the parents to follow when the child first exhibits symptoms. These guidelines might include medical management issues such as the use of corticosteroids, inhalers, and flow meters, along with patient education for identification of environmental or physical activities that trigger an attack. These guidelines can then be used to prevent emergency admissions to the hospital and promote quality of life for members with asthma. After guideline development, a sample of medical records from asthma patients is monitored for compliance. In addition, the case managers will monitor asthma patients admitted to the hospital after dissemination of the guidelines. Data supporting a reduction in the admission rate would indicate improved health status for pediatric asthma members.

The asthma example demonstrates how the case management process can be integrated with quality improvement activities conducted in the managed care organization, improving health care for members and leveraging internal human resources in the health plan.

Utilization Management

The utilization management standards section in the NCQA manual directly addresses case management. As previously stated, NCQA does not require case management but expects that the health plan will have at least utilization management activities that address medical necessity and a process for decision making for approving health care services, criteria or protocols for decision making, an appeal process for members and providers regarding utilization decisions, a process for updating criteria and involvement of physicians in criteria development, and integration of utilization management with the quality improvement program.

Managed care organizations doing case management will be surveyed as to how well the utilization management function works together with the case management process. Description and clarity between roles and responsibilities of staff in case management and utilization are imperative. Utilization management and case management need not be organizationally structured in the same department, but the expectation is that the two areas communicate effectively because both areas are involved in facilitating patient care delivery.

The NCQA will also expect to see a description of the case management process. Which members are assigned a case manager, what does the process entail, how do members and providers participate in decision making regarding coverage determinations for services, what types of criteria or guidelines form the basis for decisions in case management, how often are these criteria updated, and is information from case management used in other quality improvement initiatives? Most of these questions can be addressed in a case management program description. Exhibit 11-1 showed a recommended outline for a program description for case management. The case management program description should be reviewed and updated at least annually to remain current and should be referenced as part of the health plan's quality improvement program description.

The NCQA's standards are written from the members' perspective. The standards attempt to validate that the services provided by the managed care plan continuously improve the medical care that members receive and that administrative services are customer friendly and do not impede health care delivery. Case management can support achievement of standards compliance in both areas.

CONCLUSION

Quality improvement and case management are not mutually exclusive. Demonstration of case management outcomes in improving quality of medical care, patient education, promotive or preventive health services, and collaboration with physicians and other health care professionals provides the foundation for this statement. Recognition of this fact leads to the conclusion that whether seeking accreditation through the Joint Commission or NCQA, case management will improve survey results.

The beauty of the relationship between case management and quality improvement is simplicity of effort. If the hospital or managed care organization already has case management focusing on patient advocacy, usage of appropriate and high-quality services, enhancing communication between the health care delivery team, developing consensus among providers in the form of practice guidelines or critical pathways, acting as a change agent with physicians to improve the delivery of health care services, and working with patients in preventive/promotive health care activities and education, then quality improvement is a natural outcome. If the case management program performs all these functions well, a significant portion of both the Joint Commission and NCQA standards will have been met, reducing redundant programs and saving dollars. In preparing for the survey, all the organization needs to do is "show and tell" their case management story.

REFERENCES

1. Joint Commission on Accreditation of Healthcare Organizations. *1995 Accreditation Manual for Hospitals.* Oak Terrace, Ill: The Joint Commission Department of Publications; 1995.
2. Bower K. *Case Management by Nurses.* Washington, DC: American Nurses Association Publishing; 1992.
3. Mullahy C. *The Case Manager's Handbook.* Gaithersburg, Md: Aspen Publishers, Inc.; 1995.
4. National Committee for Quality Assurance. *Standards for Accreditation.* Washington, DC: National Committee for Quality Assurance Publications; 1995.
5. Williams T, Howe R. *Applying Total Quality Management: A Nursing Guide.* Chicago, Ill: Precept Press, Inc.; 1991.
6. Zander K. Case management series. Part II: identifying patient populations for case management. *New Definition.* 1994;9(4):1.

■ 12 ■

Strategies for Operationalizing Case Management

Magdalena A. Mateo, PhD, RN, FAAN
Cheryl L. Newton, MSN, RN, CCRN, CNRN
Barbara H. Warner, MS, RN

Health care institutions are implementing case management (CM) as a care delivery system in a variety of ways. Differences in implementation may be a result of the credentials of the person assuming the case manager role, the type of organization, and the patient population being served. Patients are managed according to diagnostic categories throughout the continuum of care (before admission through postdischarge). In this chapter, the issues and strategies in operationalizing CM in a hospital setting are presented. Although other health care professionals have assumed the case manager role, our focus is on the nurse as case manager. The critical path (CP), a tool used in CM, is briefly described. An in-depth discussion of CPs is presented in Chapter 5.

LAYING THE GROUNDWORK

Case management is a model of care in which the primary goal is to provide quality patient care in a cost-efficient manner. This goal is accomplished by establishing patient outcomes that can be met within a designated time frame through multidisciplinary collaboration. The case manager coordinates a patient's care over the episode of illness and uses a CP to monitor and determine outcomes of care.[1] The concept of CM as it relates to the organization and a proposal for implementation needs to be developed and support from staff must be obtained.

Concept Development

Concept development is an initial step that needs to occur when implementing CM as a care delivery model. During development of the concept, a determination must be made on the nature of CM: (1) Is CM replacing an existing care delivery model or is CM being adapted to an existing model? (2) Is CM being adopted primarily by the division of nursing or throughout the organization by all disciplines?

Instituting CM as a model of care throughout the organization, instead of a profession-specific model such as a nursing care delivery model, is preferable because multidisciplinary collaboration is a key factor in achieving patient outcomes within a designated length of stay (LOS). "The model must depict the way that the institution organizes to deliver patient care."[2]

During the developmental phase, it is helpful to introduce the adoption of a new care delivery model from the institution's perspective and to identify the roles of each health care discipline as staff may be concerned that their jobs will be abolished. Conducting an analysis of the work performed on a unit or within a service line when planning CM is helpful in delineating the role of staff in providing care. It is ideal to include an evaluation component in order to determine whether outcomes are attained. Examples of outcomes include decreasing charges and LOS and improving patient satisfaction. Focusing on the outcome of improved patient care and satisfaction can decrease staff uncertainty about the effect of implementing CM on their jobs.

Proposal

A proposal, written by the group recommending CM, is a viable tool that can be used to gain the support of administrators and physicians. Essential components of the proposal are (1) the rationale and logistics of implementing CM, (2) method for evaluating outcomes (including patient and staff satisfaction and cost-benefit analysis), and (3) dissemination of results.

Rationale and Logistics of Implementing CM

Included in the rationale for and logistics of implementing CM are identifying the need for CM; defining the boundaries of the case manager role—within one unit, across units, or beyond the organization; introducing the CM concept to the health care team members; and establishing the implementation process, dates, CPs, and monitoring variances.

Method for Evaluating Outcomes

Measurement of outcomes needs to be congruent with the goals of CM, which are to provide quality patient care in a cost-efficient manner that is satisfactory to patients and staff. In addition to identifying and describing reliable and valid tools that will be used to measure patient and staff satisfaction, a detailed protocol for data collection before and after the implementation of CM has to be included in the proposal. When collecting data for satisfaction of staff, it is advisable to consult with the human resources department on the process and the tool being used to ensure that items are not included that could be disputed by a staff bargaining unit (e.g., issues pertaining to salary and benefits).

Cost-benefit analysis is an important outcome to include in the proposal as it illustrates how the implementation of CM results in the delivery of quality and cost-effective patient care. Data for the analysis can be partially obtained through the medical records and fiscal departments and can be summarized in a table or graph to illustrate aspects of patient care and its costs. Exhibit 12-1 presents items that could be included in the cost-benefit analysis for a patient undergoing a craniotomy.

There are many types of costs that pertain to patient care. When determining the items to be included in the analysis, the sources of the cost must be considered. For example, costs for delivering care to a patient undergoing surgery include the following:

- place where care is provided (e.g., intensive care unit [ICU], operating room [OR], recovery room [RR])
- job titles of staff providing care
- procedures (e.g., administration of anesthesia, medications, blood draw for test)

Exhibit 12-1 Example of Cost-Benefit Analysis for a Patient Undergoing Craniotomy

Categories of Sources of Costs	Comparable Hospital	Current Care Delivery	Case Management	% Difference
Time in operating room				
Number of days in intensive care unit				
Title of staff providing care				
Equipment and supplies				
Therapies (e.g., respiratory therapy)				
Number of readmissions within 48 h of discharge				
Consultation fees				
Cost of tests and procedures				
Other costs				
Total cost				

- actual time in OR, RR
- equipment and supplies

It is essential to review the number of days patients spend in the ICU and identify reasons for a prolonged ICU stay (e.g., patient condition, bed availability, unfamiliarity of staff with patient population). A case manager could be instrumental in determining readiness of patients to be transferred to a general care unit, thereby avoiding readmission to the ICU. Other aspects of care that can be used to assess costs can be identified by considering the following questions:

- What staff–patient ratio is necessary to achieve quality care?
- What RN–ancillary staff mix is necessary to achieve quality care?
- What types of services can unlicensed care givers provide?
- Are patients charged for equipment even when they no longer need it?
- Are patients appropriately charged for supplies and equipment?
- Are therapies ordered in a timely manner?
- Are tests and procedures redundant (e.g., daily blood work is ordered even if the patient's blood values are normal)?

After identifying costs, ways CM can be used to decrease costs should be considered. In providing care to a patient who is having surgery, strategies that can be used to reduce costs are

- Decrease the patient's time in the OR by having anesthesia staff insert invasive lines (e.g., arterial lines) while the patient is in the preoperative holding area.
- Decrease the number of hospital days by doing the preoperative workup on an outpatient basis and admitting the patient on the day of surgery.
- Implement and send the preadmission risk assessment tool to patients before admission to the hospital. Questions should include items such as neurologic deficits, living arrangements, and insurance coverage.
- Identify high-risk patients for extended LOS by using the preadmission risk assessment tool. The case manager can use the tool to plan the patient's care to avoid delays in consultation and discharge. Patients who live alone may need extended care because of inability to care for themselves.

Dissemination of Results

The proposal should also include plans for communicating CM outcomes. Although results should be shared with staff after the implementation and evaluation phases, it may be necessary to provide interim reports on the progress of CM. Factors that may have affected results need to be identified when reporting interim and final findings to enhance correct interpretation of outcomes (e.g., organizational and patient acuity changes).

Support for Case Management

When an institutional model is initiated, staff who are directly and indirectly involved in providing patient care need to be included in planning, implementing, and evaluating CM as implementation will affect their roles. For example, there could be an overlap between social workers who have traditionally taken an active role in discharge planning and the case manager who will have a significant role in the discharge process.

It is essential to obtain support from administrative staff, multidisciplinary health care team members, and collective bargaining leaders (if staff who belong to a union are affected by the change to CM). Support from administration includes resources such as secretarial assistance, computer access, and funding for case manager positions. Lack of a full-time secretary and a computer can delay implementation of CM as extensive support is required in developing or adapting CPs, providing education materials, establishing the case manager job description, and monitoring variances.

Existing budgets are often the financial source for case manager positions. Case management responsibilities may also be added to the responsibilities of an advanced practice nurse or of staff nurses. Whichever method is used to acquire case manager positions, creating a new position and a job description is recommended.[3] This decreases the possibility for confusion among staff of the role of case managers.

The appointment of case managers as full-time salaried instead of hourly employees promotes flexibility in fulfilling responsibilities, such as making rounds with physicians and being available for patients and families to plan care.[3] However, assuming a salaried position requires a shift in orientation from fulfilling responsibilities for a designated shift to an overall accountability for a patient's care. When there is a nursing collective bargaining unit, the director of nursing needs to work closely with the human resources department and representatives from the bargaining unit when nurses are being considered for the case manager role. Issues that primarily have to be addressed include the role of case managers, salary (monthly or hourly), and special privileges such as working primarily on weekdays and being off on holidays.

The roles and responsibilities of most case managers include coordination of patient care for a specified diagnosis-related group (DRG) and development, implementation, and evaluation of CM. Activities under each responsibility category are listed in Exhibit 12-2.[4-6]

The support of the medical staff is crucial to the success of CM. Strategies that can be used to obtain physician support include promoting their involvement from the time CM is considered as a delivery model through its implementation and evaluation phases. It is essential to set meeting times suitable to the physicians' schedules and to conduct productive meetings within scheduled times. Discussion of data that are meaningful should be included in the meeting agenda, as well as LOS, cost, charges, and outcomes related to quality of care for their patient population. It may be helpful to compare the data to similar institutions and physician practices. Groups should be organized that have similar practices (e.g., neurosurgeons) who are currently practicing at the institution. Hospital administrators should be requested to reiterate the importance of the project and to help acquire support from physicians.[7] Other strategies are listed in Exhibit 12-3.

IMPLEMENTATION PROCESS

Implementation of CM includes the establishment of a steering committee, initiation of CPs, and presentation of education programs.

Establishment of a Steering Committee

Establishing a multidisciplinary group to serve as a steering committee enables members to begin working together. This is beneficial in the implementation phase because staff are more likely to support ideas of people who are part of their group. Charges of the committee include monitoring the implementation of CM and developing strategies for dealing with issues/problems that arise, selecting case managers, seeking staff support for CM, facilitating the development and use of CPs, and monitoring variances.

Monitoring the implementation of CM ensures that activities and time lines are accomplished. This is important when evaluating CM to determine the factors that may influence outcomes. It is also important to keep a diary of events or changes that occur during implementation so these events and their possible effects on outcomes can be considered when interpreting results. Examples of events that need to be noted include changes in staff (e.g., turnover rate, staff–patient ratio), patient acuity, and costs.

Initiation of Critical Paths

Critical paths are essential tools of CM and are used as guides to achieve the desired outcomes and facilitate discharge within the allotted LOS for a

Exhibit 12-2 Sample Case Manager Job Description

Position Summary

   The case manager assumes responsibility and accountability for the clinical management of patients within specific case groups for an episode of illness. He or she coordinates patient care during the episode of illness and facilitates discharge within the expected length of stay. The case manager ensures that specific patient outcomes are achieved and that variances are evaluated and addressed. In collaboration with members of the health care team, the case manager assists in the development, implementation and revision of critical paths.

Qualifications:

—minimum of 3 years clinical experience and specialty certification
—bachelor of science in nursing required, masters degree in nursing preferred
—licensed as a registered nurse
—self-directed with strong interpersonal skills
—effective communication skills

Roles and Responsibilities

1. Assists in the development and implementation of case management
   • Researches, organizes, and documents clinical data necessary for the development and implementation of critical paths
   • In coordination with members of the health care team, develops, implements, and revises critical paths
   • Provides support, educational programs, and clinical expertise to other members of the health care team
2. Coordinates patient care for a specific case group
   • Assesses the health status of patients assigned to their case group
   • Individualizes the critical path based on the patient's health status and unique needs
   • Reviews the plan of care with the primary physician and other members of the health care team
   • Uses resources appropriately
   • Holds members of the multidisciplinary team accountable for the case management process and intervenes as necessary
   • Promotes collaboration and communication among the multidisciplinary team
   • Ensures that specific patient outcomes are achieved
   • Identifies, evaluates, and addresses variances
   • Facilitates discharge planning within the expected length of stay
3. Provides education regarding case management
   • Serves as a resource for the multidisciplinary team
   • Assesses educational needs and provides instruction to members of the health care team
   • Assesses educational needs and provides instruction to patients and family members
   • Provides support and clinical expertise regarding critical paths

continues

Exhibit 12-2 continued

4. Evaluates the case management model
   - Develops tools (such as financial indicators, length of stay, and satisfaction) to monitor the effectiveness of the case management model
   - Collects and monitors continuous quality improvement data through variance tracking
   - Analyzes trends and reports variances to appropriate members of the health care team
   - Develops strategies to improve negative variances and promote positive patient outcomes
   - Performs ongoing evaluation of critical paths and outcomes

specific DRG. The CP is a multidisciplinary tool that guides patient care by highlighting key incidents that must occur in a timely and predictable manner.[8,9] It includes consults, treatments, diet, medications, discharge planning, patient teaching, and interventions that occur during the patient's episode of illness.[10] Critical paths can serve as a documentation tool, documenting care provided to patients and any variances that occur. However, it is only effective if it is used by the multidisciplinary team. Critical paths can also be used as an education tool for the health care team members and patients and their families by developing two versions of the CP. The patient/family version of the CP allows patients and their families to participate, provides information regarding their treatment plan, and enables them to follow their progress. Examples of CPs for the health care team and patient are presented in Chapter 5.

Exhibit 12-3 Strategies To Promote Physician Participation in the Implementation of Case Management (CM)

1. Enlist participation in activities at the time plans for CM begin.
2. Present information on outcomes that are related to quality improvement, patient satisfaction, and cost savings from settings that have successfully implemented and evaluated CM.
3. Include practices and preferences that many physicians believe promote patient satisfaction (e.g., calling patients after discharge from the hospital).
4. Implement CM on a unit where physicians in leadership roles are progressive. Promote their active involvement in leading the group to develop treatment guidelines/algorithms or pathways.
5. Ensure that medical residents, students, and staff are active participants.
6. Provide an evaluation component such as patient satisfaction and cost-benefit analysis.

Before the implementation of CM and the development of CPs, it is essential to identify patient populations who are to be case managed by assessing high-volume, high-acuity, and high-cost patients. Background information such as patient volume and acuity, LOS, patient charges, and costs can be obtained from medical records and fiscal departments.

Developing CPs is time consuming; therefore, it is important to determine if purchasing them from publishing companies or institutions is more cost effective. If it is decided that CPs will be purchased, it should be considered that these may need to be revised and adapted to reflect the current practice of the institution. It is vital to decide on a format for CPs to promote consistency within the organization.

Once CPs have been developed or purchased, one CP at a time should be implemented. Simultaneously implementing too many CPs can confuse and overwhelm staff. A pilot test should be conducted to assess the relevance and usability of the CP. The number of variances that have occurred must be evaluated as well as the number of patients who "fall off" the CP (patients who do not progress according to the CP). Feedback is obtained from the multidisciplinary team, and staff compliance is evaluated. If compliance with using the CP is low, the reasons must be determined. Is the CP too cumbersome, therefore making it difficult to use? Issues must be resolved before implementing another CP. When staff are comfortable in using one or two CPs, others can be implemented.

Presentation of Education Programs

An important strategy for operationalizing CM is to provide information to staff and patients and their families through educational programs, group meetings, written handouts, and an open house. In addition, sponsoring a regional conference that focuses on CM provides staff the opportunity to network with colleagues from other institutions.

Mandatory education programs communicate to staff the importance of CM. When conducting education programs, only the information that is necessary for staff to fulfill their responsibilities is provided. Topics should include DRG reimbursement, prospective payment system, concepts, goals, benefits of CM, and staff roles. Lengths of stay, cost, and trend data are best illustrated with graphs and tables. Presentations by multidisciplinary clinical, financial, and management staff reinforce the importance of involving all disciplines. Active involvement of the chief financial officer and finance staff in the initial orientation and ongoing education of case managers is strongly advised.[11]

The education program for case managers needs to be extensive. Information should be included on time management, priority setting, conflict resolution, and team building. Exhibit 12-4 highlights topics that can be covered in education programs for case managers. Ongoing support for case managers is provided by holding regularly scheduled group meetings that serve as a forum for discussing problems and issues and venting frustrations.

An open house for staff and patients and their families is a stimulating, fun, and social event that can be used to showcase a unit that has successfully implemented CM. Critical paths, unique strategies, and positive results such as increased patient satisfaction and quality of care, decreased LOS, and cost savings are highlighted. The event is made interesting by displaying bright-colored posters with bold prints that are easy to read. Handouts with text that is written in lay language can be used to inform patients and families about CM. These can include the definition and purpose of CM, the role of the case manager, and how to use and read their version of the CP.

A structured method of providing widespread education for staff is to sponsor a conference on CM. A call for abstracts will elicit speakers from various backgrounds. This is an excellent way to generate new ideas as well as network with others who are doing CM.

EVALUATION OF OUTCOMES

When measuring staff satisfaction, all staff (nurses, physicians, interdisciplinary, and ancillary) who provide direct care to patients should be included. In addition to using questionnaires, other types of data such as attendance records and turnover are useful. The interpretation of turnover rates includes identifying the reason(s) for a staff member's transfer and resignation to determine if they are related to CM. Maintaining anonymity of data is problematic when the number of persons within each category of staff is fewer than five; therefore, this has to be considered when managing the data.

Patient and family satisfaction is an outcome measure that is meaningful when evaluating CM because they are the recipients of the care and can therefore determine if the care they receive meets or exceeds their expectations. A dimension that could also be included is patients' abilities to assume their roles and responsibilities after discharge from the hospital. A published tool that has been used to evaluate outcomes of care is the 36-item Medical Outcomes Study (MOS) short-form health survey.[12,13] Concepts measured by the MOS survey are physical functioning, bodily pain, role limitations due to physical health problems, role limitations due to personal or emotional problems, general mental health, social functioning, energy/fatigue, and general health perceptions.

Quality of care can be measured by indicators established as part of an organization's quality improvement and management efforts. By coordinat-

Exhibit 12-4 Elements of a Case Management Outline for an Educational Program

1. Evolution of case management (CM)
   A. Trends in health care
2. Diagnosis-related groups, third-party payers
3. Concepts
   A. Multidisciplinary team
   B. Outcomes: clinical and fiscal
   C. Critical pathway
4. Goals of CM
   A. Facilitate early discharge
   B. Patient satisfaction
   C. Appropriate use of resources
   D. Promote collaborative practice
   E. Staff satisfaction
5. Roles and responsibilities
   A. Case managers
   B. Multidisciplinary team
   C. Staff nurses
   D. Physicians
6. Tools of CM
   A. Critical path
   B. Flowsheet
   C. Variance tracking tool
7. Team work
   A. Team building
   B. Collaborative practice
   C. Communication
   D. Interpersonal relationships
   E. Conflict resolution
   F. Problem solving
8. Patient education
   A. Patient readiness
   B. Evaluation
9. Discharge planning
   A. Community resources
   B. Patient home health needs
10. Time management
    A. Priority setting
    B. Organizational skills
    C. Stress management
11. Variance
    A. Monitoring methods
    B. Analysis
    C Organization of results
    D. Dissemination of results

Topics 1 to 6 to be attended by all staff.
Topics 1 to 9 to be attended by case managers.

ing this effort with those pertaining to the standards of care required by accrediting bodies such as the Joint Commission on Accreditation of Healthcare
Organizations, these outcomes can be monitored efficiently.

Length of stay is a frequently used outcome measure. Monitoring variances
from the CP can give an idea of the factors that may have affected LOS so
interventions can be directed accordingly. Aside from determining the number of days a patient stays in the hospital for an episode of illness, it is vital
also to keep track of emergency department visits or readmission of patients
for a condition that is related to a most recent hospital stay. It is also wise to
collect data on the number of days between the patient's discharge from the
hospital and the visit to an emergency department or readmission.

Intra- and interdisciplinary communications is an integral part of CM;
therefore, these have to be evaluated in terms of staff ability to work together in meeting patient care goals. Another dimension that could be monitored is participation of staff in collaborative efforts in planning, implementing, and evaluating patient care.

Comparing costs of providing care before and after implementing CM
provides data that can be used to determine if decreased costs are achieved
by the expediency in which tests, procedures, and referrals for patients are
performed. The care provided to the case managed group could also result in
only needed tests and procedures being performed.

ISSUES AND STRATEGIES RELATED TO THE CASE MANAGER ROLE

The successful implementation of CM is affected by the ability of case managers to assume their role. When selecting case managers, a criteria should
be used that includes professional and personal attributes that applicants
must possess. After case managers are selected, they should be assisted in
making the transition and enacting their role.

Selection of Case Managers

Vital personal attributes of case managers include autonomy, ability to
assume a leadership role, excellent communication skills,[14,15] capability to
deal with ambiguity, and ability to work with various people, possibly from
different institutions, in the continuum of care. Additional characteristics are
keeping abreast with the cost of health care, health care reform issues, and
advances in clinical practice. "It is the unique individual who can effectively
meet the clinical and financial aspects of patient care. They must be able to
see the challenge and opportunity in the role and be willing to sharpen the
skills that will be required for effectiveness."[11(p.14)] These criteria could be

challenged by labor union leaders who may prefer to use seniority as a basis for selection of candidates for the case manager position. Emphasizing that the ultimate goals for implementing CM is the promotion of patient care and the professional role of the nurse is a strategy that can be successfully used to foster the implementation of CM as a joint effort between the institution and the labor union.

Transition to Case Manager Role

Although case managers are responsible for a group of patients, unit staff sometimes do not perceive case managers as having the authority and the ability to enforce plans. Defining roles and responsibilities of case managers and sharing this information with staff can facilitate the transition toward CM.

It is not uncommon for case managers to focus on tasks and roles they had before assuming their new roles because they feel confident in their previous role but feel insecure as a case manager. Sometimes there is anger or jealousy from the staff on the unit when their peer has been selected for the case manager role. This is not easy for new case managers to understand or accept, and it affects relationships, formally and informally.

Enactment of the Case Manager Role

It is crucial for staff members who assume the case manager role to gain the respect of others to be successful. This can be accomplished by fulfilling job requirements, establishing open communications with the health care team, and dealing with patient care issues in a timely manner.

Multidisciplinary team members may request a new case manager to assume responsibilities that are beyond their role description. To please, an inexperienced case manager may give in to impossible requests. Consequently, the case manager is overextended and experiences "burnout." Biller[3] found that within two months, the three nurse case managers in her setting felt "overworked and unprepared." They abandoned the role because of frustration and burnout.

CONCLUSION

Although CM has been reported as an organization's model of care and as a nursing care delivery model, it has been suggested in the literature that adoption of CM by an organization is more desirable. This is understandable when one considers that the delivery of high-quality and cost-effective care, the primary goals of CM, is achieved more readily when collaborative relationships among the multidisciplinary team exists. Fostering collaborative relationships during the phases of laying the groundwork, implementing CM, and evaluating outcomes can be done by seeking the active involvement of members of the health care team. Strategies that can be used to promote activities related to operationalizing CM are featured in Table 12-1.

Case managers have a significant contribution to the success of CM; therefore, it is vital to select individuals who are capable of making the transition

Table 12-1 Phases, Issues, and Strategies in Implementation of Case Management (CM)

Phase	Issue	Strategies
Laying the groundwork	Staff support	Create a multidisciplinary steering committee Delineate role of each discipline and new roles in CM Identify roles and responsibilities of case managers Emphasize multidisciplinary collaboration versus individual staff roles
	Administrative support	Write proposal that is concise and includes description of implementation, fiscal outcomes, and patient satisfaction
	Collective bargaining unit	Seek assistance of human resources department to address roles and responsibilities of case managers, salary, selection of individuals, and incentives for assuming role
	Resources	Negotiate for financial, human, and material resources
Implementation	Workability	Implement all aspects of CM on prototype unit(s)
	Knowledge of staff	Present education programs that include relevant information on roles Provide incentives for attendance
	Selection of case manager	Specify qualifications and scope of responsibilities
	Role enactment of case manager	Clarify, redefine, and evaluate roles
	Critical paths (CP)	Develop and implement a limited number of CPs Monitor use
Evaluation of outcomes	Validity and reliability of outcome measurements	Monitor process for obtaining data
	Use of CPs to monitor care	Identify and track variances from CP Revise CP as needed

and enacting the role. Education programs can be used to orient staff and patients and their families to the CM model. Participation of staff and patients and their families promotes the attainment of CM outcomes. Outcomes of CM include an increase in staff and patient/family satisfaction, quality of care, a decrease in LOS and costs, and improved communication.

Critical paths are valuable tools for identifying sources of variances that may be increasing or decreasing the costs of providing care. Consequently, it is important that CPs reflect current practice and are properly implemented.

REFERENCES

1. Petryshen PR, Petryshen PM. The case management model: an innovative approach to the delivery of patient care. *J Adv Nurs.* 1992;17:1188–1194.
2. Fralic MF. Creating new practice models and designing new roles. *J Nurs Adm.* 1992;22(6): 7–8.
3. Biller AM. Implementing nursing case management. *Rehabil Nurs.* 1992;17:144–146.
4. Simmons FM. Developing the trauma nurse case manager role. *Dimens Crit Care Nurs.* 1992;11:164–170.
5. Zander K. Case management. Part III: case manager role dimensions. *New Definition.* 1995;10(1):1–3.
6. Smith GB. Hospital-based case management. In: *Continuing Education for Ohio Nurses 1995 Course Catalog.* Sacramento, Calif: Continuing Medical Education Resource; 1995:45–70.
7. Zander K. Physicians, caremaps, and collaboration. *New Definition.* 1992;7(1):1–4.
8. Marr JA, Reid B. Implementing managed care and case management: the neuroscience experience. *J Neurosci Nurs.* 1992;24:281–285.
9. Zander K. CareMaps: the core of cost/quality care. *New Definition.* 1991;6(9).
10. Giuliano KK, Poirier CE. Nursing case management: critical pathways to desirable outcomes. *Nurs Manage.* 1991;22(3):52–55.
11. Fralic MF. The nurse case manager: focus, selection, preparation, and measurement. *J Nurs Adm.* 1992;22(11):13–14.
12. Ware JE, Sherbourne CD. The MOS 36-item short-form health survey (SF-36): I. conceptual framework and item selection. *Med Care.* 1992;30:473–493.
13. Hays RD, Sherbourne CD, Mazel RM. The RAND 36-item health survey 1.0. *Med Econ.* 1993;2:217–227.
14. Lynn-McHale DJ, Fitzpatrick ER, Shaffer RB. Case management: development of a model. *Clin Nurse Spec.* 1993;7:299–307.
15. Tahan H. The nurse case manager in acute care settings. *J Nurs Adm.* 1993;23(10):53–61.

■ 13 ■

Training and Education Needs of Case Managers

Hussein A. Tahan, MS, RN, CNA

Case management was first implemented as a nursing care delivery model. Today, however, it has evolved into a patient care delivery system. In the past decade, case management has changed tremendously and more change will come. However, the goals of case management have remained basically the same: cost containment and high-quality patient care. The most important change in case management is in the role of the nurse case manager. Nurses as case managers are receiving acclaim, enthusiasm, and support not only from nurse executives and hospital administrators but from public leaders, insurance company executives, public policy lobbyists, politicians, and health care legislators as well.

The success or failure of case management models is in the hands of very important key players—the nurse case managers. Their success depends a great deal on their preparation, education, and training. Despite the popularity of case management delivery models, the literature is limited regarding training and development of case managers.

To date, case managers have been prepared in clinical settings. Nursing schools have not addressed the concept of case management in depth.[1] The advances in training and education continue to remain clinically based and institution specific. No full scope curriculum or nursing degree has been established yet. Formal education has been limited to either a class session or a separate two- to three-credit course. Such a course is given to graduate nursing students preparing for advanced practice roles. This chapter presents an acute care case management training program that can be adapted for preparing nurses to assume case manager roles. It also presents a tool for evaluating the performance of these nurses. The content can easily be adapted to an academic setting.

Before planning an educational program for training of nurse case managers, answers to the following questions are important.[2-4]

1. What is the job description of the nurse case manager? Scope of practice? Roles and responsibilities?
2. What should be included in a program for educating case managers?
3. What are the available resources: personnel and finances?
4. Who should teach in the program?
5. How many days are required for a successful program?
6. What is the required educational background of those eligible for case management roles?

Answering these questions is very important because they set the stage for the program, define its length, and help identify the experts needed to teach in the program.

LENGTH OF THE CURRICULUM

Most hospital programs are three to five days of didactic training and one to two weeks of precepted clinical experience/ practice. The amount of time designated for instruction is based on the scope of practice of the case manager and the required educational background and level of experience. If the case manager is to assume utilization review and social services responsibilities, then a five-day program is recommended; otherwise, a three-day program is appropriate.

DEFINING A KNOWLEDGE BASE FOR THE CURRICULUM

"Nurses assuming the case manager roles require in-depth knowledge and skills. These requirements are generic, transcending the issues of where or by whom the case manager is employed."[5] The details of the curriculum are based on the skills (Exhibit 13-1) and tasks (Exhibit 13-2) delineated in the job description of the case manager. The more responsibilities given to the case manager, the longer and more detailed the curriculum should be.

Development of a case management curriculum should reflect all elements of the case management process. Other topics might be added to the curriculum based on the needs of the organization and the nurses selected to become case managers.[1] Background education is very important when deciding on the content. If the case managers selected are not prepared on a

Exhibit 13-1 Case Manager's Skills

1. Clinical (patient care, tests, and procedures)	8. Conducting meetings
2. Decision making	9. Team building
3. Critical thinking	10. Customer relations
4. Problem solving	11. Consulting
5. Conflict resolution	12. Teaching
6. Negotiation	13. Financial analysis
7. Communication and interpersonal relations	14. Writing for publication and writing reports
	15. Public speaking

master's degree level, then detailed discussions of topics such as management, leadership, power, conflict resolution, decision making, problem solving, critical thinking, team building, running meetings, and communication should be included at length in the curriculum. However, if they were prepared on the master level, a quick overview of these topics is appropriate.

DELINEATING THE GOALS AND OBJECTIVES OF THE CURRICULUM

Case management curriculums are developed to provide nurses who are selected to assume case manager roles with the knowledge and skills necessary for success in such roles. The curriculum is a formal strategy to add to the knowledge and expertise of these nurses.

The major objectives of the case management curriculum reflecting the case management process are to:[1,3,4,6]

1. Discuss contemporary models of case management.

2. Define the role and responsibilities of the case manager.

3. Describe the relationship between case management, managed care, and health care financial environment.

4. Explain the development, implementation, and evaluation of case management models and case management plans.

5. Describe the relationship between case management and quality improvement.

6. Identify the appropriate strategies for measuring, evaluating, and assessing case management outcomes.

7. Build the leadership skills of case managers.

It is very important to include a historical overview and description of the various case management models, the subtle variations of these models, and

Exhibit 13-2 Case Manager's Most Common Tasks

1. Assessment of patients (initial and on-going)
2. Setting care-related goals (day-specific/short-term and hospitalization-specific/long-term)
3. Coordination and facilitation of tests and procedures
4. Collaboration with members of the health care team to ensure completion of patient care activities
5. Documentation of activities and outcomes of care
6. Patient and family teaching
7. Staff in-services regarding case management
8. Supervision of resource utilization
9. Discharge planning
10. Review of appropriateness of admissions and hospital stays
11. Variance identification and analysis, quality indicators and clinical indicators data collection
12. Screening patients for social services needs, home care needs, and making referrals as needed
13. Referring alternate level of care patients to utilization review and/or discharge planning
14. Coordination of services with managed care companies (HMOs, preferred provider organizations [PPOs], etc.)
15. Development of case management plans
16. Consultation as needed with physicians, specialty nurses, managed care organizations, home care agencies, home health attendant vendors, and other community resources
17. Completion of the required paper work for other health care institutions or community resources agencies
18. Facilitation of inter- and intrahospital transfers

how they relate to the particular organization. It is also necessary to discuss the process of implementing a case management model from planning through evaluation. Another important topic to include in the curriculum is the relationship among the various members of the health care team, the different disciplines involved in the model, and the impact of the nurse case manager role on patient care delivery.

CURRICULUM OUTLINE

Case management entails training and education in the skills and tasks presented in Exhibits 13-1 and 13-2. The following is an overview of the topics covered in the case management education and training curriculum.

Days 1 and 2

These two days (Exhibit 13-3) are designated for leadership skills building. As mentioned earlier, based on the level of education of the case manager, leadership building skills are either discussed in detail over a two-day period or covered in one day as a "leadership skills review day."

Exhibit 13-3 Case Management Curriculum—Days 1 and 2

Topic	Content
Communication	• Verbal and nonverbal • Strategies to improve communication • Strategies that hinder communication • Definition of behavior • Assertive and nonassertive/aggressive behavior • Components of assertive behavior • Effective listening • Dos and don'ts of effective communication
Conflict resolution/ negotiation	• What is conflict? • Sources of conflicts • Resolution of conflicts • Problem-solving and decision-making techniques • Win-win approach to conflict resolution • Techniques and strategies for successful negotiation • Situational crisis
Meetings	• Preparing the agenda • Taking minutes • Beginning and ending a meeting • Roles of leaders and facilitators • Leading and facilitating strategies • Strategies for successful and productive meetings • Strategies and skills for dealing with difficult people • Team building strategies • Formal and informal leaders
Leadership	• Definition • Qualities of a leader • Leadership styles • Types of leaders • Relationship to case management and case managers
Management	• Definition • Qualities of a manager • Types of managers • Managerial styles • Administrative versus nursing process • Accountability versus responsibility • Contingency management • Relationship to case management and case managers
Power	• Definition • Sources of power • Strategies to obtain power • Constructive versus destructive use of power • Relationship to case management and case managers • Sources of power in the case manager role

continues

Exhibit 13-3 continued

Topic	Content
Application of leadership, management, and power	• Relationship of leadership, management, and power • Relationship to the case manager role • Application to the case manager's daily activities • Leadership and managerial characteristics of case managers
Change	• Definition • Types of change (technical, structural, and people-oriented) • Theories and processes • Lewin's theory of change (freezing, moving, unfreezing) • Change agents and case managers • Effecting positive change • Strategies for making change acceptable • Strategies to undermine resistance to change • Relationship between change and case management
Reports	• Writing the report • Types of reports • Business reports • Cost analysis reports • Diagnosis-related groups (DRGs) and length-of-stay reports • Activities report • Different styles of writing reports

Some of the suggested topics to be presented during these days include change, leadership and qualities of leaders, management and qualities of managers, communication skills, problem-solving techniques, and conflict resolution. Theories behind these topics are discussed with role play when appropriate.

Although the case manager is not a traditional manager position, leadership topics are important in the curriculum. These topics help build the case manager's skills in dealing with people, solving problems that arise around patient care, and time management.

Case managers are given power by virtue of their job description and responsibilities. This makes the concept of power and how it relates to the case manager's role a very important part of the curriculum.

Another significant topic is change and change theory and process. The concept of change is discussed at length. It provides the case managers with the required knowledge to facilitate change because they function as change agents, particularly during the implementation phase of case management. This discussion provides the case managers with the strategies and skills that help effect change and ease the process.

Running meetings is a very frequent activity in the life of case managers. Strategies for successful meetings is a relevant topic for inclusion in the curriculum. This discussion provides case managers with the strategies and skills needed for dealing successfully with people.

Days 3 and 4

During these days (Exhibit 13-4), a detailed review of case management, from model design to implementation to evaluation, is shared. The discussion should start with an overview of the health care industry, issues of crisis, and current changes and their implications for case management. Health care financial reimbursement systems are discussed in detail. The case manager must know this topic well because case management delivery models were implemented as cost containment strategies in response to the introduction of the prospective payment system by the federal government in the mid-1980s. The diagnosis-related groups (DRGs) should also be a part of the curriculum, particularly in those hospitals that are located in states (e.g., New York) where the DRG system is still followed in reimbursement. Other health care financial reimbursement systems such as managed care, capitation, and third-party payers are important parts of the curriculum.

Discussion of the role of the case manager should include a detailed explanation of the scope of practice, job description, and responsibilities as well as the relationship between the case manager and each member of the health care team and how case management relates to the various disciplines involved in the provision of care. Collaboration among health care team members and coordination and facilitation of patient care activities cannot be stressed enough. It is these activities that have an effect on length of stay, cost, and quality of patient care. Case load and patient selection criteria are discussed in depth, including case examples. This discussion should include the day-to-day activities and responsibilities of the case manager in the provision of patient care.

Development, implementation, and evaluation of case management plans is another topic discussed. A detailed discussion of the process of developing these plans and the skills needed for a successful and productive process is essential.

Outcomes measurement and quality improvement processes are reviewed, with examples of the tools used to track outcomes data and clinical and quality indicators. The Joint Commission on Accreditation of Healthcare Organization's standards on improving organizational performance should be discussed in reference to case management. The responsibilities of case managers in these processes should be explained. Documentation of vari-

Exhibit 13-4 Case Management Curriculum—Days 3 and 4

Topic	Content
Health care industry	• Overview of health care • Current issues in health care • Health care crises • Health care reform • Legislation • Advances in technology
Health care financial reimbursement systems	• Prospective payment system • DRGs and length of stay • Third-party reimbursement • Per diem rate reimbursement • Medicare and Medicaid • Managed care organizations (HMOs, PPOs, etc) • Managed competition and contractual agreements
Case management	• Overview of case management • Historical background • Various case management models (primary care case management, professional practice case management, leveled practice case management, advanced practice case management) • Theoretical development of case management models • Within-the-walls case management (hospital-based) • Beyond-the-walls case management (community-based) • Strategies for physician buy-in
Case management model (specific to the organization)	(Organization-specific content) • Committee structure (steering committee, etc) • Goals • Design • Planning and implementation • Evaluation strategies • Pre- and post-data collection • Benchmarks • Expected outcomes • Role of the case manager (unit-based, free-floating) • Areas of case management coverage (inpatient, outpatient, community)
Case management plans	• Definition • Types (critical paths, multidisciplinary action plans, CareMaps®, clinical pathways, etc) • Design and format • Development, implementation, and evaluation • Relationship to length of stay and quality outcomes • Teams in charge of developing plans • Tracking of variances

continues

Exhibit 13-4 continued

Topic	Content
Case manager role	• Job description (unit-based, free-floating) • Roles and responsibilities • Tasks and skills • Daily operations (facilitation, collaboration and coordination of care, patient advocacy, patient teaching and discharge planning) • Relationship with other disciplines and members of the health care team • Relationship between the nurse manager and the case manager • Reporting mechanism/channels of communication • Case load • Patient selection criteria
Outcomes measurement	• Definition of outcome • The three core strategies in outcome measurement (assessment, monitoring, and management) • Outcome indicators, quality indicators, clinical indicators • Tracking and trending of outcomes • Definition of variance • Types of variances (patient, system, community, and health care provider) • Variance analysis, evaluation, and follow-up
Quality improvement	• Definition of quality • Customer perspective of quality • Joint Commission standards • Shewhart cycle/PDCA cycle (plan-do-check-act) • Quality improvement process (develop a team, identify quality barriers, review current process, establish root causes, target and select alternative solutions, implement solutions, reevaluate, operationalize, and normalize solutions) • Relationship between quality improvement and case management

ances on the case management plans, tracking and trending variances of care, and variance analysis are discussed in depth because these tasks are part of the case manager responsibilities.

Day 5

The last day (Exhibit 13-5) of the case manager's training and education program is designated for topics related to the case management process and strategies for evaluation of the model. Documentation is among the important topics presented. Strategies for clear and concise documentation, including hospital and Joint Commission documentation standards, are discussed. Screening

Exhibit 13-5 Case Management Curriculum—Day 5

Topic	Content
Case management documentation	• Patient's screening • Initial and ongoing assessments • Strategies for clear and concise documentation • Progress notes, critical path, action plan • Guidelines for documentation (organization-specific policy) • Joint Commission standards • Documentation of variances • Referrals and consultations
Legal implications of case management	• Liability, negligence, fraud, malpractice • Risk management issues • Current legal implications • Role of the case management plans in court/lawsuits • Patient bill of rights and advanced directives
Patient and family education	• Health care teaching needs assessment • Teaching process • Health behaviors • Attitude versus belief • Theories on patient education (health belief model, social learning theory, adult learning theory) • Strategies for effective teaching and learning • Joint Commission patient and family education standards
Discharge planning	• Overview of discharge planning • Initial and ongoing needs assessment • Social work and home care referrals • Screening for high-risk patients • Collaboration among health care providers
Case management evaluation strategies	• Cost analysis/cost accounting systems • Research • Patient satisfaction • Staff satisfaction • Benchmarking • Length of stay/DRGs review/financial data • Pre- and postimplementation data collection • Outcome indicators, clinical quality indicators
Practice sessions	• Case studies • Case discussions • Role play • Writing reports • Documentation • Developing case management plans

of patients on admission for inclusion in the case manager's case load and initial and ongoing assessments are also discussed. The responsibilities of the case manager, staff nurse, and the various members of the health care team regarding documentation in the medical record and the case management plan are also shared with related examples and exercises.

Patient and family teaching is an important topic included in the curriculum. Because reduction in length of stay is a major goal of case management and patients are discharged earlier, patient and family education becomes more and more important. Health care needs of patients and families are assessed at the time of admission, a teaching plan is then constructed and executed carefully throughout the hospitalization. Details of patient teaching including strategies, processes, theories, and standards are discussed. Strategies for maintaining patient's compliance with the medical regimen and preventing readmission to the hospital are also discussed. Patient and family education is an integral aspect of the case manager role. It is made clear to the case managers during education how important patient teaching is to the success of the case management model. Case examples are presented to ensure better understanding of this role.

Discharge planning is presented with special emphasis on the relationship between case managers and the social work and home care departments. The case manager is made aware of how to (1) assess a patient and plan the discharge starting from time of admission; (2) arrange for community resources such as home care, visiting nurse service, or nursing home; (3) differentiate between low-risk and high-risk patients; (4) conduct financial screening and obtain approval for resources; (5) apply for Medicaid coverage when appropriate; and (6) make referrals to appropriate disciplines and personnel when needed. This session, if possible, is best conducted by a representative from the department of social services and home care. Case presentations and discussions are a significant method for better understanding discharge planning and how it relates to the case manager role.

Legal implications of case management models are a timely topic on the last curriculum day. As case management becomes more popular, so do the legal concerns of health care providers. This session should include risk management, patient advocacy, and advanced directives. It should also include some discussion of negligence, fraud, malpractice, and liability in patient care. Inviting a lawyer from the legal and risk management department is worthwhile. Current literature on legal aspects of case management programs should be shared with discussions of real court examples to relieve any risk management concerns case managers might have.

How to evaluate a case management model is the last topic presented. Emphasis on the role of case managers in the evaluation process is important. Aspects of evaluating the model (e.g., research, patient and staff satisfaction, length of stay, financial analysis, and clinical quality indicators) are discussed, with special notation of the responsibilities of case managers in data collection.

Finally, it is extremely important to allocate some time for an open discussion about the case management model, case studies, and role play related to the topics discussed in the program. These methods of learning provide better understanding of the role of case managers and opens a forum for questions and answers about any unclear areas. It is also important to designate some time for new case managers to meet with experienced ones to have a first-hand dialogue on what it is like to be a case manager.

PRECEPTORSHIP PROGRAM

Mentoring case managers before they assume their independent roles is an integral part of the training. Developing a case management preceptorship program is not an easy task. It requires a multitude of resources, management support, and clear, consistent expectations of all involved. The use of preceptorship to facilitate the orientation and development of new nurses is well documented in the literature.[7-14] Although no documentation has been found that relates preceptorship to the training and development of case managers, the same concepts that apply to training of staff nurses are very appropriate to be applied to training case managers. Case management preceptorship programs are important strategies that link the didactic educational experience to practice. They provide opportunities for the novice case manager to resolve inaccuracies in role conception and integrate theory and practice in an actual work setting under the supervision of an expert case manager.

The primary responsibility of a preceptor is to facilitate learning,[11-13] particularly in the skills and tasks presented in Exhibits 13-1 and 13-2. The preceptorship experience is carried out on a one-to-one basis and over a predetermined period of time—usually two weeks on average. The length of the preceptorship program should be flexible and sensitive to the needs of the individual case manager.

The responsibilities of the preceptor include planning, teaching, role modeling, and evaluating the performance of the novice case manager. It is crucial for the nurse manager to meet with both the preceptor and preceptee on a regular basis to discuss their experiences, provide support and guidance, and make recommendations and modifications as needed.

It is also important to assign the novice case manager to spend some time observing other expert case managers in the institution, regardless of their areas of practice. Although specialties are different, approaches to case management are basically the same. This assignment exposes case managers to different case management styles, broadens their experience, and helps them decide which style is more appropriate for them to apply when they become independent. Preceptorship programs usually bring the case managers group together and provide a networking environment and support system, especially to those new in the role.

PERFORMANCE EVALUATION OF CASE MANAGERS

The Joint Commission, in the "Management of Human Resources" chapter of the *1995 Accreditation Manual for Hospitals,* stresses the importance of orientation, in-service education, and competency of staff.[14] As nursing administrators introduce case management and nurse case managers to the organization, they are obligated to make sure that training and education programs are in place to address orientation and establish competency of nurses who assume the new roles.

The establishment of case management training and education programs based on the curriculum presented in this chapter is a perfect way of complying with the Joint Commission standards. This program provides a mechanism for orientation and in-service education for case managers.

Competency of nurse case managers can be evaluated in reference to the skills and tasks delineated in the job description. Competency is defined as a "nurse's actual performance in a particular situation. It describes how well that individual integrates his or her knowledge, attitudes, skills and behaviors in delivering care according to expectations."[15]

Nurse case managers' competencies need to be evaluated on hire via licensure verification, educational background, work history and experience, previous performance evaluations, and reference checks. They are then evaluated at three months, six months, and one year. Each specialty area requires the development of a separate set of task-related competencies that is based on the population served and the extent of patient care delivery. The competencies related to the case manager's leadership skills are basically the same regardless of specialties. Those can be developed based on the skills listed in Exhibit 13-1.

Competency assessment of case managers also requires an annual performance evaluation (Exhibit 13-6). The tool is presented only as an example for nursing administrators to adapt to their organizations. It can be used after it is modified for a particular institution in relation to the scope of practice of case

Exhibit 13-6 Case Manager Performance Appraisal Tool

Key Performance Area	Relative Weight	Performance Expectations	Performance Level Achieved*	Comments
Functions as an effective advanced practitioner	20%	1. Identifies patients based on the established criteria and follows them from admission until discharge. 2. Assesses the physical, psychological, emotional, and social needs of the patient and family. 3. Documents assessment data and communicates relevant information to the health care team. 4. Identifies patient's actual and potential problems during hospitalization. 5. Establishes goals and plans and implements nursing care. 6. Uses internal and external resources to meet patient and family health care needs. 7. Ensures continuity of care and availability of resources. 8. Implements and individualizes the case management plans appropriate for the patient's diagnosis. 9. Ensures patient safety.		
Coordinates and facilitates patient care during hospital stay	25%	1. Facilitates scheduling of tests and procedures and follows up on and expedites results. 2. Communicates the patient's plan of care to the nursing and other staff. 3. Reviews with the health care team the case management plan for the day, for the hospital stay. 4. Refers patients as needed to other disciplines or specialty personnel (e.g., enterostomal nurse, nutritionist, home care and physical therapist). 5. Reviews the discharge plan with the health care team.		

continues

Exhibit 13-6 continued

Key Performance Area	Relative Weight	Performance Expectations	Performance Level Achieved*	Comments
		6. Communicates pertinent information regarding hospitalization with the related insurance companies/managed care organizations.		
Evaluates the provision of care	10%	1. Evaluates effectiveness of interventions and implementation of the case management plans.		
		2. Monitors expected outcomes of care and clinical quality indicators after interventions.		
		3. Evaluates patient's responses to care.		
		4. Evaluates appropriateness of care and length of stay as allocated by the DRGs.		
		5. Collects data based on the pre-established evaluation strategies of the case management model.		
Demonstrates skills in patient and family teaching	15%	1. Assesses patient's and family's health care needs.		
		2. Plans and implements and evaluates patient and family teaching activities provided by the health care team.		
		3. Evaluates patient's and family's level of health knowledge in preparation for discharge.		
		4. Provides self-care instructions for patient and family regarding health care needs, medications, treatments, and equipment.		
		5. Evaluates instructions given and teaching plans as well as patient outcomes and responses to teaching.		
Develops/revises case management plans	15%	1. Collaborates with the interdisciplinary team on developing new case management plans and/or revising old ones.		

Exhibit 13-6 continued

	15%	

		2. Meets with other case managers to discuss new plans.
		3. Follows up on the implementation and evaluation of the case management plans.
		4. Coordinates in-service education sessions for the medical, nursing, and other staff members regarding the use of case management plans in the provision of care.
Demonstrates excellence in leadership skills and professional performance	15%	1. Holds self accountable for delivering care that is safe, effective, and consistent with the organizational policies, procedures, and standards.
		2. Uses effective and excellent communication skills with patients, families, health care team, and other staff.
		3. Demonstrates effectiveness in critical-thinking, problem-solving, and decision-making techniques.
		4. Acts as a role model and expert clinician.
		5. Participates on patient care committees.
		6. Belongs to professional nursing organizations.
		7. Submits appropriate patient care and self-performance reports to immediate supervisor.
		8. Demonstrates effective public speaking and professional writing skills.

*Key to performance level achieved: 1 = does not meet expectations, 2 = meets expectations, 3 = exceeds expectations.

managers, policies and procedures, and standards of care and practice. The performance areas for evaluation presented in this tool are developed based on job description, roles and responsibilities, and the day-to-day activities of case managers.

CONCLUSION

Education and training of case managers is crucial to the success of case management models. The curriculum outline for training and education of case managers can be used as a guide when establishing similar educational programs. Although this curriculum is hospital based, it provides baseline information needed to develop a university-based case management curriculum that may offer either a certificate or a nursing degree. When considering this curriculum, one should know that it is malleable and can be adjusted to the particular needs of the organization. Any modifications should be made based on the individual institutional scope of practice of nurse case managers, selection criteria, job description and roles and responsibilities, the organizational structure, policies and procedures, and standards of care and practice. Consideration of these issues is a key to the success of the educational program.

It is crucial to the success of the program to identify key people in the organization who have the knowledge and experience in the various topics included in the curriculum and who are capable of teaching. These people act as the program's faculty and subject matter experts. Because case management models have an impact on the function of hospital ancillary departments, the curriculum developed should be flexible enough to be modified to meet the educational needs of various disciplines other than nursing.

REFERENCES

1. Cohen EL, Cesta TG. *Nursing Case Management: From Concept to Evaluation*. St. Louis, Mo: CV Mosby; 1993.
2. Lynn-McHale DJ, Fitzpatrick EL, Shaffer RB. Case management: development of a model. *Clin Nurse Specialist*. 1993;7:299–307.
3. Cline K. Training: hospitals find success in individualized programs. *Hosp Case Manage*. 1993;1:74–77.
4. Zander K. Managed care and nursing case management. In Mayer GG, Maden MJ, Lawerenz E, eds. *Patient Care Delivery Models*. Rockville, Md: Aspen Publishers, Inc.; 1990: 37–61.
5. Bower KD. *Case Management by Nurses*. Kansas City, Mo: American Nurses Association, 1992.

6. Rohrer KS, Poppe M, Noel L. Staff preparation for managed care. *Nurs Adm Q.* 1993;17: 74–78.

7. Kolb DA. *Experiential Learning: Experience as a Source of Learning and Development.* Englewood Cliffs, NJ: Prentice Hall; 1984.

8. May L. Clinical preceptors for new nurses. *Am J Nurs.* 1980;80:1824–1826.

9. Everson S, Panoc K, Pratt P, King AM. Precepting as an entry method for newly hired staff. *J Continuing Educ Nurs.* 1980;16:44–46.

10. Redland AR. Mentors and preceptors as models for professional development. *Clin Nurse Specialist.* 1989;3:70.

11. Hill AS. Precepting the clinical nurse specialist student. *Clin Nurse Specialist.* 1989;3:71–74.

12. Modic MB, Bowman C. Developing a preceptor program: what are the ingredients? *J Nurs Staff Dev.* 1989;2:78–82.

13. Davis LL, Barham PD. Get the most from your preceptorship program. *Nurs Outlook.* 1989;37:167–171.

14. Joint Commission on Accreditation of Healthcare Organizations. *The 1995 Accreditation Manual of Hospitals.* Oakbrook Terrace, Ill: Joint Commission; 1995.

15. Joint Commission on Accreditation of Healthcare Organizations. *Nursing Competency Assessment: Regaining Control of the Process.* Oakbrook Terrace, Ill: Joint Commission; 1993.

■ 14 ■

Roles of the Professional Registered Nurse in Case Management and Program Direction

Donna McNeese-Smith, EdD, RN
Gail Anderson, MN, RN, CPHQ
Cheryl Misseldine, BSN, RN
Gabriele Meneghini, MN, RN

Modern health care in America has often been delivered in a fragmented, uncoordinated manner. Patients are frequently cared for by multiple specialists focused on a single disease or body system. These specialists, experts in the diagnosis and treatment of a disease process, rarely consider the total health of a patient or family. Health care may be of a lesser priority until wellness becomes threatened by illness. The care given by one expert might not be coordinated with the care given by another. Some treatment may actually be counterproductive to the overall health of the patient and family.

Mark[1] described three underlying dimensions of nursing practice models that must be considered to reduce fragmentation: integration of care, coordination of care, and continuity of care. She recommended that care systems be designed to maximize these dimensions. In this chapter, these terms are defined as follows:

1. Integration of care—the consistency between planning and delivering a patient's care

2. Coordination of care—the degree that the plan of care is carried out by all care givers

3. Continuity of care—the extent that the plan of care is continued in other settings.

Case management is designed to maximize this integration, coordination, and continuity of patient care. Additionally, case managers in many settings have the opportunity to focus on illness prevention and health promotion and to move the locus of control to the patient and family. The original goals of primary nursing—responsibility and accountability of a primary nurse involved with a patient and family in care decisions at the point of service—can be met in this care delivery model.

Case management is being implemented in many settings and systems including insurance companies, HMOs, ambulatory care, community health care clinics, home and long-term care settings, and acute care. The job description and foci may vary in each of these settings or systems, but the roles and necessary skills are very similar. This chapter discusses the roles and skills used by the registered nurse (RN) in the position of professional case manager. Additionally, it presents roles and skills used by the director in implementing a case management program (Exhibit 14-1). These roles and skills were identified by examining the practices of case managers in both acute care and community settings.

ROLES OF THE CASE MANAGER

Case management programs are implemented to manage care and control cost while maintaining or improving quality. Not all hospitalized or ambulatory care patients require case management services. Patients with a consistent and predictable treatment course may be managed by the clinical staff, using critical pathways or a plan of care. Registered nurse case managers are a resource and

---

Exhibit 14-1 Roles of the RN Case Manager

In Case Management	In Program Direction
Case Finding/Screening	Care Coordination at the Program Level
Clinical Roles	Financial Management
Assessment	Outcomes Management
Planning	Project Management
Implementation	Resource
Care Coordination/Resource Manager	Leadership*
Evaluation	Ethical Practitioner*
Patient Advocate/Facilitator	
Negotiator	
Outcomes/Quality Manager	
Utilization/Resource Manager	
Educator*	
Political Activist*	

*Refers to both case manager and director.

role model for the direct care clinician. The goal of this role function is to integrate the case management philosophy and practice at the point of service.

Case Finding/Screening

Different models of implementation may have an effect on the manner in which patients are referred for case management. Case managers may select their clients from a broad-based client population or from specific groups of patients (i.e., by diagnosis or presenting problem such as high-risk pregnancy, diagnosis-related group [DRG], physician, or payer group). Typical patient populations referred for case management services include:

- catastrophic illnesses or injuries
- chronic medical conditions
- complex service needs (multiple health care providers)
- complex discharge needs
- lack of financial and/or social support
- high-risk patients—prone to complications, high use of resources, extended length of stay (LOS), and/or readmissions
- psychologically and/or cognitively challenged patients

Community health care clinics may refer patients who are also homeless, indigent, emotionally challenged, and substance abusers. These patients are at greater risk for acts of violence, often resulting in emergency department (ED) visits. Overcrowding in shelters creates health problems as well as increased stress. This group has distinctive needs and accesses the health care system differently from those in a stable environment. Difficulty in procuring food, clothing, shelter, and money is a major concern that often results in neglect of health problems. Critical indicators of a need for case management should be identified (i.e., four or more clinic visits or two ED visits for the same diagnosis; hospitalization without previous clinic visits). Providing continuity of care to this transient population is both frustrating and a challenge. A comprehensive and multidisciplinary approach is required to improve the health status of the homeless and manage the costs.[2] Critical components in a successful system are the prediction of population needs, demographics, identification of high-risk behaviors, and epidemiology.

Clinical Roles

In many settings, case managers are RNs who function in an expanded role. Case managers are clinical and systems experts who coordinate the timely delivery of health care services to meet an individual's specific health care needs in a cost-effective manner. Case managers work in collaboration with physicians and other health care team members to assess the needs of an individual and family, facilitate the development of an interdisciplinary plan of care, coordinate services across service sites, evaluate the effectiveness of services, and modify the plan of care and/or system to improve the process of care.

In some case management models, case managers dedicate a percentage of time to providing direct care. Although providing direct care can limit the case load of a case manager, several advantages result:

- Case managers retain clinical skills.
- Case managers can evaluate and improve the integration of case management at the point of service.
- Implementation of the model is based on realistic expectations.

The case manager clinical role can best be described using the steps of the nursing process.

Assessment

Assessment is an ongoing, continual process that occurs with each patient/case manager interaction. During the assessment process, the case manager strives to gain an understanding of the patient, his or her family, and health care beliefs and practices. Using interviewing and communication skills, the case manager may assess:

- physical, psychological, developmental, and spiritual level of functioning
- cultural factors that may influence health care practices
- coping abilities
- social support
- health care resources
- educational needs
- environmental factors
- expectations and goals

Through analysis of data, strengths and problems are identified, and with mutual planning with the patient/family and medical team, a plan of care begins to unfold.

Planning

Using the assessment data base, clinical expertise, and a holistic approach to care, the RN case manager collaborates with the patient/family, physician, and members of the health care team to develop an individualized compre-hensive plan of care. Clinical expertise is especially beneficial during the plan-ning phase as the RN case manager understands the patient population, treatment patterns of the medical/health care teams, and expected outcomes along the continuum of care. Also beneficial is the knowledge of common complications: expected time of occurrence, early signs and symptoms, treat-ment goals, and interventions.

After careful analysis of all data, an interdisciplinary plan of care is devel-oped. Components of this plan are:

- problem statements and/or nursing diagnosis
- mutually agreed-on goals
- essential interdisciplinary interventions
- anticipatory monitoring and preventive interventions for complications
- educational processes/outcomes
- discharge outcomes

In acute care, discharge planning is initiated on or before the day of ad-mission. As care progresses, constant efforts are made to ensure that the discharge plan supports the optimal level of physiologic, cognitive, and psy-chological functioning.

Throughout the hospitalization or continuum of care, the plan becomes a means of monitoring and evaluating the care process and outcomes. The plan is continually modified to reflect the individual patient condition and preferences.

Implementation

Implementation of the plan of care involves the provision, delegation, and coordination of planned care activities. Through communication and collabo-ration, the RN case manager and the nursing staff work as a team to provide all aspects of nursing care.

Care Coordination/Resource Manager

Care coordination and resource manager are two of the hallmark role functions of a case manager. By understanding the total process of care, the case manager works as a liaison to link the patient with necessary resources. Dwindling community resources are having an effect on the ability to provide care. Creativity in the acquisition of resources that meet the needs of the client/family is necessary. For example, eyeglasses, dental services, and drug and alcohol detoxification programs are difficult to locate for people with no funds. Methods of finding resources include networking, subscriptions to professional journals and to on-line computer networks, and appealing to community organizations such as churches and vendors.

Knowledge of the client's benefit structure is crucial to providing and procuring appropriate services. Needed community services include legal, financial, nutritional, personal care, home health, and mental health services, durable medical equipment, detoxification and drug rehabilitation programs, women's health, skilled nursing facilities, and housing.

Using a collaborative approach, communication is vital between the interdisciplinary team as well as with community agencies to ensure quality care, timely interventions, coordination of services/resources, and client satisfaction. Necessary tools include information systems, software programs, outcome studies, resource guides, access to medical records, voice mail, beepers, and fax machines. One way to maintain multidisciplinary communication is through conferences that provide an opportunity to discuss a variety of cases, share problems, and brainstorm solutions.

Through frequent interaction with the patient and family, the case manager provides education regarding the care delivery process. (Education is discussed later in this chapter.) Issues of control confront case managers daily, constraining the provision of adquate services. It is the client who ultimately controls decisions such as keeping or cancelling appointments, complying with prescribed treatment plans, or seeking services elsewhere if not satisfied. Many clients are occupied with survival, not wellness and prevention. Often a lack of a permanent address and telephone make it difficult to follow up with patients or even access them into a primary care setting. Another obstacle for clients with limited funds is lack of transportation to clinics for follow-up visits. A taxi voucher system or van transport system can alleviate this problem. The diabetic patient, living in a shelter with limited funds for food; the asthmatic patient living on the street; the chronic obstructive pulmonary disease patient who does not stop smoking; or the alcoholic patient who uses the ED for primary care are all challenges to the case manager. Continual coordination and educational efforts between patient/family and the health care team enhances continuity of care, decreases fragmentation and duplication of services, and optimizes patient self-care abilities.

Evaluation

The established plan of care is used as a means to monitor and evaluate the care process. Using the critical pathway (or plan of care in many nonacute settings), process and outcomes are evaluated at specified time frames. If patients vary from the process or goals, investigation and analysis occur. The plan of care is evaluated to determine if it is realistic. The case manager may arrange an interdisciplinary health care team meeting to evaluate and revise the plan of care. Problem solving, creativity, critical thinking, and leadership abilities are essential throughout this process.

The effectiveness of the plan and patient response to interventions are continually monitored. The ongoing relationship between the case manager and patient facilitates the detection of subtle changes in the patient condition. Early detection and intervention are essential to minimize or prevent complications and negative outcomes.

As care is evaluated, patient, clinician, and system variances are identified. A process must be established to link this aspect of case management with the quality management program. Reporting, analyzing, and trending variances will contribute to the continual improvement of the care process.

Patient Advocate/Facilitator

One of the most important elements in the case management process is the client relationship. This relationship begins at the point of referral and extends to other care delivery settings. The goal of the relationship is to maximize outcome, minimize cost, and promote independence in health and wellness.

The case manager/client relationship is built on trust, respect, rapport, and communication, a partnership to establish patient goals to ensure optimal wellness. The client is always the central focus of the case management process. At the point of entry, assessment reveals the client's beliefs, values, support, and resources. The case manager gains an understanding of the client's perspective or reality. It is within this reality that the case manager becomes an instrument through which care is advocated, negotiated, and coordinated. The challenge is to facilitate the client's integration into the health care system, medically and structurally, and to assist the client through the maze. Many clients are unsophisticated and unable to move through the system without assistance. Also, access to primary and preventive care is deficient in various areas. Many clients have no primary care providers and use the nearest ED as their primary care site. This misuse of ED services imposes a financial strain on an already burdened health care system. The community health care clinic may be the client's first link to accessing a comprehensive health care delivery system. Frequently, patients have multiple complex problems necessitating many referrals. The ambulatory care setting becomes the primary treatment site for coordination of required services.

The case manager gains an intimate understanding of the client and family as the relationship matures. As care is being negotiated, the case manager represents the client's needs and desires to other members of the health care team. Frequently, the case manager coordinates meetings between the client/family and members of the health care team to exchange information and develop future action plans. Throughout the relationship, the case manager fosters and supports the informed decision-making process of the client and family.

Within acute care, client advocacy extends beyond the hospital doors. Case managers may identify high-risk patients who require continued contact after discharge. Throughout the LOS, the case manager anticipates clients' needs to ensure continuous provision of quality care. She or he communicates with future care providers to validate they have the necessary knowledge and skills to provide care and to promote a smooth transition from the acute care hospital. Benefits of this continued advocacy and care may include:

- support of client and care giver
- early recognition/intervention of problems
- decrease in readmission to an acute facility
- timely access to additional community/health care resources
- reinforcement of the educational process
- health promotion

Advocacy is one of the key role functions of the case manager. The case manager becomes the liaison between client, providers, and payers, keeping the care on schedule and on track.

Negotiator

Negotiation is one of the subtle skills acquired by successful case managers. At times, case managers must negotiate with reluctant or hostile clients for limited space and services, with payers and providers, and with vendors for durable medical equipment. A useful set of skills includes mirroring, pacing, questioning, leading, and bargaining. Some strategies that can be helpful in this process are to:

- establish rapport
- identify existing agendas
- clearly state objectives/goals
- be completely honest
- know your subject and have your facts
- use active listening
- be attuned to verbal and nonverbal cues
- create a win-win situation

Rapport is essential to ensure that the prescribed plan of care is understood and followed. After negotiation, a contract is important to ensure that all parties have a clear understanding of the goals, plan of care, and expectations of each participant.

Outcomes/Quality Manager

Process and outcomes management is an integral part of the organization's case management program and the quality improvement system. Established links between quality management and case management are necessary to measure the effectiveness, efficiency, and outcomes of the care provided.

One way in which the case manager facilitates this quality management component is in monitoring and evaluating patient progress through use of the critical pathway. Pathway-based monitoring and evaluation of process and outcomes are interdisciplinary, with the case manager providing leadership in the design, implementation, and evaluation of the critical pathway.

Case managers are responsible for coordinating the development of critical pathways using current research, standards of care, and best practice patterns. Case managers always work with the medical staff and health care team to negotiate and define, for specific patient populations, the process of care and desired outcomes.

A distinct role of the case manager is integration of the critical pathway into the day-to-day care delivery process of the direct care clinician. The pathway is used by the entire interdisciplinary team and connects the process of care to outcomes by establishing time-specific goals along the continuum of care. This connection enables the direct care clinician to consistently implement the process as well as to monitor and evaluate outcomes of care concurrently. Immediate actions can be taken when variances from the pathway have an effect on the outcome of care. Variance analysis is a critical element of the organizational goal to improve continually quality and efficiency.

Another method to measure the effectiveness and quality of care is the establishment of an interdisciplinary, pathway-based monitoring system. As it is not possible to monitor every element of a critical pathway, critical events in the care process that have an effect on outcome should be defined. References used to identify these events include patients/families, physicians, current research, standards of care, third-party payers, and the entire health care team. As critical events are defined, indicators are established to assess, measure, and improve the care process.

Case managers play an instrumental role in developing indicators as well as participating in data collection and analysis. The case manager is also instrumental in the development and implementation of documents that support the care process (i.e., protocols, standing orders, documentation systems, and patient education materials).

An example of this process occurred when a physician, case manager, and interdisciplinary health care team reviewed the literature, standards, medical records, and best practice patterns for the cardiac surgery patient. The team supported the care process by developing a critical pathway, an activity protocol, a weaning protocol, and educational materials. Based on their review, the team decided to measure the following aspects of care:

- number of hours intubated
- morning laboratory results printed by 7:00 A.M.
- chest x-ray on viewer by 7:00 A.M.
- patient education materials/instruction provided
- activity progression
- patient/family proficiency in care

An important outcome of case management is customer satisfaction. Patient and family satisfaction is an essential outcome to measure; physician, team members, and other involved agencies are also important customers. Case managers work closely with the health care team to assess, monitor, and analyze the delivery systems, care process, and patient response continuously to improve the organization's performance.

Utilization/Resource Manager

All health care systems, but particularly hospitals, are a resource-intensive environment. In addition to being advocates of the client, case managers must be advocates of the system, actively negotiating solutions to problems confronting health care.[3] This commitment involves the examination of the health care delivery process at every level of the organization.

In the acute care setting, case managers work closely with the utilization review staff or may be responsible for utilization review functions. At a minimum, case managers need a working knowledge of reimbursement practices, as they have accountability for both financial and clinical outcomes.

Throughout the LOS, resource utilization is monitored. The critical pathway is one tool that can be used to monitor the use of resources. Time-specific, expected resource utilization patterns are detailed on the critical pathway. If ordering patterns vary from the critical pathway, case managers and the clinical staff monitor to ensure resources are necessary and are being used effectively.

The entire health care team should be alert to and recognize resource-intensive orders. Examples of these include daily laboratory tests, repeat radiologic procedures, and intensive care unit care. Each shift, the clinical staff should evaluate and address the continued necessity of these resources. One of the most resource-intensive areas in the hospital is the operating room.

Typically, critical pathways have not yet detailed the process of care or resource utilization in this area. As case management models are extended to include such areas, opportunities exist to improve efficiencies and outcomes while significantly decreasing cost.

High-quality, efficient documentation is essential for optimal reimbursement. On admission, documentation must reflect the need for acute care (severity of illness) and have a corresponding treatment plan (intensity of service). To maximize reimbursement, the case manager and utilization manager work closely with physicians and the health care team to ensure that essential information (e.g., complications, comorbidities, and procedures) is documented. Throughout the hospital stay, the case manager is keenly aware of the required documentation that would support the need for continued stay.

Case managers combine their advocacy and utilization management roles to effect an individualized, cost-effective discharge. Some patients may have continued medical needs that can be provided at a lower, less expensive level of care (e.g., subacute care, skilled nursing, rehabilitation, or home health). To facilitate an appropriate referral, case managers must have knowledge of the wide range of resources and services offered outside the acute care facility. The case manager and the discharge planner collaborate with the physician, patient/family, health care team, and third-party payers to negotiate and customize a timely discharge plan to meet the individualized needs of the patient and to optimize recovery. At times, it may become necessary to negotiate for benefits with the third-party payer for the special needs of a patient. The case manager can be instrumental in explaining the clinical and financial advantages of the proposed plan.

In a resource-scarce environment, all members of the health care team must be committed to resource management. Care delivery processes must be examined at all levels to ensure cost-effective patient care management. As a leader of the health care team, case managers strive to optimize patient outcomes while protecting health care resources.

Educator

A fundamental role function for the RN case manager is that of an educator. The case manager has a twofold responsibility in education: one as a patient educator, and the other as a staff educator. Both responsibilities offer specific challenges.

Goals of the case manager/client relationship are to maximize outcomes, minimize cost, and support independence in health and wellness. A clear understanding of the disease entity, in language that is understood by the patient, is critical. With the diversity of patients, cultural sensitivity is critical in the delivery of health education and care. Patient/family education is particularly challenging as hospital LOS decreases and patient acuity increases. Preoperative hospital stays are virtually nonexistent. Patients arrive for complex surgery just hours before entering the operating room. Patients are being discharged earlier and usually require some form of continued care. Timely provision of patient education is critical to the management of the hospitalized patient.

Prime opportunities are sought to provide the patient and family with thorough and understandable information (i.e., clinic visits, prehospital appointments). To ensure comprehension, appropriate teaching methods must be used, in a language understood by the client. His or her reading level and how he or she processes information are important to assess. By picking up verbal cues and nonverbal language, the case manager can determine how information is being processed—visually, auditorially, kinesthetically, or "by doing." Materials can be presented in a manner that benefits the client, such as by video, in written form, through discussion, or by having the client write or perform a process. Many facilities present information that cannot be easily understood by the client, thus rendering it ineffective. The focus of community-based settings must be on health promotion with an emphasis on preventive health and wellness teaching at the client's level of understanding. Patient education occurs with almost every patient/case manager interaction. Patients are requesting printed information to supplement the educational process. Interdisciplinary educational protocols are created to supplement the critical pathway. Case managers are a resource either to develop or select supporting educational materials. Educational outcome indicators should be established to measure the effectiveness and quality of the patient educational effort.

Continual staff education is essential as the case management care delivery model is a dynamic evolving process. For optimal success in implementing a case management process, a commitment is required by staff at every level of the organization. The case management model must be integrated in the organization's day-to-day care delivery process. Each employee should be responsible and accountable for supporting and participating in the case management process. To gain this level of support, specific areas of integration may include:

- philosophy and strategic plan of the organization
- job descriptions
- performance appraisals
- clinical ladder

- documentation tools
- quality management

As the case management process evolves and is integrated throughout the hospital, continual education is provided. Examples of forums in which education can be provided include:

- physician in-services
- hospital and nursing orientation
- interdisciplinary in-services
- one-to-one coaching
- departmental in-services
- community agency in-services
- university/educational classes

Case managers play a key role in the agency and communitywide education process. They must be creative, knowledgeable about educational theory and principles, and have strong presentation skills. As a case manager interacts with the interdisciplinary team, he or she must be a team player, a motivator, and a catalyst, yet have enough flexibility to step back continually and examine the care delivery process.

Political Activist

The goal of a case manager is to effect positive change, improve quality, and promote healthy communities. The importance of community investment and involvement must be recognized as a necessary component to the redesign and refocus of health care. Health care professionals must take a leadership role in the administrative and legislative forums of government.[4] They must work with political and professional groups to create change. This can be accomplished by developing health policies that reflect the unique needs of the community. Case managers need to monitor legislation, participate in lobbying efforts, and write letters to political leaders to ensure the voice of the community is heard and its needs reflected. They can also make the legislators and community aware of community needs by giving speeches, participating on advisory boards and discussion panels, writing articles for professional journals, and teaching community workshops and adult education classes.[3]

ROLES OF THE CASE MANAGEMENT DIRECTOR

The next section of this chapter discusses the roles and skills used by an effective case management director.

Care Coordination at the Program Level

At the program management level of case management, coordination of care is essential. Coordination is involved in:

- planning for standardization of care for like diagnoses and/or procedures
- implementation of the plan
- monitoring of care and evaluation
- continuous quality/performance improvement
- celebration of success and communication to all

The backbone of a progressive and aggressive acute care case management program is the use of *selected* critical or clinical pathways. At a private, nonprofit church-owned hospital, critical pathways are developed by quality/performance improvement teams consisting of all the disciplines involved in the care of the selected patient grouping (i.e., the case manager, nursing, physicians, respiratory therapy, pharmacy, physical therapy, social work, and discharge planning). All the principles of building quality teams are used in the development and subsequent monitoring of performance standards. For example, a cardiac surgery team was chartered after the analysis of hospitalwide DRG financial performance for the previous year and an overture by the cardiologists and cardiac surgeons to work cooperatively with administration to achieve a competitive edge for this product line. The team met one hour weekly for 12 weeks to design the critical pathway, multidisciplinary patient care plan, teaching plan, patient/family critical pathway, and patient education materials. They have met quarterly since pathway implementation to monitor the performance and recommend improvements.

The role of coordination at the program level is essential to set organizational goals, establish teams, guide pathway development and implementation, oversee case management at the clinical level, and strive continuously for maintenance of gains and improvements. At the example hospital, it is considered essential to involve all disciplines that care for the patient when developing critical/clinical pathways. Although this at times violates one of the "principles" of quality improvement teams (i.e., keeping the number of team participants at a manageable 10 or less), it has proved to be a key for success at the time of implementation. Common sense and knowledge of human nature tell us that involvement at the outset of any project provides for buy-in and is motivating to the participants. As evidence to this basic principle, team data analysis at times demonstrates an improvement in the LOS and cost measures as soon as the team starts to meet, not necessarily when the critical pathway is implemented. Likewise, data outcomes are frequently the best when the team is meeting intensively.

Involvement is not meant to be limited to the employees of the medical center but applies to the physicians as well. It is essential to involve medical staff from the outset. Otherwise, acceptance is often delayed and implementation is difficult. Actions that contribute to physician participation include:

- follow-up of all overtures to be involved
- using personal direct contact at all times
- sharing data openly
- selecting clinically respected case managers
- communicating

All team members are important to the success of endeavors. Involvement and participation are key to team success. Involvement and participation are achieved through skillful coordination.

One aspect of program coordination frequently overlooked is the ongoing maintenance required to continue a vital program. Critical pathways, patient care and teaching plans, and patient education materials need continuing improvement; teams require infusions of enthusiasm to maintain high levels of achievement. In some specialties, the medical regime changes as rapidly as the team can respond (e.g., transition of chemotherapy to the outpatient setting, aggressive coronary angioplasty versus cardiac surgery). Critical pathways and case management methodologies need to change in a coordinated and timely manner to be proactive rather than reactive.

The last, but very important, step of coordination is celebrating and publicizing the successes of the program. Case management must demonstrate success by measuring clinical outcomes and cost savings, giving credit to those who accomplished these successes, and publicizing these to everyone, particularly administration. Staff must receive credit and a sense of accomplishment to remain enthusiastic; administration must believe that the program is cost effective to continue to provide the financial resources to support the program.

Financial Management

Today's case manager needs to understand clearly that one essential role is that of financial manager. All health care environments are faced with doing more with less, and clinicians take pride in accomplishing better care for less cost. To achieve this mission, *financial analysis* is a must. To accomplish financial analysis, *data* are critical! The options for data access are variable, depending on the organization. If information systems/finance support personnel are available and can be counted on to supply data per an established schedule and as needed, the case manager and program director can use their energies in analysis of the data. If support personnel are limited and/or overloaded, then a minimum of one member of the case management team must have approval to access and the necessary skill to retrieve it. Otherwise, it will be impossible to evaluate the priorities for and contribution of case management in the financial arena.

The surgical team provides an example of the role of "financials" or financial data. Development of a critical pathway for hip surgery patients was selected as a goal when the program management/case management director reviewed the top DRGs, specifically volume, cost, loss, and LOS in relation to Health Care Financing Administration (HCFA) averages. Hip surgery was selected along with nine other diagnoses to be the developmental priorities for the year.

When the surgical team met, requests for data included cost, charges, LOS, admission source, disposition, attending physicians, surgeons, cost of surgery, HCFA and corporate comparisons (LOS, cost, physician data per DRG from the hospital-owned corporation), day of surgery correlations with LOS, and time window of preoperative antibiotics. Outcomes measures selected by the team included LOS and cost per discharge. Timely provision of data allows the team to conduct their analysis. Measurement of progress is not possible without objective ongoing data. Financial outcomes are critical in a managed care environment.

Financial analysis must identify and track predictors of cost and predictors of problems. Cost predictors may include:

- surgical intervention
- surgeries involving prostheses
- procedural intervention (e.g., cardiac catheterization, percutaneous transluminal coronary angioplasty [PTCA], PTCA with stent placement)
- comorbid conditions/complications (e.g., methicillin-resistant Staphylococcus aureus [MRSA])
- high drug costs (e.g., new chemotherapeutic or antiemetic agents and hematopoietic agents)

Problem predictors may include:

- comorbid conditions/complications (e.g., MRSA, cardiovascular accident, pneumonia; immobility)
- long presurgical admissions
- extended intubation times

Outcomes Management

One of the greater challenges with case management program coordination is the determination and measurement of clinical outcomes. Although it may be somewhat easier to select process measures that reflect quality care, the collection and analysis of data are frequently manual and labor intensive. Then, if the measurement indicates 100 percent compliance, the cost of measurement provides little benefit in the improvement of care. Still, if the outcome is essential to the quality of care, the measurement should be repeated intermittently to ensure continued compliance (e.g., hemoglobin and hematocrit obtained within 30 minutes of admission of the patient with gastrointestinal bleeding).

Financial and LOS outcomes are relatively easy to measure over time due to the historical importance of computerized financial data and subsequent availability of a substantial financial data base. Quarterly presentation of cost, LOS, and quality outcomes to the clinical improvement teams is a combined responsibility of the case and program managers.

Process and outcome measures and goals are determined by the clinical improvement teams at the example hospital. The pulmonary clinical improvement team, for example, selected the following outcomes to measure the performance of their pneumonia critical pathway:

- laboratory work drawn within 2 hours of admission
- sputum obtained within 2 hours of admission
- respiratory therapy induced sputum specimen if sputum not obtained within 2 hours of admission
- antibiotic in ED
- intravenous antibiotics started within 2 hours of admission
- chest x-ray performed in ED or within 4 hours of admission
- case manager makes initial contact within 24 hours of admission
- physician review/change antibiotic by day 3
- sputum culture and sensitivity on chart within 72 hours

In addition, each case manager tracks variances at an "overview" rather than at the detail level. In other words, the case manager notes the overriding reason(s) the patient did not proceed per the critical pathway guidelines rather than which critical events on the pathway were not met. An example was the recent identification of a delay in transferring patients to the transitional care unit due to several factors. The scope of the problem was identified through variance analysis.

Project Management

Implementation of an organizationwide case management program is the ultimate in project management. Steps of program implementation are:

- identification of case management as an important goal of the organizational strategic plan
- choice of a case management director, strategically placed to maximize administrative, clinical, and financial support (perhaps using an overall quality improvement team task force to direct the process)
- identification of existing organizational strengths on which to build
- selection of a case management model
- determination of priorities and goals (based on program and financial analysis)
- development of an implementation strategy
- development of critical pathways via clinical improvement teams
- education of participating staff
- approval and publicity of the process
- trial of the critical pathways
- ongoing measurement of outcomes and determination of variances
- evaluation and problem solving and continuous improvement
- celebrating and publicizing accomplishments

Indeed, it is essential to develop a critical pathway for the project management of the case management program. For the program to be successful, it requires nurturing and coordination by a dedicated and skilled individual and preferably several champions. The roles of coordinator and champion must include roles of "change agent and catalyst."

Raven and French[5] describe the importance of using both organizational and personal power to achieve organizational goals. It is essential that the case management director be positioned to receive legitimate power within the organization and that organizational support comes from all areas of administration, finance, and clinical practice. Additionally, the director and case managers must have the skills to generate personal power, both expert and referent (to be well liked) to achieve support from patients, families, physicians, and staff.

A full-time case management program coordinator can manage approximately five clinical teams on an intensive meeting schedule at one time, more or less depending on support. At the example hospital, eight clinical improvement teams are organized: cardiac/cardiac surgery, oncology, pulmonary, neonatal intensive care unit, perinatal, medical, surgical, and detoxification. A psychiatric clinical improvement team is included in the strategic plan. The case management department also does its own financial analysis. The number of critical pathways and associated tools one program coordinator can handle is approximately 20. The format and amount of detail included will contribute significantly to the complexity of this task. The sample hospital has 25 critical pathways and associated tools designed with minute detail.

Resource

The case management program director serves as a resource for case managers and clinical staff, as well as administration and the medical staff. This role is of primary importance early in program development. With expertise in their individual clinical areas, the case managers assume the clinical aspects of the resource role, to free the program director to support the overall program and pursue additional opportunities for improvements and expansion of the program.

Leadership

The individual case manager must function in a leadership role, whether it is as a patient advocate or in the implementation of a new quality improvement team. This role is even more critical for the program director as this individual must be able to provide a vision, direction, and practical implementation of a new system of care. The essential leadership behaviors have been defined in the research of Kouzes and Posner.[6] These behaviors, applied to case management, are

- *Inspiring a shared vision*—The leader (and champion) must describe the vision for case management, using vivid language, energy, and enthusiasm. Second, the leader must involve everyone in that vision. This vision must be a part of the organizational strategic plan and show the benefits of case management.
- *Challenging the process*—The leader must be able to take risks, try new ideas, encourage suggestions, network with other leaders, use feedback from the customers (patients, families, physicians, and other care givers), seek new ways to keep patients healthier, reward new ideas, constantly learn and grow, and seek opportunities to take case management to a higher level.
- *Enabling others to act*—The case management leader must build trust and focus on multidisciplinary teamwork, decentralize decision making

to the point of service, share power, involve and educate everyone, use excellent communication skills, and provide support and follow-up.

- *Modeling the way*—To build trust, the case manager must be clear about the values and standards of case management and be a consistent role model. The leader must expect these standards of everyone including administration and physicians, show others how to do the job, be sure case management occurs 24 hours a day 7 days a week, and jump in and help others when the load is heavy. The effective leader must also be able to break this momentous project down into manageable, measurable tasks.

- *Encourage the heart*—Lastly, the case management leader must celebrate accomplishment, praise everyone for their work, especially the direct care staff, and provide team rewards. The leader must provide support when individuals or teams are experiencing difficulty and build the self-esteem of all. Lastly, the champion must publicize the accomplishments of case management on an ongoing basis to keep up enthusiasm and ensure the continued support of administration.

Ethical Practitioner

The most frequent negative feelings about case management come from health care professionals who fear that case management is a system created to prevent patients from gaining access to care. These individuals frequently seem to have a horror story to relate about this "prevention of quality care." Every RN involved in case management has an ethical responsibility to ensure that case management is used to coordinate and maximize care delivery to provide both quality of care and excellent patient outcomes as well as cost-effectiveness.

EDUCATION OF THE RN CASE MANAGER

Case management has grown so quickly that there are insufficient well-prepared individuals for this role. Many resourceful individuals have gained on-the-job training to enable them to step into this role. However, many organizations are establishing educational standards for the position of a bachelor of science in nursing or a graduate degree. The best preparation is a strong background in a clinical area and broad preparation in finance, utilization review, the management of systems, management information systems, interpersonal skills, and leadership. Personal characteristics must include self-direction, being a team player and a problem solver, and having strong interpersonal relationships, creativity, and persistence. The program director must also be strong in financial analysis, a generalist, a change agent, a project manager, comfortable speaking in group settings, a strong leader, and should have a graduate degree. At the University of California, Los Angeles (UCLA), some of the nursing administration graduates are enjoying positions of leadership in case management. Other advanced practice nurses, such as clinical nurse specialists, are also choosing to obtain the finance and systems management skills to function in case management roles. Workshops at UCLA, offering this preparation to skilled clinicians, have been very popular.

GRADUATE PROGRAMS FOR CASE MANAGER PREPARATION

Graduate programs to prepare case managers as an advanced practice role should develop curricula that educate graduates in all areas previously discussed. Graduates should have a broad background so that they are able to function in acute care, community, and nontraditional settings including schools, insurance companies, or integrated care delivery systems. They must be able to cross boundaries and be change managers. Additionally, many must be able to be political leaders and educators, qualified to provide direction in the tumultuous years to come.

CERTIFICATION/CASE MANAGEMENT ASSOCIATIONS

Why become certified? Although not a substitute for an advanced degree, certification offers competence-based credentials that are nationally recognized. At this time, the American Nurses Association does not certify case managers. The following information is provided by the two certifying associations discussed.

One method for certification is to become a Certified Professional in Healthcare Quality (CPHQ).[7] The CPHQ program is a voluntary certification program administered by the Healthcare Quality Certification Board. The program was founded in 1984 and operates under the sponsorship of the National Association for Healthcare Quality. The CPHQ examination is the only accredited certification program in the field of health care quality, utilization, and risk management. Accreditation by the National Commission for Certifying Agencies in Washington, D.C., a division of the National Organization for Competency Assurance, gives superior credibility to the CPHQ program. To become CPHQ all of the following requirements must be satisfied.

1. Educational Requirements
   • Possess a minimum educational preparation of an associate, baccalaureate, masters, or doctoral degree in any field, or be a registered

nurse or licensed practical nurse, or accreditation in medical records technology

2. Employment Requirements

   • Possess a minimum of 2 years of full-time experience or the part-time equivalent (4,160 hours) in health care quality, utilization, case and/or risk management activities

3. Certification Examination

   • Pass a comprehensive examination that assesses knowledge and understanding of regulations, certification requirements, program development and management, and quality improvement concepts as well as departmental management skills

   • Demonstrate a commitment to excellence by his or her desire to become a certified professional

Information can be obtained from the Certification Board Executive Director, c/o HQCB, P.O. Box 1880, San Gabriel, Calif. 91778, (818) 286–8074, (800) 346–4722, or FAX (818) 286–9415.

A second method of certification is sponsored by the Commission for Case Manager Certification. Case management is recognized as an area of specialized practice that includes practitioners from a variety of professions. As a result, the credential is designed to serve as an adjunct to other professional credentials in health and human resources.

Case management certification is achieved by satisfying specific educational and employment requirements and passing the CCM examination. The CCM examination is based on a body of knowledge that encompasses laws, public regulations, and the delivery of case management services as practiced within the United States. For more specific information and requirements, contact the Commission for Case Manager Certification (CCMC), 1835 Rohlwing Road, Rolling Meadows, Ill. 60008. Telephone: (708) 818–0292.

CONCLUSION

The future of case management certainly will involve expansion to other settings and to areas that involve a high concentration of costs, such as the operating room. Case management will have a greater focus in the ambulatory setting as reimbursement systems pay to keep patients well rather than reimbursing illness care only. Case managers and program directors must continue to be ready to embrace change and lead the process of expanding case management concepts when there is a need. Mullahy[9] reminds case managers to watch for doors that will close and doors that are opening and not to be so focused on the closing doors and "what might have been" that opening doors and new opportunities are missed. Case managers must be about designing care that provides integration of patient services, a coordinated plan of care, and continuity of care so that patients receive the highest quality of health possible for a cost that is reasonable and attainable.

REFERENCES

1. Mark BA. Characteristics of nursing practice models. *J Nurs Adm.* 1992;22(11):57–63.
2. Cousineau MR, Lozier JN. Assuring access to health care for homeless people under national health care. *Am Behavioral Scientist.* 1993;36:857–870.
3. Wagner JD, Menke EM. Case management of homeless families. *Clin Nurse Specialist.* 1992;6:65–71.
4. O'Grady TP. Building partnerships in health care: creating whole systems change. *Nurs Health Care.* 1994;15(1):34–38.
5. Raven BH, French RP. Bases of social power. In: Cartwright D, Zanders A, eds. *Group Dynamics: Research and Theory.* 2nd Ed. New York, NY: Harper & Row, 1960:607–623. Discussed in Hellriegel D, Slocum JW. *Management.* 6th ed. Reading, Mass: Addison-Wesley Publishing Co.; 1992.
6. Kouzes JW, Posner BZ. *The Leadership Challenge: How To Keep Getting Extraordinary Things Done in Organizations.* San Francisco, Calif: Jossey Bass, Inc.; 1995.
7. Healthcare Quality Certification Board. *Certification Program for Healthcare Quality Professionals.* (1994 brochure available from JLM Associates, P.O. Box 1880, San Gabriel, Calif. 91778).
8. Certification of Insurance Rehabilitation Specialists Commission. *Certification Guide.* (1994 brochure available from CIRS, 1835 Rohlwing Road, Suite D, Rolling Meadows, Ill 60008).
9. Mullahy CM. The case manager is the catalytic collaborator in managed care. *J Care Manage.* 1995;1(1):7–9.

■ 15 ■

Alternate Case Management Models

Karen A. Clark, MS, RN

Many health care organizations have adopted case management as their model for the delivery of health care services for clients. Case management activities differ from setting to setting, depending on the focus of the provider. However, in all instances the central premise is coordination and delivery of quality health care.

The prototype of today's case management approach was established during the early history of community service coordination. In the 1900s, the public health nursing literature discussed approaches to identifying and coordinating medical and social resources within the community for specific populations.[1] After World War II, the model evolved and progressed as it was used to coordinate the provision of long-term services to discharged psychiatric patients.[1]

The coordination of services model took a major step with the enactment of the Community Mental Health Act of 1963. As a result of this law, patients left the state mental institutions and returned to the community. It became necessary to provide a coordinated system to avoid fragmentation of services.[2] This model was also very useful in the provision and coordination of services for the elderly. The early case management of these two client populations provided the foundation for today's case management models.

The term *case management* began to appear in the early 1970s in social welfare and nursing literature.[3] Other terms are commonly used today, such as *case coordination, service integration, continuing care coordination, continuity coordination, managed care,* and *utilization management.*[4] Although the names are different, these systems share the overall goals of decreasing health care fragmentation and enhancing client services.

Case management system classification is generally determined by who is purchasing or who is providing the service.[5] Purchasers are found in both the private and public sectors. The private sector includes HMOs, preferred provider organizations, private insurers, and self-insured employers and private individuals, among others.[5] The public sector includes health departments, home health care agencies, public hospitals, and Medicare and Medicaid payers.

The providers of this service are called case managers. They may be clinical nurse specialists, nurse practitioners, masters-prepared social workers, or physicians. They work independently or in teams.

Various models exist for applying case management to a health care delivery system. One of the most familiar models is the acute care nursing case management model. This is a client-centered approach to care instituted during episodes of acute illness. The focus is on defined outcomes of quality and resource utilization, as well as nursing accountability.[6] This model was presented earlier in this book. The following are some alternate case management models found outside of acute care facilities (Table 15-1).

PRIVATE CASE MANAGEMENT

Private case management covers those services contracted by individuals and/or their families or subcontracted by other groups. This model of management is popular because of concern over rising health care costs and the confusion that often accompanies the choices consumers must make. Entrepreneurial health care professionals identified the needs of this market segment and quickly moved forward to assist clients through the complex maze of today's health care options.[4] Because private case managers are paid privately by the client, they may continue to support clients after reimbursement issues would normally terminate other services.[7]

The case manager in this model is usually a clinical nurse specialist or masters-prepared social worker. This individual provides the client with the guidance needed to differentiate among health care options and the knowledge to make informed choices.

The role of the private case manager has three main functions:

- *Coordination* involves assessment of clients' strengths, needs, and resources. The challenge is to match those findings with available services. Central to this function is the necessity for the case manager to build a network of professional resources. This allows interdisciplinary and interagency cooperation and permits the case manager to locate the most appropriate services for clients. It also allows the identification of gaps in available services. This function includes follow-up, case monitoring, and some provision of services.

Table 15-1 Alternate Models of Case Management

	Private	Social/ Community	Primary/ Institution	Vendor/ Gatekeeper
Setting	Across all settings	Agencies, clinics, health departments	HMO, hospitals, home care	Insurance companies, self-insured employers, third-party payers
Services provided	Advocacy, coordination, counseling	Case finding, advocacy, assessment, planning, monitoring, resource linking, counseling	Gatekeeping, cost contain-ment, monitoring, resource linking	Cost contain-ment, gatekeeping, resource linking
Case manager	CNS, RN, MSW	MSW, CNS, nutritionists	RN, CNS, MSW, nurse practitioner, physician	RN, CNS, MSW, physician
Client	Individuals/ families, subcontracted by other groups	Focus on well individual, supportive services, mental health, aging, special needs children	Medicare clients, HMO participants, high-risk or specialty population clients	Focus on catastrophic illnesses, high-risk pregnan-cies, preterm infants
Cost/funding	Out of pocket or paid by agencies for specialty populations	Tax supported, grants, no out of pocket	HMO or insurance companies, Medicare or Medicaid	Insurance companies, third-party payers

- *Advocacy* is that part of the role that allows the case manager to assist the client in identifying broad goals and setting measurable objectives. The focus is on identifying client strengths and assisting him or her to use those strengths to accomplish the desired objectives.[8] Another im-portant role for the advocate is helping the client assume responsibility for progress. This supports the principle of client self-determination.[9]
- *Counseling* expands the role of the case manager to include a holistic approach to clients. With the repeal of the Medicare Catastrophic Bill in 1989, many people with major disabilities or debilitating illnesses were moved away from inpatient settings and into the community.[5] This

societal change has created a need for economic, family, social, and life planning counseling services from the case manager for these clients who still have profound needs for assistance.[10]

Fees for private case management are generally paid by the individual client, the client's family, or by agencies on behalf of specific patient populations. In some instances, there is limited purchase of services for low-income geriatric clients by government agencies.[7] These fees range from approximately $200 to $400 for the initial assessment. Follow-up services typically cost $50 per hour.[7]

An example of private case management is the Interventions Case Management Model. This model is coordinated by Interventions, an Illinois nonprofit corporation that provides treatment services to substance abusers.[11] This program operates on the premise that clients are more likely to be successful if barriers to recovery can be reduced at the time the client is motivated to seek help. The case manager assesses each client and develops an individualized plan. The manager then overlays the individual plan with available community and private resources to customize care. If the client has no insurance and is unable to pay part or all of the costs incurred, the case manager has access to agency-designated indigent funding until public services become available. These case managers are very active in relapse prevention and relapse interruption and provide continuity for clients for up to three years.

Preliminary data from the assessment of the Interventions model have demonstrated a decrease in the amount of time required to obtain needed services.[11] The future application of private case management to populations such as this appears promising.

SOCIAL/COMMUNITY-BASED CASE MANAGEMENT

Social/community-based case management focuses on the identification and recruitment of well individuals who have a potential need for health care services or access to support services. As deinstitutionalization occurs, an additional priority is anticipating the needs of those clients who are moving back into the community. These clients encounter service delivery problems for themselves and their families that can be ameliorated by community-based case management.[9] Community-based programs designed to meet the needs of these clients are often managed by health departments or agencies set up by the federal government.

The various programs available are usually organized around a specific client population. Programs for the aging, migrant children, special needs children, persons with human immunodeficiency virus (HIV), chemically dependent people, and those with mental health problems are primary examples of these client populations.

Case managers for community programs are traditionally masters-prepared social workers, clinical nurse specialists, nurse practitioners, and occasionally nutritionists. There is a great deal of independence in the role for these managers. The main functions are the same as the private case manager: assessment of need, linking with appropriate resources, and coordination of client care. The long-term nature of the manager–client relationships requires excellent teaching and coaching skills to help individuals and their families participate in the plan of care. Fiscal management skills are also needed as these managers are often accountable for apportionment of limited funds within the various programs. They frequently must ration funds to allow access for the greatest number of clients.[10]

Much community-based work has been performed in the area of mental health and drug rehabilitation. One such program is the Linkage Program in Worcester, Massachusetts. This program was created as a communitywide, bilingual/bicultural case management system to merge primary care and substance abuse treatment programs that specifically address the problem of HIV among intravenous drug users.[12]

The Linkage Program addresses the universal problem facing community-based health care, that of coordinating multiple organizations, each one having its own boundaries and structural differences. In this model, case managers are identified in each of the participating agencies. They function as a network to link the appropriate resource with the client's need. The entry point for clients is through any of the case managers. Ongoing management is passed from one case manager to another as clients' service needs change. Although cost-effectiveness has not been measured, it appears there is a reduction of service duplication by community organizations when an effective community network is in place.[12]

An innovative community program in Santa Cruz County, California, provided dental care to children of migrant and low-income families. It represents a prime example of coordination of community resources to provide needed services to a client population. The case manager was a clinical nurse specialist who coordinated the identification of clients. Service was provided by 16 volunteer dentists and the community college dental hygiene program. Parents were required to accompany the child and participate in preventive dental education. This program was funded by a grant of $5,000 from the Community Foundation. It has been recognized as a model of accessing community resources to provide needed care for low-income children.[13]

Community-based case management plays a major role in many cities in early development programs for special needs children. Case managers assist families to manage the health care needs of these children, and they teach parents how to find methods to meet their child's educational and environmental needs. Managers identify problems of poverty, transportation, functional illiteracy, and lack of basic essentials. Community-based case managers also face the challenge of limited financial resources and uneven distribution of services in providing community-based case management.[14]

An example of a large community-based case management model is AID Atlanta, located in metropolitan Atlanta, Georgia. This model is funded by the Robert Wood Johnson Foundation as an acquired immunodeficiency syndrome (AIDS) demonstration project. Sites at six locations are staffed by case managers trained to close the gap between the need for medical care and social services available in the community.[15] Social workers, nurses, pastoral counselors, and therapists form an interdisciplinary team to work in partnership with clients. There are multiple entry points into the program based on the particular need and level of acuity of the client. Case managers share resources and information when dealing with complex individual profiles and clients are expected to be full participants in their plan of care. A client council functions to assist case managers in the identification of systems problems and the development of client-focused solutions.[15] The program's success comes from its ability to provide management services based on the level of client need and its ability to coordinate these services to prevent duplication.[15]

Another unique model of community-based case management is the Nursing Center. It is located in Brooklyn, New York, and is operated by the College of Nursing, State University of New York Health Science Center, in conjunction with Heights and Hill Community Council, a nonprofit social work agency.[16] Nursing graduate students serve as case managers for an elderly, low-income population with chronic health problems. Undergraduates assist in the provision of direct care.

Each case manager follows approximately ten clients. He or she provides assessment of physical and functional health including the identification of risk factors such as medication mismanagement, social isolation, and home environment dangers.[16] The manager directs the interdisciplinary plan of care and supervises home visits to the clients. When necessary, he or she oversees transition of the client to other levels of care as needed, such as nursing homes or inpatient hospitalization.[16] This model has the dual benefit of providing students with necessary community experience while providing preventive health care for clients. This approach to prevention and early detection of health care problems reduces the need for more expensive late-stage intervention.

Although case management seems appropriate for managing clients in the community, it is not without drawbacks. Issues of quality of care and service gaps remain. The problems of interagency collaboration is a continuing challenge in the light of changing funding, different cultures, and program capacities. Excessive paperwork, created in part by the governmental interface, impedes the system and siphons off funding needed for client care.[17] Success or failure of most of the models appears, unfortunately, to be inexorably linked to funding.

PRIMARY CARE CASE MANAGEMENT

Primary care is a case management approach based on the medical model. System entry is through the primary care physician or nurse practitioner. It begins when clients present to physicians' offices, hospital emergency departments, or HMOs with a health problem. Case management is often performed by an interdisciplinary team consisting of nurses, physicians, and social workers.

Primary case management focuses on gatekeeping, cost containment, monitoring, and coordination of services.[5] This model is evolving and frequently provides discharge planning services, including long-term follow-up in the community.[2] This hospital-to-community model allows case managers to follow the movement of high-risk clients between acute care and long-term care settings.[18]

The Arizona model is a multidisciplinary illustration of the extended program. Case managers are responsible for clients with chronic health problems, or those with end-stage disease, during and after their hospitalizations. Relationships between these clients and case managers are long-term, lasting from several months to several years. In these cases, there is a documented reduction in subsequent hospital admissions when compared with clients not in a case management system.[2]

The HMO model is being used by some employers in the northwestern United States. It is designed to help people with occupational injuries successfully return to work.[19] Clients are triaged by a primary care physician or clinic nurse and assigned to a case manager. These case managers are occupational health nurses who use their assessment skills to monitor treatment and establish rehabilitation plans. Other team members assist the client to adhere to managed care organizational guidelines, answer modified work restriction questions, and handle claims and billing paperwork. It is anticipated that this case management approach facilitates good working relationships with area employers while improving the quality of care for the injured worker.[19]

VENDOR/GATEKEEPER MODEL OF CASE MANAGEMENT

In the vendor/gatekeeper model, the case manager functions much like a purchasing agent. His or her job is to locate vendors who will provide appropriate client services at the lowest cost. Some companies or independent case management centers have found a niche consulting for insurance companies and HMOs to provide these services. Vendor case managers analyze the service market and negotiate terms and price on behalf of the payer or HMO.

As gatekeepers, these managers are expected to provide direct or indirect cost savings by restricting client access to high-cost services such as emergency departments and acute inpatient services and avoiding admissions to detoxification units.[20] Control is exerted through the requirement for preauthorization regarding the length and type of service the client may access. The success of this strategy is directly related to the availability of appropriate alternatives. To be most effective, the case manager must perform this gatekeeping function as an independent, remaining separate and distinct from the provider delivery system.[21]

Catastrophic care is a major cost for insurance companies and therefore one of the first areas selected for the application of case management. Clients with high-cost problems, such as chronic conditions, high-risk pregnancies, and AIDS, have been efficiently handled through case management. The financial impact of case management in these cases is very convincing. Northwestern National Life's Life/Health Reinsurance Division reported savings of $32 million in four years from the case management approach to its catastrophic medical cases. The company's figures show savings of more than $30,000 per case in high-risk pregnancies. Additional costs were reduced for care for preterm babies by 28 percent. AIDS patients' costs were reduced by more than 30 percent through the use of case management.[21]

Critics argue that the vendor/gatekeeper model is a very limited approach to case management. However, its use is expected to rise with the arrival of capitated reimbursement structures and the emphasis on cost containment.

CONCLUSION

The cost of health care continues to escalate in the United States. Health care expenses are projected to increase as much as 19 percent by the year 2000.[22] At the same time, the public is exerting increased pressure on our government to provide legislation that will redirect federal, state, and local resources to provide a wider range of human services, including health care.[9] Mandates for fiscal responsibility, program accountability, and measurable outcomes will be increasingly expected.

Ethical conflicts are a continual dilemma for case managers. Those who work in primary care or vendor/gatekeeper models must balance client advocacy with cost containment.[5] Private case managers have the charge of increasing client independence, which by definition results in decreasing the need for their services.[5] Those working in the social/community arena must often confront the dilemma of the good of the many versus the good of the individual. Reasonable strategies are necessary to support ethical decision making by case managers. In many cases, these strategies remain to be developed. It is expected that these issues will ease somewhat as case management models are refined.

Alternate case management models appear to have the potential to make a significant impact on quality of care while at the same time containing spiraling health care costs. Outcomes research, however, is needed to demonstrate the actual link between these elements. Although the case management approach is increasing in popularity, nurse researchers are just beginning to examine the issues that are involved in the use of this model.[18] A comprehensive program of theory-based research using scientific designs is needed to understand and evaluate case management.[18]

REFERENCES

1. Grau L. Case management and the nurse. *Geriatr Nurs.* 1984;5:372–375.
2. Lyon J. Models of nursing care delivery and case management: clarification of terms. *Nurs Econ.* 1993;11:163–169.
3. Bower K. *Case Management by Nurses.* Washington, D.C.: American Nurses Publication; 1992.
4. Secord L. *Private Case Management for Older Persons and Their Families. Practice, Policy, Potential.* Excelsior, Minn: Interstudy, Center for Aging and Long Term Care; 1987.
5. Brault G, Kissinger L. Case management: ambiguous at best. *J Pediatr Health Care.* 1991;5:179–183.
6. Weinstein R. Hospital case management: the path to empowering nurses. *Pediatr Nurs.* 1991;17:289–293.
7. Gerber L. Case management models: geriatric nursing prototypes for growth. *J Gerontol Nurs.* 1994;20(7):18–24.
8. Rapp R, Siegal H, Fisher J. A strengths-based model of case management/advocacy: adapting a mental health model to practice work with persons who have substance abuse problems. *NIDA Res Monogr.* 1992;127:79–91.
9. Roberts-DeGennaro M. Generalist model of case management practice. *J Case Manage.* 1993;2:106–111.
10. Malloy S. Defining case management. *Home Healthcare Nurse.* 1994;12(3):51–54.
11. Bokos P, Mejta C, Mickenbert J, Monks R. Case management: an alternative approach to working with intravenous drug users. *NIDA Res Monogr.* 1992;127:92–111.
12. McCarthy E, Feldman Z, Lewis B. Development and implementation of an interorganizational case management model for substance users. *NIDA Res Monogr.* 1992;127:34–49.
13. Good M. The clinical nurse specialist in the school setting: case management of migrant children with dental disease. *Clin Nurse Specialist.* 1992;6:72–76.

14. Steele S. Nurse case management in a rural parent–infant enrichment program. In: Smith S, ed. *Issues Comprehensive Pediatr Nurs.* 1991;14:259–266.

15. Sowell R, Meadows T. An integrated case management model: developing standards, evaluation, and outcome criteria. *Nurs Adm Q.* 1994;18(2):53–64.

16. Fielo S, Crowe R. A college-managed nursing center offers training in case management for nursing students. *J Case Manage.* 1993;2:147–152.

17. Bergen A. Case management in the community: identifying a role for nursing. *J Clin Nurs.* 1994;3:251–257.

18. Lamb G. Conceptual and methodological issues in nurse case management research. *Adv Nurs Sci.* 1992;15(2):16–24.

19. Leigh B. Case management in a health maintenance organization: improving quality of care. *AAOHN J.* 1993;41:170–173.

20. Ridgely M, Willenbring M. Application of case management to drug abuse treatment: overview of models and research issues. *NIDA Res Monogr.* 1992;127:12–33.

21. Wolfe G. Cooperation or competition? Collaboration between home care & case management. *Caring Magazine.* 1993;10:52–60.

22. Lescavage N. Nurses, make your presence felt: taking off the rose-colored glasses. *Nursing Policy Forum.* 1995;1:18–21.

■ 16 ■

Relationship Building in Developing the Continuum of Care Concepts

Rhonda M. Anderson, MPA, RN, CNAA, FAAN

In the early 1990s, Hartford Hospital was faced with the challenges of the ever-changing illness care environment. Until that time, the State of Connecticut had escaped the managed care influence that had penetrated states such as California and Minnesota. Hartford Hospital's executive leadership staff were watching the nationwide changes and trends. Managed care contracting had increased. The number of citizens enrolled in HMOs was increasing nationwide. The growth from 1990 to 2000 was projected to be 23 million new enrollees.[1] This growth was leading to the development of integrated delivery systems with a community-based primary care focus. Shortell et al.[2] have researched the success factors of integrated delivery systems. System design shifts the emphasis from the hospital and keeping its beds full to a model that encompasses primary care providers, population-based planning, and facilities or services offered in less expensive sites. Outcomes based on health status seem to be the measurement tool for success or failure. The design of this new system of care, if it is architecturally sound, will allow the managed care goals in our country to be realized.

In the late 1980s, the Northeast seemed to still be spared from aggressive managed care penetration, but the signals of movement to New England in the early 1990s were very clear as one assessed the Massachusetts marketplace. Because Hartford is the insurance capital of the world, leadership people at Hartford Hospital knew the managed care missile would be redirected toward Connecticut after it hit Massachusetts. In recognition of its destiny and that it would not be spared, the executive team at Hartford Hospital embarked on a plan to develop the changes necessary to move from an illness model to a wellness model. The plan was to develop a system of care, an integrated delivery system, that was efficient and effective in patient care management.

305

To contribute effectively to the integrated delivery system, Hartford Hospital developed a new model of care that included the following important elements:

- critical paths
- health care teams
- patient care coordinators (case managers)
- outcomes measures

These elements, when organized into a new system to provide care, support the managed care companies' goals to decrease cost, maintain quality, and have the patient in the right level of care at the right time.

To begin organizing care differently, critical pathways were developed for many patient populations. At Hartford Hospital, critical pathway was defined as a tool that contains information on the timing and sequence of major therapeutic events needed to achieve agreed-on progressive patient outcomes for a specific type of patient.

In selecting patient populations for critical pathways, high-volume patient groupings by diagnosis-related group (DRG) were identified. Other criteria used in the selection of the critical path were:

- percentage of geriatric patients in that DRG
- complexity of the social problems encountered with patients in that DRG
- difficult to manage patient populations

Other variables in the critical path selection process are the present length of stay, the present cost of the cases, the opportunity to decrease the cost and length of stay, and the opportunity to manage the patient population effectively using the continuum of care.

To develop a critical path, a multidisciplinary group of providers reviewed the charts and care given to the past 50 patients of that DRG. They then determined what components of care should be rendered at what interval in the patient's episode of illness. They created a new hospital expected length of stay, as well as the pre- and posthospital transition for the patient's pathway. Demand management was identified on the prehospital side of the path to determine how patients might be managed without hospitalization. The Health Care Advisory Group, out of Washington, D.C., has identified demand management as one success factor in managed care.[3] Their research has shown that only to reengineer the inpatient acute care side without developing new screening approaches for demand of hospitalization will not improve the cost savings to the health care system.[4]

Another aspect that leads to successful management of patients is lower-cost care settings.[5] In the research conducted by the Health Care Advisory

Board, it was cited that lower-cost settings save a significant number of the dollars spent on care. Two types of settings, home care and institutional, made up 51 percent of the potential savings they were able to determine through their review of the successful new models.[5] Between demand management/care avoidance and lower-cost care settings, 83 percent of the savings can be realized.[5]

The essence of a critical path was that a multidisciplinary group of providers would develop the path. They used the benchmarking technique to gain new insight to the path of care to be designed. They would be responsible for effectively contributing to the patient care management once the path was implemented. This multidisciplinary group of providers is known at Hartford Hospital as a health care team. The team members and construct of the team vary based on the patient population. The disciplines most significantly contributing to the patients' outcomes and who have a significant number of interventions with the patient population make up the health care team. There is, however, always a nurse, physician, and patient care coordinator (case manager) for each health care team. A participant whom the team likes to have in these developmental and planning meetings is one from the agency to which this patient will transfer after discharge. If a Visiting Nurse Association or long-term care representative, or both, is a part of the critical path planning process, better decisions can be made as to length of stay and transition of patient to another level of care. An additional benefit from their participation is their readiness to accept patients once the path is operational. Many patients are going to the home setting needing more complex tasks performed for them than home care nurses have been doing in the past. Because of the agency involvement in path development, they have staff prepared with new skills to ensure the quality of patient care is not compromised in the new setting.

The team develops the pathways, monitors their effectiveness, revises them when necessary, and invites the third-party payers to participate in setting global objectives for the patient population.

Patient care coordinator is the title of Hartford Hospital's case managers. Zander[6] defines case management as an integration of services for the achievement of specific clinical, financial, and satisfaction goals. Hartford Hospital's position description for its patient care coordinator has the following expected performance outcomes:

- The clinical and fiscal health care outcomes for a specific population are a shared responsibility with the health care team.
- Patients are satisfied with care as evidenced by scores on the patient satisfaction tool and other feedback from primary health care providers.

- Admission through postdischarge placement reflects appropriate cost-effective decisions based on patient care needs.

Coile,[1] in his predictions, identifies that nurse case managers will coordinate care and delegate assignments to nonregistered nurses. The nurse case manager as a knowledgeable worker, one who assimilates data, manages care on a critical path, and helps achieve cost and quality outcomes, is the one with value-added status in the health care organization of the future. This individual will also be key in relationship management, a valued skill in today's health care environment.

RELATIONSHIP BUILDING

Many of the industries' present leaders purport that relationship building is one of the key leadership skills needed in this decade. As one reviews the environmental forces that are influencing the care delivery system and the nurse's role as a case manager, it becomes obvious that building successful relationships serves as a basis for positive outcomes for patients. The relationships are many, but this section of the chapter concentrates on four important relationships and describes the significance of each in respect to case management.

CONSUMER RELATIONSHIPS

The first relationship of importance is the consumer relationship. For too long, the consumer of illness care has been a passive recipient of care services. Clinicians have been assessing and planning the care of patients much of the time without the patient's input, knowledge, or buy-in. What happens when patients are involved? Clinicians generally find out that patients have much more knowledge about themselves and their response to illness or their beliefs about healthy life styles than the clinician has about them. This new discovery helps clinicians develop a more effective plan of care than when they isolated their approach through use of assumptions.

Transitioning clinicians' thinking to building respectful, useful relationships with the consumer should be a result of improving the patient-centered model of care. The relationship building should be centered around partnership concepts. It also should be shifting from an illness focus to a wellness focus. There are two aspects to this transitioning process. One takes place with consumer groups, the other with the individual patient.

Consumer groups, those with like interests or disease processes, should have forums or focus group opportunities to give input to the health prevention and system of care being designed for them. They should be encouraged to construct the design that is simple for them to access; one that provides them information on how to manage their own health effectively and, if they have a need to use the illness services, how to be a partner in accessing the services and reaching appropriate outcomes. The case manager can play a significant role in convening these focus groups and gathering the information. Through use of the information, the case manager influences the health care team, critical path, and institutional systems to reflect necessary changes.

In the work a case manager does with an individual consumer, the emphasis centers on mutual goal setting. This process establishes the partnership for the case manager-patient relationship. Discussion can take place about how each partner will contribute toward the mutually agreed-on outcomes of the health/illness experience. Each partner also becomes a learner and a teacher. The patients share their experiences in managing their health or chronicity. The case manager provides education to enhance and improve the patients' ability to manage themselves and builds that education on the patients' current way of managing themselves.

TEAM RELATIONSHIPS

The second relationship necessary to succeed in this new health care environment is that of the case manager and multidisciplinary team. The case manager has two significant opportunities to build successful relationships here. One opportunity is with the entire team. Generally, the case manager has the accountability to give leadership to the team. To do so effectively, good facilitation skills are needed. The case manager should be able to guide the group to work toward mutually agreed-on appropriate outcomes for an individual patient or a patient population.

Through use of continuous quality improvement techniques, the case manager can also help the team members improve their individual protocols, which, in turn, contribute to the total critical path improvement managing various patient populations. Groups or teams sometimes have members in them who hinder the group process. Some members do not participate; others may be uncooperative, disruptive, or domineering. The case manager needs to be skillful at converting these behaviors to helping roles. This transition requires behaviors that clarify, provide information, initiate discussion, encourage others to participate, or help to build consensus. If this transition can occur, each individual member will contribute to the group as it becomes a productive health care team.

A second opportunity in working with the team is the one-to-one relationship building. As the coordinator of the patient's care, it is important for the case manager to oversee and coordinate effectively the linkage of all internal resources for any given patient. If the case manager has not established respectful, trusting, open, effective communication with individual team members, the smooth coordination of care and services most likely will not occur. In turn, the individual team member must realize respect and respond to the role and function of the case manager. That function is to coordinate all providers' interventions so that the patient receives efficient coordinated care.

PAYER RELATIONSHIPS

The third significant area of relationship building is with the payers or managed care companies. Generally, these companies are looking at dollars that have been spent on individual patients or a group of patients. They are also determining how and where they will allow the future dollars to be spent. If a real paradigm shift is to occur, the emphasis cannot be only on dollars. The development of an effective system of care that has incentives for the consumer to stay well is important. Shared financial risk by payer and provider is an important principle on which to build contractual relationships. The case manager should invite participation of the managed care company in mutual determination of goals and outcomes of care for various populations. An example would be if an HMO is expecting women who have an uncomplicated pregnancy and birth to be in the hospital only 24 hours, then the mutually agreed-on process to attain the goal might be as follows:

1. All uncomplicated deliveries have a home visit for baby and mother 24 hours after hospital discharge. (Provided by the HMO.)
2. All uncomplicated deliveries have their first return to the HMO physician 2 weeks after delivery.
3. All babies are followed by the pediatrician's office through telephone follow-up for 2 weeks postdelivery.
4. All prenatal classes reinforce the goals and educate the family to their role in postdischarge care of mother and baby.

All the goals and outcomes should be incorporated into the protocols of care. The case manager must coordinate the work of the care providers accordingly and, periodically, consult the managed care companies about their level of satisfaction with the cost/quality results of a given patient population. Patient satisfaction results should be reviewed jointly so that a goal or the processes might be improved when necessary.

CONTINUUM OF CARE PROVIDER RELATIONSHIPS

The last relationship to be built and cultivated is that with various providers across the continuum of care. Those types of providers are selected by the case manager and health care team based on patient population need, payer direction, or patient choice. The charge to the team is to build effective transitions for patients to the most appropriate levels of care at the appropriate time. Generally, subacute facilities, long-term care facilities, and home health care providers are the posthospital relationships that need to be pursued. The physician's office staff, HMO clinicians, and clinic clinicians are the prehospital relationships to build. For each individual patient, the case manager may negotiate the effective transition of that patient through each component of the continuum. For patient populations, the case manager, hospital management, or the health care team may negotiate with facilities to partner with them to care for this group of patients. If the role of patient care coordinator is developed and operationalized effectively, the system of care for the client will meet the goals of the new health care environment.

To complete the Hartford Hospital successful elements of care model, outcome measures for each patient population were developed. There was a shift in focus with this model from quality indicators, which were generally process oriented, to true outcome measures.

The old quality indicators measured morbidity, mortality, and infection rates. Rarely was the quality of life or functionality of the individual measured or even identified. If patient satisfaction was an indicator, the general questions centered around satisfaction with the hotel services. All those measures listed above were fine measures in an illness system and helped us look at the hospital-related issues that could have been of concern for care givers. Our present review should not ignore those measures, but in addition, the increasingly important outcome of patients' response to illness should be reviewed. These additional measures should be evaluating functional health status. How patients adapt to their illness and its effects on their functional ability is the measurement that is most meaningful. Have the clinicians given the patient and the family the knowledge, information, and tools to respond effectively to the physical or mental challenge caused by some disease and/or social process? If our new health care system is measuring the level of health in our citizens and trying to improve on that baseline level, then functional outcomes are the appropriate yardstick.

In orthopedics at Hartford Hospital, the new system of care has been implemented. The four components—critical pathways, health care team, case management, and outcomes measurements—have really enabled the paradigm shift from providing illness care to managing hospital care in the context of a total episode of illness. The patient population selected in orthopedics was total joint replacement. Both total knee and total hip replacement were the first critical paths developed. These both met the criteria listed earlier, a large percentage of patients older than the age of 65 with long lengths of stay and charges exceeding the DRG payments.

In developing each pathway, it was decided that the patients could be partners in their care if they were included early in the process through outpatient education programs. The case manager and a nurse educator designed classes for the patients so that they knew what was going to happen to them each day of their stay. A handout (i.e., a patient education pathway that parallels the critical pathway) is given to the patient during this class. The physical therapist is an integral team member in this process. The exposure of the patient, early in the process, to a therapist who demonstrates and explains what ambulation will be occurring postoperatively is a catalyst for improved outcomes and better compliance to the expected pathway. Patients who attended the classes had a much better and predictable postoperative course. Those who did not attend tended to respond less quickly to the designed postoperative care and discharge time frame. Our data show that those patients attending the preadmission classes were 53 percent in 1993 and 58 percent in 1994. Women were the higher percentage of attendees. Table 16-1 compares length of stay for those patients participating in the class and those not attending. Those attending class have a lower length of stay each year. They also seem to be more satisfied due to their increased knowledge of what is happening and their participation in their care.

Many relationships had to be established by the case manager. A health care team was established and the members' relationships cultivated. Because the patient population was elderly, a geriatric nurse specialist joined the "typical team" of nurse case manager, orthopedic physician, social worker, physical therapist, and dietitian. This person was invaluable in helping describe appropriate expectations for these patient populations. The team identified each day's interventions and patient expectations. They crafted the ideal length of stay for each path. They also asked previous patients for their input to the proposed path. They negotiated a short time in a subacute facility with continued physical therapy intervention as a transition location between acute care and home.

Table 16-1 Class Effect on Length of Stay (LOS)

Procedure	Required LOS	
	1993	1994
Total hip replacement		
LOS with class	6.75	5.97
LOS without class	7.73	6.34
Total knee replacement		
LOS with class	6.88	5.69
LOS without class	7.88	6.52

After the proposed prehospital, hospital, and transition plan was pathed, the team discussed it with all the orthopedic physicians. After incorporating their comments and finalizing expected outcomes, the path was implemented. It was recognized by all participants that the path would need to be improved after data was collected, analyzed, and discussed. Some additional results are found in Table 16-2. Success factors in this model are:

1. organized, coordinated health care team with a case manager as the leader
2. patients as respected partners who have knowledge about and influence on their process of care leading to achievable agreed-on outcomes
3. decreased hospital demand and use of resources, leading to improved cost per case
4. functional health outcome measures that help the team monitor the quality of care and improve areas when appropriate

The orthopedic team is trying continuously to improve their system of care, critical path, and outcomes of care. They are presently working with payers to refine the goals of hospitalization for these two patient populations. They are starting a three-month, six-month, and one-year review of functional health status indicators for each patient population to determine how their process of care influences patients' abilities to restore their health.

This entire change process was not implemented in a short period of time. Preparation for the changes and incremental change took about three years. Staff education and preparation, as well as constant communication, were essential to the success of this change.

At Hartford Hospital, the case manager role was not easily accepted by staff nurses and in some cases was not embraced by any member of the health care team. Some staff wanted the case manager to do just the discharge planning for patients. Other staff thought case managers were a barrier to their collaboration with private attendings. Others thought case man-

---

Table 16-2 Cost and Length-of-Stay Outcomes

	Required LOS	
Procedure	1993	1994
Total hip replacement		
Average length of stay	6.96 days	5.09 days
Average charges	$16,545	$14,904
Total knee replacement		
Average length of stay	7.0 days	5.55 days
Average charges	$15,014	$14,387

agers should just be data collectors for variance reporting. However, in orthopedics, this role seemed to flourish in a value-added way. Staff and case manager are colleagues and enhance each other's practice. The tone and expectation was set for everyone by two key leaders in orthopedics, the nurse manager and orthopedic chief. Because of their support, expectations, coaching, and continuous improvement approach to developing the new system of care and roles to function in that system, the patient has benefited. The model for them has been a winner.

REFERENCES

1. Coile RC. Nursing trends 1995–2000: advanced practice nurses, case management, and patient-centered care. *Health Trends.* 1995;7:18.
2. Shortell SM, Gillies RR, Anderson DA, Mitchell JB, Morgan KL. Creating organized delivery systems: the barriers and facilitators. *Hosp Health Services Adm.* 1993;38:447–466.
3. Health Care Advisory Board. *The Grand Alliance, Vertical Integration Strategies for Physicians and Health Systems.* Washington, DC: The Advisory Board Company; 1993.
4. Health Care Advisory Board Governance Committee Annual Meeting: reengineering care to lessen length of stay. In: *The New American Medicine: Survey of Clinical Reform at the Frontier.* June 1995;137–142.
5. Health Care Advisory Board Governance Committee Annual Meeting: understanding the source of savings by underlying theory. In: *The New American Medicine: Survey of Clinical Reform at the Frontier.* June 1995;126–127.
6. Zander K, ed. Case management series, IV: who could be case manager? *New Definition.* 1995;10:1.

SUGGESTED READING

Aiken IH, Salmon ME. Health care workforce priorities: what nursing should do now. *Inquiry.* 1994;31:318–329.

Allred CA, Arford PH, Michel Y, et al. A cost-effectiveness analysis of acute care case management outcomes. *Nurs Econ.* 1995;13:129–136.

Argyris C. Good communication that blocks learning. *Harvard Business Rev.* 1994;72:77–85.

Curtin LL. Learning from the future. *Nurs Manage.* 1994;25:7–9.

Devers KJ, Shortell SM, Gillies RR, et al. Implementing organized delivery systems: an integration scorecard. *Health Care Manage Rev.* 1994;19:7–20.

Ellis MA, Newson T, Sudela K. Teaching parents self-care: a manager's vantage point. *J Pediatr Nurs.* 1992;7:152–153.

Kaluzny AD, Ricketts AD, Zuckerman HS. *Partners for the Dance: Strategic Alliances in Health Care.* Ann Arbor, Mich: Health Administration Press, 1995.

Lamb GS. Early lessons from a capitated community-based nursing model. *Nurs Adm Q.* 1995;19(3):18–26.

Lutz S. Hospitals continue move into home care. *Modern Healthcare.* 1993;23:28–32.

Perry J. Has the discipline of nursing developed to the stage where nurses do "think nursing"? *J Adv Nurs.* 1985;10:31–37.

■ 17 ■

Physician/Nurse Collaboration in Case Management

Rella A. Adams, PhD, RN, CNAA
Pam M. Warner, RN, CPHQ
Eric G. Six, MD, FACS, APQAURP
Ben M. McKibbens, MHA, FACHE

Collaborate is derived from the Latin word *collaborare*, which means "to labor together."[1] *Collaboration* is defined by Webster as "to work jointly with others."[2]

After defining *collaboration*, it was necessary for the authors to understand the sequence of events that enabled them to collaborate and develop nurse/physician case management and restorative care paths. There are few articles that describe collaboration between staff nurses and physicians or administrators and physicians. We found collaboration between administrators and physicians must be based on trust and mutual respect. Trust and respect are developed by working through difficult situations and finding mutually agreed-on solutions.

We discovered that collaborative behavior was initiated and strengthened through the physician/nurse liaison committee, in which the chiefs of staff and medical director worked with the senior nurse administrator to resolve clinical issues and develop the clinical areas of the hospital. The physicians and administrator had mutual respect for each other's clinical knowledge. This respect provided a common bond for communication and problem solving. Over a period of five years, we were able to collaborate and agree on solutions regarding complex issues and implement changes vital to our survival in the managed care environment.

Our first successful initiative was restorative care paths. Nurse case management soon followed as a second successful strategy. Since the implementation of nurse case management, we are planning the integration of physician case management. These successful programs are possible solely through collaboration between physicians and nurses.

COLLABORATION: A CONCEPT ANALYSIS

There are four essential elements of collaboration: attributes, antecedents, consequences, and empirical referents. For collaboration to occur, certain defining attributes and antecedents are necessary[3] (Table 17-1). The attributes describe the cooperative endeavor or joint venture aspect of collaboration based on shared power and authority. This power is based on expertise and/or knowledge and not on title or function. The persons involved are aligned by common purpose, planning, and joint decision making. Antecedents, such as persons with inherent personal qualities, which are individual readiness and confidence in their own ability, group dynamics, and environmental factors, are also necessary to support collaboration. Environmental factors include a flat organizational structure, visionary leaders who support autonomy, creativity, shared values, effective group dynamics, and commitment to mutually agreed-on goals.

The consequences are felt by the individual, group, organization, and the consumer (Table 17-1) The individual's self-worth, competence, and importance are reinforced. The group's professional cohesiveness, collegiality, and mutual respect are enhanced. The organization benefits from increased productivity and effectiveness, as well as employee satisfaction and retention. The consumer of health care receives the positive outcomes that can be achieved by a collaborative team of health professionals.

Empirical referents are structures and processes that result when the components of attributes, antecedents, and consequences are present. We consider restorative paths an empirical referent and have added it to Table 17-1. If all the above components are present in the environment, it appears that case management is the collaborative methodology by which restorative care paths would be created.

MODEL OF CLINICAL COLLABORATION

At Boston's Beth Israel Hospital, a small group of nurses and physicians pioneered a collaborative model on a hospital unit.[4] They overcame the difficulties in achieving collaboration between nurses and physicians that result from barriers such as gender, class, educational preparation, status, income, and stereotypical differences. They learned that collaboration had to be approached as a value system, not an organizational design. It is a philosophy of caring, commitment, and trust. Collaboration between nurses and physicians represents total integration. The staff at Beth Israel thought their model of collaboration improved both patient care and provider satisfaction.

The main components that Beth Israel's nurses and physicians found necessary for successful collaboration were fewer providers practicing consistently over time; nurses taking responsibility for tasks and functions formerly

Table 17-1 Elements Essential for Collaboration

Defining Attributes	Antecedents	Consequences	Empirical Referents
Joint ventures	Individual readiness (e.g., prior experience)	Supportive and nurturing environment	Multidisciplinary rounds, standards
Cooperative endeavor	Understanding and acceptance of one's own role and expertise	Reinforces confidence, self-worth, and importance	Restorative Paths*
Willing participation	Confidence in one's ability	Promotes "win-win" attitude and sense of success and accomplishment	Use of "we" versus "I" statements
Shared planning and decision making	Recognition of the boundaries of one's discipline	Esprit de corps	Dialogue between members of team
Team approach	Effective group dynamics including excellent communication skills, respect, and trust	Interprofessional cohesiveness	High scores on collaborative practice scales
Contribution of expertise	Environment with team orientation	Improved productivity and effective use of personnel	
Shared responsibility	Organizational values include participation and interdependence	Increased employee satisfaction	
Nonhierarchical relationships	Visionary leaders supportive of autonomy	Improved patient outcome	
Power is shared; based on knowledge and expertise versus role or title			

Summary of defining attributes, antecedents, consequences, and empirical references.
*Restorative care paths added by authors of this chapter.
Source: Reprinted with permission of the *Journal of Advanced Nursing,* 1995, 21, pp. 103–109.

completed by ancillary services; and involvement of experienced nurses and physicians. After one year, there were fewer patient care errors and omissions, the care delivered was unified and expedient, and patients' functional ability was better preserved and restored. Unexpected transfers to intensive care units were less frequent, and patients were less confused and apprehensive. Statistical analysis of the values that promoted collaborative behaviors showed that nurses reported changes in attitudes that supported collaboration. The physicians' response regarding these values showed a trend toward more collaborative attitudes, but it did not reach statistical significance on a collaborative practice measurement tool.[4]

PHYSICIAN/NURSE LIAISON COMMITTEE

Physician/nurse collaboration has been the foundation of a variety of important projects at Valley Baptist Medical Center. We have built on the success of these collaborative efforts to nurture and develop further strategies to be competitive in the ever-changing health care environment. The essential component of our collaborative efforts is the physician/nurse liaison committee. We did not envision these collaborative effects with the initial formation of the committee, but in retrospect, they clearly fit within the theoretical model for collaboration by Henneman et al.[3]

Within the structure of the physician/nurse liaison committee, collaboration occurs between the senior vice president of nursing and the chiefs of staff, medical director, medical board liaison, and performance improvement director. The senior vice president of nursing and the chief of staff are cochairpersons. They develop the agenda based on issues pertaining to performance improvement, utilization review, risk management, and innovations in patient care. All issues are addressed in a timely, unbiased, concerned manner. The committee has been meeting monthly for the past five years and continues to be most effective.

We also deal with complaints of unacceptable staff behavior that affect patient care or the orderly operation of the medical center. Most inappropriate behavior can be improved with education, dialogue, or letters to personal files. In the past five years, physician offenders have either modified their behavior or resigned. This collaborative effort at addressing difficult issues has resulted in trust and a functional dialogue and understanding among participants. It has driven progress and the ability to deal with other complex clinical and management problems as they occur.

The results achieved by the physician/nurse liaison committee enable us to work collaboratively on projects that are easily integrated into the patient care system through many continuous quality improvement projects. For example, the committee was not only the impetus for development of the case management plan, but it helped us coalesce the elements essential for collaboration in producing the empirical referent—the restorative care path.

FROM MANAGED CARE TO CASE MANAGEMENT

As hospitals reorganize for the new era of health care, they downsize by layoffs or attrition of higher-salaried employees first. Usually these employees are registered nurses (RNs). However, there are specialty groups of RNs who remain in demand, such as nurse practitioners, nurse midwives, certified registered nurse anesthetists, and nurse case managers.

Nurse case managers are involved in health and wellness assessment, restorative care paths, utilization management, performance improvement, informatics, and coding/billing. The concept of physician case managers is currently being planned by the chief executive officer, medical director, and senior vice president of nursing for introduction into the physician/nurse liaison committee for further development and implementation. A physician case manager, working collaboratively with a nurse case manager, is a specialist who represents a product line such as neurosurgery, orthopedics, or cardiology and oversees treatment protocols and outcomes from the restorative care paths for his or her own patients as well as those of colleagues. The physician case manager will be responsible for continuing education of colleagues related to evaluation of aggregate patient data and resource and outcome management and will assist in the development of innovative programs within the product line.

The nursing and medical professions contribute their own unique care components to the health arena by means of the medical and nursing models. The classical medical model emphasizes the diagnosis and treatment of diseases, whereas the nursing model emphasizes holistic care, prevention of illness, and health promotion. In our case, the whole, meaning the integration of both models, would be greater than the sum of its parts. The combined collaborative model of case management would "fit" any area where health care is administered. What could be more ideal and workable than the integration of the two models of care, each one contributing its own uniqueness? Physicians and nurse case managers form a team defining patient-centered, quality-driven, cost-effective care. They systematically evaluate and coordinate care across a continuum for high-risk, complex patients. This risk can be defined as an integration of both financial and clinical outcomes affecting patient care.

In the collaborative environment, communication, shared values and responsibilities, cooperation and teamwork, and mutual respect and trust between the medical and nursing professions has provided a basis from which to develop our case management plan. This collaboration is necessary in the new era of health care.

COLLABORATION IN CASE MANAGEMENT

Collaboration between case managers and physicians at Valley Baptist Medical Center demonstrates a true partnership that is necessary to improve process, outcome, and resource management. A defining attribute for collaboration between physicians and case managers is mutual respect for each other's clinical knowledge. The senior vice president of nursing, the administrative director, and the medical director agreed that the case managers must be RNs who have clinical expertise in advanced practice in their assigned area. This knowledge and experience facilitates the identification of variances within restorative care paths through medical record review and/or patient assessment. The process provides credibility for nurses when reporting findings to physicians. In fact, their judgment is valued and seldom questioned by physicians.

Nurse case managers are initially involved with patients before admission, or they otherwise review all cases as soon as possible after admission and continually follow the progress of patients through discharge. Using variance screens that show deviations from the restorative care paths and that have been jointly developed with the medical staff, the case manager identifies potential opportunities to improve patient care and brings these to the attention of the physician. This collaboration results in an immediate plan for resolution. One example is an abnormal serum potassium that has not been addressed in the progress notes or through additional treatment orders. When brought to the physician's attention, he or she will document the needed assessment and intervention so the appropriate diagnosis-related group (DRG) assignment can be made. We have supported nurse case managers documenting factual information on physician progress notes to clarify the record and justify treatment changes. The documentation and revision of the DRG improves reimbursement to the medical center and eventually to the physicians in the form of statistics. These statistics are reviewed by insurers for the purpose of deciding whether to offer physicians managed care contracts. The appropriate and timely treatment of the abnormality also improves patient care by speeding recovery and reducing the length of stay, resulting in satisfaction for the patient and the health care team. To enhance the restorative pathway system, we have developed hospitalwide protocols for variances such as hypokalemia, hyper/hypoglycemia, and heparin use.

The clinical variance screens used by the case managers are categorized by clinical, disposition, patient/family, treatment, systems, and physician variances. The clinical variance screen is presented in Exhibit 17-1. The clinical variance graph is presented in Figure 17-1. When variances are identified and not resolved on a one-to-one basis with the practitioner, the issue is brought to the attention of the physician director of that specialty. In cases in which

Exhibit 17-1 Clinical Variance Screen

A. Premature admission for tests/consults _____

B. Premature admission for preoperative day _____

C. Diagnostic test unrelated to documented diagnosis _____

D. Abnormal test result not addressed in record _____

E. Potential delay in evaluation and treatment _____

F. Potential delay in discharge _____

G. Readmission for same diagnosis _____

H. Retrospective review _____

I. Other _____

variances are identified, after peer review of the medical record the physician is issued an educational letter. An example of this is an order for a diagnostic test unrelated to a documented diagnosis. One of the most common tests ordered is a mammogram. In the past, it was considered entirely appropriate to order a routine mammogram on a middle-aged hospitalized woman. It

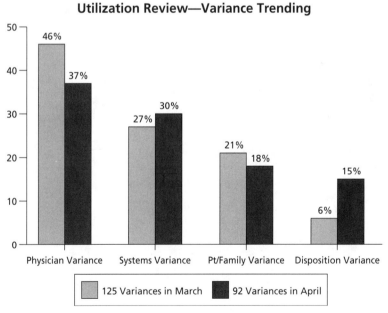

Figure 17-1 Clinical Variance Graph

was convenient for the patient, it was reimbursed by the insurance company, and it resulted in quality care because the physician knew the patient had complied to an annual screening. This is no longer possible with managed care because mammography is not reimbursed as an inpatient procedure. If the mammogram order is identified before testing, the nurse case manager can often avert the procedure through collaboration. Physicians who are unaware of the ramifications of ordering this procedure will be sent an educational letter by the peer review committee (Exhibit 17-2). Physicians welcome this information, and repetition does not occur. There are additional educa-

---

Exhibit 17-2 Example of Peer Review Committee Letter

DATE:

TO:

RE: Diagnostic Test Unrelated to Documented Diagnosis

CASE: Patient Name:

        Account Number:

        M.R. Number:

        Admission Date:

        Discharge Date:

        Room Number:

This patient had a _____ mammogram _____ during hospitalization and the test appears to be unrelated to the admission diagnosis. If possible, please document in the medical record the necessity of this test being performed as an inpatient.

Unless documentation can relate this examination to the reason for hospitalization, it is cost effective to perform this test, and any other tests that do not relate, as an outpatient.

This letter is intended to be educational to assist you in maintaining your profile for managed care contracting. No reply is necessary.

We will also provide a trending report on a quarterly basis.

Thank you for your cooperation.

Sincerely,

Medical Director

---

tional letters that address other variances, such as potential delays in evaluation and treatment, abnormal diagnostic test results not addressed in the record, and potential delays in discharge, readmission, and admission classification, such as inpatient status versus short stay observation. Written by a colleague, the letters have a friendly format and offer education and assistance to physicians to avoid quality issues and to improve their profile as they compete for managed care contracts.

We realize our current system has outlived the antiquated traditional medical staff committee structure of utilization review. We are in the process of developing physician case managers, each an expert in a particular product line. This could only be planned in the presence of a strong physician/nurse collaborative environment with the physician/nurse liaison committee.

DEVELOPMENT OF RESTORATIVE CARE PATHS

Our case management system supports the development of diagnosis-specific restorative care paths. Initially, the research and first drafts were facilitated by the case managers through collaboration with the multidisciplinary health care team. Final revision was the responsibility of the medical and nursing staffs. The orthopedic product line for hips and knees was our first effort because it represented high-volume, Medicare-reimbursed DRGs. Length of stay and resource use were two major concerns.

Two nurse case managers and the nursing unit manager of the orthopedic unit facilitated the development of restorative care paths for total joint replacements. Three orthopedic surgeons, who practice independently, do more than 550 total joint procedures each year. Motivating these three individuals and the nursing staff to collaborate as a team was a challenge. The nurses demonstrated to the surgeons the similarity of their practice patterns so that one restorative care path for total hip replacement and one for total knee replacement was possible through collaboration. The practice patterns were outlined, side by side, on a pathway. Slight variations were accommodated through a "checklist" format. When each surgeon understood that it was unnecessary to change his or her practice to accommodate another's practice, he or she agreed to a trial period for use of the restorative care path. The restorative care path is presented in Exhibit 17-3.

The case managers and nursing staff created a well-organized and effective preadmission testing and teaching (PATT) process to reduce the preoperative length of stay. They demonstrated to each orthopedic surgeon how patients could be taught in a group because practice patterns and expectations were similar. All this was accomplished through physician/nurse collaboration. The PATT outline is presented in Exhibit 17-4.

Exhibit 17-3 Restorative Care Path

KEY: ✓ = Completed; N/A = Not Applicable; 0 = Variance	Initial	Signature/Credentials	Initial	Signature/Credentials
PAGE 1 of 2 VBMC 1612-004-1294				
DRG: 209/210 ELOS: 4 days DX 1: ☐ Total Knee Arthroplasty ☐ Total Hip Arthroplasty				
		Case Manager		RN

Special Considerations:

	Pre-Admit/Date:	Day 1/OR/Date:	Day 2/POD 1/Date:
	RN Review	RN Review	RN Review
Consults:	___ Identify/notify family MD ___ Diabetic education ___ Dietitian ___ Notify anesthesia	___ Inform family MD of pt on floor post-op	⟶
Tests:	___ CBC, Chem-8, pro time, PTT, UA ___ CXR, ECG ___ Pulmonary function if indicated ___ T&C ___ units for surgery on ___ ___ Call MD/surgeon for abnormals	___ Obtain lab reports from O.P. ___ Stat x-ray in RR prn ___ Lab work in RR stat ___ Stat glucometer if DM	___ CBC, pro time

Exhibit 17-3 continued

| Assessments and Evaluations: | _____ Complete data base
_____ List allergies
_____ List home meds
_____ Check permit for

_____ Blood: ❑ Autologous
           ❑ Blood bank | _____ Encourage bilateral ankle
      dorsiflexion of 2° while awake
_____ Neurovascular checks _____ q 4 h
_____ CMS checks
_____ Vital signs: q 15 min × 1 h, q 30
      min × 2 hr; q 1 h × 4 h, then q 4
      h until stable | _____ ⟶
_____ ⟶
_____ ⟶
_____ Vital signs q 4 h |
| Activity: Safety
(PT, PPI) | _____ Pre-op assessment
_____ Orient to environment
_____ Identify PPI level
_____ See patient teaching plan | _____ Bed rest
_____ Apply monkey bars & trapeze to
      bed
_____ Turn q 2 h

                    PPI_____ | _____ Knee
_____ CPM application 0–40"

_____ Hip
Begin gait training in afternoon
Patient up in chair (knee/hip)
Up in chair
ROM slings
                PPI_____ |

Note: The example of the restorative care path for total hip represents only page 1 of 2 pages.
Source: Courtesy of Valley Baptist Medical Center, Harlingen, Texas.

Exhibit 17-4 Preadmission Testing and Teaching—Total Joint Replacement

Policy:	Patients scheduled for elective surgery will receive preoperative testing and teaching as an outpatient at least 72 hours before surgery.
Purpose:	To maintain quality care, ensure complete patient preparation, reduce length of stay, improve outcome, and increase satisfaction through a multidisciplinary approach.
Procedure:	1. Patient is scheduled by the physician's office through the admissions office.
	2. Telephone contact is made to the patient by case manager to verify appointment.*
	3. All scheduled patient and family members arrive at 8:00 A.M. on Thursday morning.
	4. Case managers greet patients and arrange laboratory, x-ray, ECG testing as needed.
	5. Admission data base assessment is completed by case managers.
	6. Group teaching begins at 10:00 A.M.
	—Case managers
	—Anesthesia
	—Physical therapy
	7. Case managers allow for questions and give final instructions before dismissal.
	8. All preoperative data are analyzed by the case manager and abnormalities are reported to the surgeon.
	9. The medical record is assembled and ready for the A.M. admission on the day of surgery.

*Patients are told to bring medications. Primary language spoken is verified to individualize teaching because Spanish is available.
Source: Courtesy of Valley Baptist Medical Center, Harlingen, Texas.

When the PATT process was ready for implementation, the case managers and the nurse coordinator held an educational luncheon for all the orthopedic surgeons' office managers. These office managers influence their physicians to support changes in the medical center's patient care process that are beneficial to patients. The office personnel enjoyed the luncheon, participated in the education session, and mutually agreed to do their best to make the PATT program a success. In fact, one office manager was so impressed that she made a telephone call to the senior vice president of nursing to praise the case managers and the nurse coordinator.

The diagnosis-specific, rather than physician-specific, restorative care paths and the PATT process have been in place for one year. The orthopedic multidisciplinary team has demonstrated a reduction in length of stay from 8.9 to 5.1 days for total hip replacement and from 9.2 to 4.7 days for total knee replacement. The success of this project can be attributed to physician/ nurse collaboration through case management.

Having learned from this experience, we have subsequently developed other multidisciplinary restorative care paths along equally collaborative lines. One example of this is the stroke protocol. This consists of stroke algorithm, stroke orders, and a stroke restorative care path. It also involves the patient's care and progress through admission in the emergency department, primary care physician, specialist referral, and subsequent rehabilitation.

The stroke protocol was developed collaboratively by representatives from rehabilitation, case managers, dietary, speech pathology, emergency department, and physicians. All these professionals are experts in their respective areas, mutually trusting and respecting one another. Protocols were generated to be practical, cost effective, educational, and flexible with favorable patient outcomes as the goal. (The stroke protocol is presented in Appendix 17-A.)

The stroke protocol naturally led to a carotid endarterectomy product line. Among the strategies, one was to review carefully itemized billings for multiple patients who had surgery, searching for the "ideal" treatment plan. By reviewing cost, length of stay, standing orders, and physician routine orders with a multidisciplinary collaborative group, each willing to accept and contribute critique, we were able to relearn and revise our thinking. For example, we discovered that:

1. Standing orders developed years ago, even though revised annually, were very cost ineffective and deserved more careful scrutiny.
2. Routine orders must be carefully reviewed. Without cutting corners that may jeopardize patient care, a set of minimum orders can be created to fit the ideal patient. These orders must be flexible according to clinical indications.
3. Physicians and nurses must work collaboratively with each patient/family, and these clinicians must be willing to pay closer attention to the patient than ever before.
4. Case managers must be involved in PATT, along with the primary care physician, internist, and surgeon. All these professionals must concentrate on a preselected but flexible restorative care path reinforcing patient expectations and improved outcomes.
5. The plan can be successful through correlation of cost-effectiveness and patient outcome if physicians, case managers, and all staff members work collaboratively, pay attention to detail, and are flexible with individual patients and trust each other's judgment.

We are fortunate to be able to work with each product line electively, developing clinical pathways for the ideal patient, and molding our own restorative care paths without managed care organizations providing nonclinical judgments that focus solely on cost.

CONCLUSION

Administrators and clinicians in health care institutions face the new business of managed care with trepidation. We know there will be changes that include using fewer human and material resources and adjustments to increased competition. As we strive to become more efficient and cost effective, there will be sacrifices and trade-offs. Decisions made by health care leaders will differ as the external and internal variables are analyzed at a micro and macro level for business. The financial and clinical sectors of the health care institution must become interdependent. Physician/nurse collaboration in case management is one step leading to the integration of fiscal and clinical outcomes. The future is just beginning.

REFERENCES

1. *Webster's Third New International Dictionary.* Springfield, Mass.: Merriam-Webster, Inc.; 1986.
2. The New Merriam-Webster Dictionary. Springfield, Mass: Merriam-Webster, Inc.; 1989.
3. Henneman EA, Lee JL, Cohen JI. Collaboration: a concept analysis. *J Adv Nurs.* 1995;21: 103–109.
4. Pike AW, Alpert HB. On the scene. *Nurs Clin North Am.* 1994;18:10–15.

Appendix 17-A
Stroke Protocol

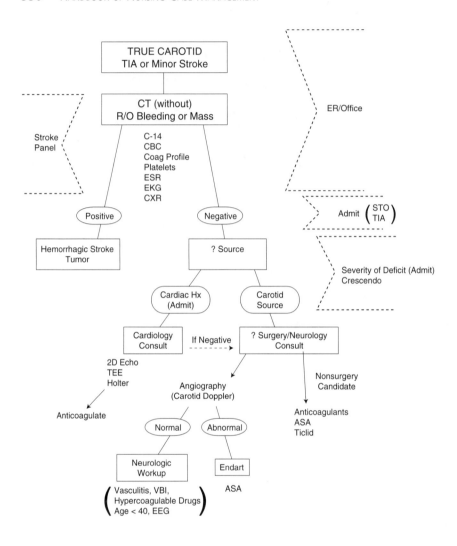

Figure 17-A-1 Algorithm for Management of TIA or Minor Stroke. *Source:* Courtesy of Valley Baptist Medical Center, Harlingen, Texas.

Exhibit 17-A-1 Admission/Daily Orders—Minor Stroke/TIA

DAY 1—ADMISSION DAY

1. Neurology Consult (specify) _____ MD
2. Cardiology Consult (specify) _____ MD
3. Neuro signs every two (2) hours.
4. Bedrest, elevate head of bed 30 degrees.
5. NPO (no food, fluids or medications) until bedside dysphagia test done per nursing. Diet consistency to be recommended by Nursing after dysphagia test within the following nutritional parameters: _____
6. ❑ Alternating pressure stockings
   ❑ TED stockings—thigh high
7. Spot pulse oximeter - if O_2Sat <92%, use oxygen per protocol.
8. IV—LR at _____ cc/hour.
9. I&O every eight (8) hours.
10. F/C
11. Turn every two (2) hours.
12. Suction prn.
13. Medications:
    _____
    _____
    _____
    _____
    _____
    _____
14. BP parameters: _____
    _____
15. Lab: _____
    _____
16. Radiology: _____
    _____
17. Social Service to evaluate.
18. Physical Therapy to evaluate.
19. Occupational Therapy consult for evaluation.
20. Speech and Language consult for evaluation.
21. Ensure the following tests were completed in ER:
    CBC, platelets, pro time, PTT, Sed Rate, Chem 14, EKG, Chest X-Ray, CT head with/without contrast if needed.

Date _____ Time_____

_____ MD

continues

Exhibit 17-A-1 continued

DAY 2

1. Neuro signs and v.s. every four (4) hours.
2. Saline Lock IV.
3. Dangle, progress to chair BID per nursing—monitor BP.
4. Physical Therapy to treat and progress activity as tolerated.
5. Occupational Therapy to treat and progress activity as tolerated.
6. Speech Therapy to treat and progress activity as tolerated.
7. Diet consistency per S/LP in collaboration with RD if dysphagia symptoms present.
8. If continued NPO, insert N/G tube and begin N/G feedings per dietitian's recommendations.
9. Docusate sodium & casanthranol 100 mg/30 mg P.O. or N/G BID.
10. Lab: _____
Date _____ Time_____
_____ MD

DAY 3

1. Chair TID per nursing at meals.
2. D.C. foley, offer bedpan/urinal every 2-4 hours.
3. Check for BM. Bisacodyl Supp. 10 mg rectally, if no BM.
4. Repeat CT with and without contrast.
5. Weigh patient if not eating.
6. Rehab to evaluate.
7. Discharge Planning.
8. Lab: _____
Date _____ Time_____
_____ MD

DAY 4

1. Social Services / Discharge Planning to review options with patient/family.
2. Progress to ambulation.
3. Lab: _____
Date _____ Time_____
_____ MD

DAY 5

Discharge: ❑ Rehab   ❑ Home   ❑ Nursing Home
Date _____ Time_____
_____ MD

Source: Courtesy of Valley Baptist Medical Center, Harlingen, Texas.

Exhibit 17-A-2 Restorative Care Path—Minor Stroke/TIA

KEY: ✓ = Completed; N/A = Not Applicable; 0 = Variance	Initial	Signature/Status	Initial	Signature/Status
PAGE 1 of 2 VBMC 1615-034-0595				
DRG: ELOS: DX 1:				
			Case Manager	
				RN

Special Considerations: Admit to: ☐ Telemetry ☐ Non-Monitored Bed

	Day 1 Date:	Day 2 Date:	Day 3 Date:	Day 4 Date:	Day 5 Date:	Expected Outcomes
	RN Review	RN Review	RN Review	RN Review	RN Review	
Consults	Neurology Cardiology Surgery		Rehab to evaluate			Consults complete
Tests:	Ensure stroke panel was done in ER		Repeat CT Scan with and without contrast			Lab results within expected norms
Assessments & Evaluations:	Visual field assessment per nursing Bedside dysphagia test per nursing	Observe for increase temp or signs of pneumonia	Check for BM →	→	→	Assessments complete No evidence of pneumonia Prevention of constipation VS & NS within expected norms
	VS & NS q 2 hrs	VS & NS q 4 hrs	→	→	→	

continues

Exhibit 17-A-2 continued

	Day 1 Date: RN Review	Day 2 Date: RN Review	Day 3 Date: RN Review	Day 4 Date: RN Review	Day 5 Date: RN Review	Expected Outcomes
Activity: Safety (PT, PPI)	Bedrest × 24 hrs with HOB elevated 30°	Dangle/chair bid per nursing, monitor BP	Dangle/chair tid per nursing at meals	→	↑	Tolerates activity as ordered
	Turn q 2°	Turn q 2° when in bed ↑	↑	↑	↑	Skin integrity intact
	PT to eval	PT to treat & progress	↑	→ Ambulation	↑	Progressing with transfers and ambulation
Treatment (OT, Speech, Resp., Blood, Dressing Changes, Catheters, Drains, Pain Management, etc.):	OT consult for eval	OT to treat & progress	↑	↑	↑	Progressing with self-care and communication skills
	Speech & Language consult for eval	S/LP to treat & progress ↑	↑	↑	↑	
	F/C prn	↑	D.C. F/C - BRP q 2–4 hrs	↑	↑	Voiding sufficiently
	Suction prn	↑	↑	↑	↑	Maintaining adequate oxygenation
	Spot pulse oximeter— if O$_2$ < 92%, use O$_2$ per protocol					
	I&O q 8 hrs	↑	↑	↑	↑	I&O within expected norms
	TED stockings—thigh high	↑	↑	↑	↑	Absence of DVT
	If impaired swallowing: • Position at 60–90° for meals					

Exhibit 17-A-2 continued

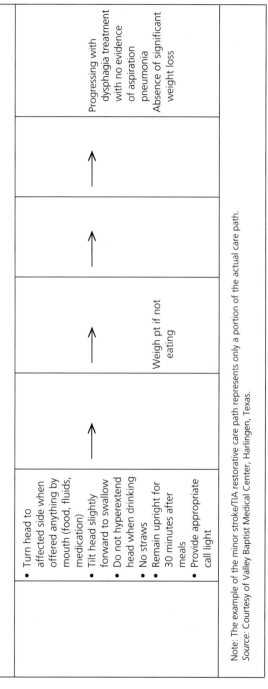

• Turn head to affected side when offered anything by mouth (food, fluids, medication) • Tilt head slightly forward to swallow • Do not hyperextend head when drinking • No straws • Remain upright for 30 minutes after meals • Provide appropriate call light	→	→	→	→
	Weigh pt if not eating			Progressing with dysphagia treatment with no evidence of aspiration pneumonia Absence of significant weight loss

Note: The example of the minor stroke/TIA restorative care path represents only a portion of the actual care path.
Source: Courtesy of Valley Baptist Medical Center, Harlingen, Texas.

■ 18 ■

Managed Care and the World of Capitated Payment

Leanne M. Hunstock, MBA, MEd, RN, CS, CNAA

Although many foreign countries have long histories of government-sponsored medical care and universal health care coverage for citizens, these are relatively new phenomena for the United States. The major thrust for health care reform has been as a direct result of the spiraling health care cost this nation has borne over the past 30 years. In 1950, health care spending comprised only 3.8 percent of the gross domestic product (GDP). Without significant reform, expenditures are projected to reach approximately 18 percent by the year 2000 and a staggering 32 percent of the GDP by the year 2030.[1] The forecasters are divided on the potential effect of reform. Some say that the Hawthorn effect is in part responsible for the reduction in health care inflation. In 1992, health care price inflation stood at 7.4 percent and fell to 5.4 percent in 1993.[1] This descending shift in the inflation of costs causes some to declare that health care cost is making the needed adjustments without outside intervention.

EVOLUTION OF MANAGED CARE AND THE CAPITATED PAYMENT SYSTEM

Currently, the health care market reflects four major reimbursement structures:

1. Fee-for-service and cost-based reimbursement is based on a charge or cost for service.
2. Per diem reimbursement is based on a contracted daily rate.
3. Per case reimbursement is a fixed rate based on a procedure, diagnosis, or other pricing factor that is used in determining the per case rate.

4. Capitation is a reimbursement system that is based on a predetermined and negotiated amount of money per covered person to be paid for a specific period of time that will not vary over the course of the contract based on volume of services provided. The capitated payment system dominates the health care marketplace and puts the provider(s) in the capitated arrangement "at risk." The term *at risk* refers to the potential for financial loss that the provider(s) bears if the costs exceed the fixed contracted income.

Managed care and capitation have evolved through some significant changes in the health care industry over the past two decades. The health care provider-consumer relationship has been changing rapidly and radically since the 1980s when the cost-based reimbursement system drove up demand for services. During this turbulent period, the supply of services flooded the market while rising costs were reimbursed as charged. When the services outpriced themselves, the market had to adjust. The largest adjustment came when Medicare, the major purchaser of health care services, determined that costs were an untenable burden and were continuing to rise at an accelerated rate. High demand for alternative lower-cost treatment models such as the ambulatory, nonresidential, and primary practitioner office settings drove the growth of such services. Reform of the Medicare reimbursement system, particularly for inpatient hospitalization, served as a catalyst for many of the changes in the private sector's third-party reimbursement stream. Medicare's restructuring of its reimbursement policies influenced the private sector to contract with providers who met pricing criteria. Contracting restricted consumers in their choice of physician and hospital and exposed the commercially insured consumer to limitations previously experienced only by early HMOs and military plans. The competition for contracts drove competitive pricing down and drove competition for new service development up to capture full-service contracts and avoid carve-out contracts, which covered only specific services such as obstetrics or mental health.

Hospitals created large marketing departments with large budgets in an effort to attract the fee-for-service patients who were free to choose their physician and hospital. This population included Medicare patients and the commercially insured, who could choose their provider and hospital despite some limitations imposed through contracting. Hospital-based customer-oriented services and programs sprang up to capture market loyalty to specific hospitals and physicians. These programs provided a variety of free health prevention, education, assistance with insurance claims, and even recreational services to its members. Public relations departments evolved into sophisticated health care marketing divisions and became a professional specialty. In many cases, the marketing department evolved into a contracting department. The contracting, marketing, and finance departments spawned a health care hybrid division called the managed care division. This flurry of activity and rapid turbulent change has continued to drive changes in the health care industry.

EVOLUTION OF INTEGRATION

The transition from a free-market, open, charge-based, reimbursement system to a managed care system is evident at all levels and in all regions across the country. The degree of integration of delivery systems and maturity in managed care is highly variable and evolves along a developmental continuum. Integrated delivery systems are being developed in many markets in an attempt to deliver high-quality, cost-effective, and appropriate medical care.

In the 1980s, the most visionary hospitals and provider entities began to enter an arena previously dominated by investor-owned hospital chains, religiously affiliated hospitals, and a very few pioneer HMOs. They began to identify other organizations with whom they could partner to establish provider networks or loosely affiliated groups of providers who could offer a marketwide contracting group. Formal alliances were cautiously formed. This approach evolved into the integrated delivery networks (IDN) or integrated delivery systems (IDS), which took the provider network configuration to the next level and expanded the affiliations to include clinics, long-term care facilities, and a variety of additional service selections to provide the contractor with a "one-stop shopping" opportunity. The one-stop shopping feature was intended to provide convenience for the patient, better management of utilization, reduction of service duplication, and better management of information across the continuum. This integration should lead to better efficiency, a better quality of care, and lower cost.

The IDN/IDS is probably the most sophisticated level of integration to date, incorporating the physician and other professional providers into the network. This configuration allows the hospital and provider to join together and to reduce cost by administering their own claims and utilization review collections. Another alternative is for the IDN/IDS to function essentially as a subcontracted provider for HMOs and other health plans. A 1994 survey of hospital and health network leaders found that 71 percent said their organizations belong to or are in the process of organizing IDSs. Eighty-one percent reported that their hospitals would not operate as stand-alone institutions within five years.[2] Integration focuses accountability into a single point at the network level. The integrated network has been recognized by the Joint Commission on Accreditation of Healthcare Organizations as an important and separate designation for accreditation.[3] The IDN/IDS can take many forms and configurations depending on the market, the need for services, and the sophistication of the individual entities in understanding the benefits of aligning of both the services and the financial incentives.

STAGES OF MARKET EVOLUTION

The nation continues its evolution on a continuum with various regions of the country evolving into more mature managed care markets. This market evolution was chronicled through a study performed by the University Hospital Consortium and APM, Incorporated Management Consultants. The evolution of managed care markets is illustrated by four primary stages with a fifth stage recently identified as the stage IV markets evolve to a new level (Figures 18-1 through 18-3).

The stage I market is *unstructured,* with hospitals, physicians, employers, and HMOs operating independently in a fee-for-service payment system. Pur-

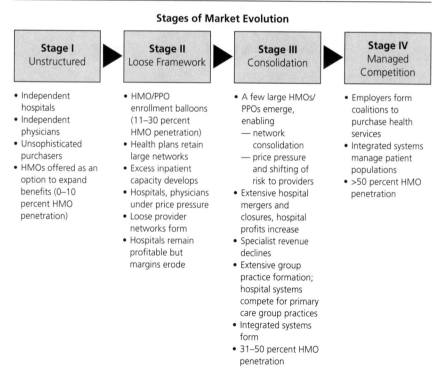

Figure 18-1 Stages of Market Evolution. *Source:* Courtesy APM Inc. © 1992, University Hospital Consortium and APM Incorporated Management Consultants.

Stages of Market Evolution

	Characteristics	Provider Pricing	Basis for Health Care Purchasing
Stage I **Unstructured**	• Independent hospitals, physicians, employers, and HMOs	Fee-for-service	• Encounter, cost of claim • Volume
Stage II **Loose** **Framework**	• Lead HMOs or PPOs emerge, loose provider networks and weak hospital affiliations form • Excess inpatient capacity develops • Hospital discounts widen	Discount, per diem	• Encounter, cost of claim
Stage III **Flux and** **Consolidation**	• Lead HMOs/PPOs achieve critical mass, begin to consolidate; hospital systems form; aggressively recruit/compete for primary care group practices • Selective contracting by major purchasers • Development of large multispecialty, primary care, and IPA groups • Development of large multispecialty, primary care, and IPA groups • Specialist practices underused; discounts increase • Beds closed as hospitals seek to eliminate excess capacity	Per diem, per case, physician capitation	• Cost per covered life per health plan • Integration
Stage IV **Managed** **Competition**	• Purchasers contract with integrated hospital/physician systems to provide comprehensive services to their beneficiaries • Shift of financial risk to primary medical groups/provider networks • Very strong incentives for beneficiaries to use contract network (extensive channeling) • Capitation model becomes prevalent	Stage III plus capitation	• Beneficiary health status, total health care costs

Figure 18-2 Stages of Market Evolution—Characteristics. *Source:* Courtesy APM Inc. © 1992, University Hospital Consortium and APM Incorporated Management Consultants.

chasing of care is based on the number of each type of encounter, cost of the claim, and volume. This market type is throughout the Midwest and the eastern United States.

The stage II market is described as a *loose framework*. This is the predominant market stage for most of the country, with the greatest concentration in the Midwest and the south central and southeastern portion of the nation. In

MARKET EVOLUTION UPDATE

I. Unstructured	II. Loose Framework	III. Consolidation	IV. Managed Competition
Galveston	Louisville	Orange, CA	San Diego
Nassau	Miami	Milwaukee	Minneapolis/St. Paul
Omaha	Fort Worth	Portland	Los Angeles
Syracuse	Cincinnati	San Francisco/Oakland	Worcester
Little Rock	Dallas	San Jose	
Gainesville	Tampa/St. Petersburg	Detroit	
Birmingham	Columbus	Sacramento	
Chapel Hill (Triangle)	Atlanta	Denver	
Charleston, SC	Jacksonville	Boston	
Newark	Orlando	Madison	
Harrisburg	Cleveland	Tucson	
Middlesex, NJ	Hartford	Salt Lake City	
Shreveport	St. Louis	Riverside/San	
Winston-Salem	Baltimore	Bernardino	
Augusta	New York City	Phoenix	
Columbia, MO	Kansas City	Seattle	
Greenville, NC	Ann Arbor	Providence	
Morgantown	New Orleans	Washington, D.C.	
Iowa City	Indianapolis	Houston	
Charlottesville	Richmond	Albany	
	Toledo	Chicago	
	Lexington	Ft. Lauderdale	
	Oklahoma City		
	San Antonio		
	Nashville		
	Pittsburgh		
	Philadelphia		
	New Haven		

Figure 18-3 National Market Classifications Update. *Source:* Courtesy APM Inc. © 1995, 1993, 1992, University Hospital Consortium and APM Incorporated Management Consultants.

---

this market, HMOs or preferred provider organizations (PPOs) begin to emerge as a key force in the market, using their large enrollments to leverage price and contracting. Inpatient utilization levels off, and excess inpatient capacity develops. Pricing pressure produces larger physician and hospital discounts as margins erode.

In the stage III market, *consolidation* begins to emerge as the leading HMOs and PPOs achieve critical mass and begin to consolidate. At the same time, hospitals form systems and networks. Physicians consolidate into group practices, and while hospitals aggressively recruit and compete for primary care groups and practitioners, pricing is based on per diem, per case, and physician capitation through the PPO. The cost per a covered life is the basis for health care purchasing and the availability for integrated services to be provided through a single transaction or contract. This market is emerging in the Pacific Northwest, northern California, the eastern seaboard, and the south Florida regions of the country.

The stage IV market is one in which *managed competition* and capitation are prevalent. There are only a few markets that have reached this level of evolution. They are San Diego and Los Angeles in Southern California, Minneapolis/St. Paul, Minnesota, and Worcester, Massachusetts. In these markets, purchasers contract with integrated delivery systems to provide comprehensive health care services to their beneficiaries. The integrated hospital and physician systems contract with the purchasers to accept financial risk for managing service utilization. Capitation or contracting for a set fee to provide comprehensive care for the specific population is the prevalent model. Capitation shifts the financial risk to the provider network and the primary care group.

More recently, a fifth stage in the managed care market evolution has been identified (Figure 18-4). This stage is characterized by some significant transition discomforts, such as the unraveling of capitation and unsustainable prices, reimbursement based on approved treatment protocols, and the lack of support for education or research. These transition discomforts will drive restructuring of the delivery systems to an end stage. In this stage, we will see networks and insurers forming partnerships, cost reductions resulting from duplicate network management will increase shared margins, and specialists will move into primary care resulting in primary care physician overcapacity. We may also see the academic health center holding an advantage in new technology that reduces utilization, and very large systems will sustain education and research support at a low cost.

SUCCESS FACTORS IN THE WORLD OF CAPITATED PAYMENT

Success in capitated markets requires organizations to meet a new set of competencies. According to Reynolds, "The key to successful integration is to strike a balance between the three essential players: physicians, hospitals and health plans. The equilibrium between these elements must be maintained through common management and financial incentives so they can appropriately match medical resources with the needs of payers and patients."[2]

With the integrated delivery system, there is a new level of complexity. The system must develop an appropriate panel of providers, a broad continuum of services, coverage of the regional market, acceptance of capitated reimbursement, and management of their risk through managing expenses and resource utilization. Coordinating patient care and medical services within an

Transition Discomforts		End Game (of Stage V)

- Unraveling of capitation and unsustainable prices/excess capacity (beds and specialists) finally wrung out
- Daily make/buy decisions on carve-out contracts
- No insurance for unapproved protocols
- No support for education or research

- Networks with market share force true partnerships with insurers
- Duplicated network management costs become shared margins
- Each provider focuses on unique competencies
- Specialist delivery of "primary" chronic/high-risk care—PCP overcapacity
- Academic health center advantage in new technology that decreases PMPM cost
- Very large systems sustain education and research support (at very low unit cost)
- Government intervention on education costs?

Figure 18-4 Stage V? *Source:* Courtesy APM Inc. © 1995, University Hospital Consortium and APM !ncorporated Management Consultants.

operating unit and across care settings such as the hospital, the physician's office, and the home requires the management point to be with the primary physician who is most often the patient's only consistent provider. One challenge of this complex joint effort is a single point of accountability for quality care and financial performance. This requires the components or operating units such as hospitals, physician offices, primary care providers and specialists clinics, pharmacies, laboratories, and other diagnostic services to understand the relationship among themselves and their counterparts. The relationships depend heavily on a foundation of a primary care physician gatekeeper model, because the physician's decisions influence resource utilization. The provider(s) must manage successfully the financial resources received in all settings.

USING CASE MANAGEMENT EFFECTIVELY TO MANAGE CLINICAL RESOURCES

Without a solid system of managing the patient and services in the least intensive and least restrictive setting, the resources, particularly in a capitated reimbursement system, can be quickly consumed. Because capitated reimbursement requires control over resource utilization, a means for managing these resources is necessary. Bower[4] defines case management as

> a clinical system that focuses on the accountability of an identified individual or group for coordinating a patient's care (or group of patients) across a continuum of care; insuring and facilitating the achievement of quality, clinical and cost outcomes; negotiating, procuring and coordinating services and resources needed by the patient/family; intervening at key points (and /or when significant variance occurs) for individual patients; addressing and resolving patterns in aggregate variances that have a negative quality-cost impact; creating opportunities and systems to enhance outcomes.[4]

Case management systems are commonly built on a framework of standards, outcomes, and protocols. The protocols and interventions are designed to reach those predetermined outcomes that are derived from consensus-based standards. A case management system can make a significant difference in managing and coordinating the clinical resources available for the patient.

At Stanford University Hospital in Palo Alto, California, the case management system is credited with saving the hospital nearly $15 million between 1990 and 1992.[5] The Stanford model places an emphasis on utilization review and discharge planning and features strong interaction between the clinical staff and the financial staff.[5]

Case management is enhanced when a comprehensive approach that includes the thorough understanding of the organization's clinical resource utilization and, subsequently, the organization's management of that resource utilization in the most effective and efficient manner is in effect. Zander[6] suggests that case management can provide a framework for organizational restructuring. This process is described as reengineering from current practice to best practice and finally to ideal practice as a means to improve care, practice, and operations continuously.[6] The search for and incorporation of targets for best practice and ideal practice into the case management system may be determining factors for reimbursement contracting in the future. In the early development phases, most case management approaches are limited to the use of critical pathways or other tools to assist various care givers to coordinate and sequence the care-based current practice in one or two settings. In the capitated environment, the scope of case management needs to reflect the scope of the delivery system and services provided under the contract. The ability of the case management system to provide a well-integrated and seamless utilization and care management function will be critical to the successful utilization of resources. Case management across all care settings within an IDS/IDN is a model for managing resources that is not yet fully evolved but may become the prevalent approach in the industry due to the ability to align with the two large utilization sources, the primary physician and the hospital.

The next level of clinical resource management augments case management with population-based care management that targets more than disease states, seeking to prevent common conditions from exacerbating out of control. Lumsdon[7] describes "disease management" as another dimension of case management that reflects the industry's effort to involve all disciplines. In this case, the use of terminology such as disease management appeals more to physicians who are sometimes reluctant to use other approaches. The objective in disease management is to focus on the key access point of the continuum, the physician. This enables patient case scrutiny based on disease management protocols before use of the most expensive utilization level in the continuum, the hospital. Although similar in process to case management's critical pathway, the disease process approach is physician driven and comes at a time when managed care is shifting from a cost or price focus to a quality focus and true outcome management. The issue of quality in managed care calls again for a sophisticated interplay of quality drivers and indicators that are measured across the integrated network continuum. The coordination alone of the data for all the areas the industry measures has become so burdensome that the data lose their impact. Data can only be useful once they are analyzed, reconfigured, and measured by function across the continuum and focused at the access to care points such as the physician's office, the hospital, the educational arena, home care, and within the health plan itself. In the new scenarios, there is also a need to examine the patient's experience within the plan, network, and systems, including coordination of services, communication, and care planning. Additionally, mechanisms for ensuring the integrity, validity, and confidentiality of patient-related data must be designed and implemented across the continuum.

MODEL FOR INTEGRATION, CAPITATION, AND SUCCESSFUL OUTCOMES

Friendly Hills Health Care Network is a successful, fully integrated health care network located in Southern California. Friendly Hills is a large provider in the Medicare managed care market. It is innovative in care planning and provision, as well as early intervention. For example, they initiate early access to services as a preventive measure to reduce usage of high-cost services. The network manages resources through the use of five geriatric nurse practitioners who visit patients in nursing homes several times a week, thus reducing physician visits, emergency department visits, and hospitalization. In addition, there are four clinical nurse specialists whose roles cross seven access points of care—primary prevention, ambulatory, acute hospitalization, tertiary, home care, long-term care, and hospice care. The network also uses assessment information from its own HMO and other HMOs it contracts with to identify high-risk patients or recently hospitalized patients. The initiative is taken to have the patient seen by a physician to assess the patient and determine prevention strategies.[8] By adopting early intervention strategies and a managed care product that provides all the levels of care required for their population, Friendly Hills Health Care Network is able to manage successfully its fully capitated resources.

CONCLUSION

The future of managed care looks bright for those entities that have adopted a strategy exemplifying the following key success factors:

- a strong value for the quality of long-term relationships among the core components of health system; the physician, the health plan, and the provider entities
- a broad and comprehensive network of providers or services that are linked through a strong centralized monitoring, control, and communication system
- their own HMO or health plan or strategic alliances that emulate this relationship for the purpose of securing patient flow
- total quality management culture with a clear and appropriate, functional process-oriented quality indicator system that evaluates and improves important functions and processes across the full continuum and within each component
- alignment of financial and clinical systems and resources with appropriate incentives for prevention and utilization management
- a value for quality outcome, prevention, and health maintenance in the community
- a comprehensive system for clinical resources management that is used by a multidisciplinary team and is reflective of best practices and other benchmarks in the field

REFERENCES

1. Solovy A. Taming the tiger, the economics of health care reform: an H&HN study. *Hosp Health Networks.* 1994;68:26–34.

2. Reynolds JX. Cited by: Bartling AC. Integrated delivery systems: fact or fiction. *Health Care Executive.* 1995;10(3):7–11.

3. Sandrick K. Network & numbers, is accreditation slow to change with the times? *Hosp Health Networks.* 1995;69(11):56–57.

4. Bower K. Care over the continuum: nursing case management for continuous quality improvement. Presented at the meeting for American Organization of Nurse Executives: April 27, 1993; Orlando, Fla.

5. Bean B, ed. Is case management the answer to coping with managed care? *Hosp Case Manage.* 1993;1:104–105.

6. Zander K. CareMap systems and case management: creating waves of restructured care. In *Reengineering Nursing and Health Care: The Handbook for Organizational Transformation.* Blancett S, Flarey D, eds. Gaithersburg, Md: Aspen Publishers, Inc.; 1995:203–222.

7. Lumsdon K. Disease management; the heat and headaches over retooling patient care create hard labor. *Hosp Health Networks.* 1995;69(7):34–36.

8. Cerne F. Rehabbing medicare, is managed care a cure-all or just a crutch? *Hosp Health Networks.* 1995;69(8):23–26.

■ 19 ■

Working with Managed Care Networks: Strategies for Success

Marilyn D. Harris, MSN, RN, CNAA, FAAN
Sharon A. Lynch, MSN, RN

Providing home care services to clients who are enrolled with managed care health insurance companies creates unique issues and challenges for both clinical and administrative staff of home care agencies. Clinical issues are related to understanding what managed care is and how it affects the way home care staff must adapt to provide reimbursable services to clients. Improved verbal and written communication between the payer case manager (PCM) and the home care case manager (HCCM) is the key to a successful collaborative relationship.

Administrative issues deal with both cost and quality of patient care. Acceptable reimbursement methods must be negotiated. A data collection and evaluation system must be in place to track, measure, and report patient outcomes. Agency administrators must be able to sort the available data to meet the needs of the home care agency's administrative staff and to respond to requests of third-party payers for enrollee-specific outcomes.

MANAGED CARE VERSUS CASE MANAGEMENT

Although frequently used interchangeably, case management is not the same thing as managed care. "Managed care is a system of cost-containment programs; case management is a process. A global term *managed care* consists of the systems and mechanisms utilized to control, direct, and approve access to the wide range of services and costs within the health care delivery system. Case management can be one of those mechanisms, one component in the managed care strategy."[1] Managed care is designed to enhance cost-effectiveness by eliminating inappropriate service.[2] The level of reimbursement for a client is set prospectively sometimes to the financial liability of the provider home care agency. Examples of reimbursement methods include

348

capitation, discounted charges, per diem, and case rates. "This is what is meant by the 'provider at risk' terminology commonly associated with discussions of managed care."[3]

True case management is the coordination of resources to meet the needs of the client, and it is the responsibility of health care providers to ensure that these needs are met.[4] To the providers of home care, case management has always been a part of the total nursing process: assessment, planning, implementation, revising, and evaluation. With health care reform, home care is emerging as the primary site for the most cost-effective delivery system of health care. This positions the family system as the focal point for delivering health care.[5] Much family education will need to be done by the HCCM to make this alternate site of care a reality. Education can help clients and families change to more positive health behaviors and life styles.

At any given point during the client's transition through the health care system, more than one case manager (CM) might be involved (e.g., the PCM and the HCCM). Each CM's different perspective can be a source for conflict. An alliance between providers of care and payers needs to evolve with the common goals of strengthening and supporting the family unit and using community resources.[6]

The PCM typically wants quality patient care but with financial restraint. The role of the PCM is to assist clients in obtaining services in the most cost-effective manner. The HCCM wants quality patient care; cost is secondary. The conflict occurs due to each one's different perspective. Perspectives of different CMs vary, but their functions within the process are similar. The challenge is to balance client advocacy/quality with appropriate resource allocation.[5]

There are two different types of case management in home care: clinical (HCCM) and fiscal (PCM). To understand managed care from the vantage point of both the PCM and the HCCM, one of the authors interviewed a nurse who left her home health agency to work as a PCM in a managed care company. After a few weeks, this nurse resigned from her position with the managed care company and returned to her former staff nurse position with a home health agency. The following is an excerpt from that interview:

> I left my position in home care in search of another challenge. At that time, I believed that case management in a managed care company would enable me to help patients by giving me the authority to institute care and services, assisting home care nurses in decision making, and overseeing total patient care. As I experienced case management, I realized that I missed patient contact. I felt distant from the aspect of home care that I enjoyed the most, total patient care. I was not prepared for the attitudes that prevailed with reference to cost control. As

a case manager, I dealt only with numbers. I had only basic knowledge of the patient and at times had to interrogate the client's nurses to gain more knowledge of the patient. I guess, due to my home care background, I wanted to know too much, which became time consuming. I resented doing cost reports each week to show how much money was saved caring for the patients at home as opposed to being in the hospital. At the time, I did not see the relevancy in this with reference to quality care. In many cases, indifference prevailed among staff of the managed care company. I missed being with the patients and the coordination of care required of the clinician. In my experience, managed care case managers dealt with numbers, not patients. Cost seemed too often more important than quality. It did not take long to realize that I could not continue in the position of PCM.

This nurse's experience can be summarized as follows: "Managed care as used by insurance companies and increasingly by the federal government, reduced to its simplest form, is finding an excuse not to pay or to delay in making payments. What this means in simple terms is that dollars are becoming more important than people."[7]

ADVANTAGES AND DISADVANTAGES OF CONTRACTING WITH MANAGED CARE COMPANIES

In home health care, there are advantages and disadvantages associated with contracting with managed care companies that are identified by the administrative, supervisory, business, and visiting nurse staff.

Advantages
- Payment is known in advance.
- There are service limits on clients who demand more service than is required.
- There are established contracts for servicing clients.
- Health care is cost efficient.

Disadvantages
- Payer case manager may not authorize payment for needed services as assessed by HCCM.
- Physicians may not order what PCM has authorized.
- Increased staff time is required for multiple telephone calls to PCM.
- Documentation requirements are increased for each PCM (no standardization of what is needed—each payer is different).

- Increased supervisory time is required to appeal denials of care when client referrals are received from hospital discharge planning nurses or social workers without preauthorization by the PCM.
- Payer case manager and HCCM duties are duplicated (e.g., telephone calls to physician).
- Increased time is needed to educate staff related to each payer's specific requirements. Some insurance payers require precertification and provide specific authorization numbers before the first visit. Other payers want a telephone call after the first visit at which time visits are authorized for the first two weeks. Telephone reauthorizations every two weeks or once a month are required for approval of continued service. Some payers do not require precertification authorization numbers.
- Increased time is associated with the billing process when supplemental materials such as copies of the chart must be submitted with bills.
- Different coverages are related to supplies (e.g., supplies may be billed separately, included as part of visit cost, or supplied by the managed care company).
- Ethical issues are related to balancing cost-containment versus patient advocacy.

In addition to all the HCCM needs to remember in the care of the client, the HCCM now has to add insurance rules and related paperwork for payment to the body of knowledge. Because there are so many types of payers (state, private, preferred provider organizations, HMOs) and each has its own rules and possibly its own forms, it is almost impossible to know and remember all this information without constant cues.

At the Visiting Nurse Association (VNA) of Eastern Montgomery County, a department of Abington Memorial Hospital, there is an insurance advisor in the business office who helps clarify what the professionals need to complete for the VNA to be reimbursed for services provided. Staff education related to payment sources begins with the orientation of new employees and continues with ongoing staff development programs. Formal sessions as well as verbal and written memoranda are used to share current information with all staff.

ROLE OF THE HOME CARE CLINICAL CASE MANAGER VERSUS PAYER CASE MANAGER

The challenge for HCCMs is to make sure they have a collaborative, not an adversarial, working relationship with the PCM.[6] The most effective working relationship is one in which both parties focus on the health care needs of the client. This requires accurate assessments by both case managers of medical/ nursing needs and the patient's personal needs and desires. The HCCM has essentially seven functions: (1) assessment, (2) planning care to be provided, (3) interdisciplinary and interagency/intraagency coordination, (4) organizing and staffing, (5) resource allocation, (6) implementation of the plan of care, and (7) evaluation/quality assurance measures to ensure that standards of care are met. The PCM has functions that are different from those of the HCCM: (1) assessing eligibility, (2) validating plan of care presented, (3) coordinating benefits if two or more payers, (4) defining payment system, and (5) conducting program evaluations and provider audits.[2]

STRATEGIES FOR CULTIVATING A SUCCESSFUL RELATIONSHIP

Negotiating for patient care is one important strategy. "Home care interests [providers] must be on the alert and demand that all home care services be delivered in conformance with the highest quality standards by licensed agencies through trained and supervised personnel."[8] It is difficult for case managers to be cooperative and competitive at the same time. There are two basic types of negotiation: cooperative (everybody wins) and competitive (only one wins). There are three criteria for negotiation to occur.

1. The issue must be negotiable.
2. Negotiators must be interested in both taking and giving.
3. Negotiating parties must trust each other as both have needs to be met.[9]

The PCM and HCCM need to be proficient in negotiation skills for the good of the patient. Here are some criteria to determine the success of negotiations:

1. Is the progress worthwhile for both parties?
2. Do both parties feel self-respect was maintained?
3. Did both parties leave with positive feelings?
4. Were both parties sensitive to the needs of the other during the process?
5. Did both parties achieve most of their objectives?
6. Would either party be willing to negotiate again with the other?[9]

One can imagine how disastrous it would be for patient care if one of the parties did not want to talk to the other again because of negotiation problems. Home care agencies could lose a contract if their HCCMs were rude or unreasonable. Thus, skillful, professional communication is necessary along with accurate documentation for the ultimate benefit of both the client and agency.

Verbal communication is a second strategy for success. Administration had initial communication that resulted in your home health agency meeting the criteria for participation in the plan. From an administrator's vantage point, this new or continuing relationship must be cultivated and nurtured on an ongoing basis. Frequent one-on-one communication with the PCM is not only required but essential. It can also be time consuming and stressful. The administrator must work with the HCCM and PCM to develop mutually beneficial communication patterns. There are many demands on the time of both the PCM and the HCCM providing care to the patient. In many instances, the patient's primary nurse/HCCM is the best person to have this communication.

At the VNA, the HCCM has the primary responsibility of managing all clients' care in the assigned case load. Administration prefers to have the HCCM call the PCM to give clinical reports because the HCCMs are the nurses who have seen the patient in the home. They can give accurate clinical and home environment information that provides a clear picture and could have an effect on the care at home. Frequently, family and a safe environment play a large role in whether the patient can be maintained at home. The HCCM who saw the patient is in the best position to answer questions posed by the PCM. The HCCM is literally the "eyes and ears" for the physician and PCM in the home. For example, one plan has prearranged times when the PCM calls the VNA office. This schedule is known to the staff. All HCCMs who need to talk to that PCM that day inform the receptionist so that each HCCM can be paged when his or her turn comes to present patient updates. The VNA nurses do not sit and wait for many busy signals, nor does the PCM play telephone tag with the VNA staff. Although voice mail messages are authorized in some circumstances and do have a role in communication, there is no substitute for the personal contact with the patient's PCM.

At the VNA, the HCCMs get to know the different PCMs. We make available lists of names and telephone numbers of certain PCMs, obtained from the payer companies. Supervisors distribute, or have a book of, frequently used names and numbers at each nurse's workstation. When a new PCM is responsible for clients, that information is added to the current list. Some PCMs also call when a new PCM takes over existing cases to provide for continuity of care.

The HCCM needs to be aware of limited resources imposed by the managed care payer to plan within those boundaries. The home care supervisor gets involved only when there is a problem between the HCCM and the PCM. For example, if the HCCM and the supervisor determine that a client needs more care at home than the PCM will approve, an appeal can be made to the medical director of the PCM if necessary. This often involves the patient's physician writing letters of medical necessity to justify the care.

"At times, indications for ongoing care may run contrary to the recommendations of an external entity performing utilization review (for example, peer review organizations, insurance companies, managed care reviewers). If such a conflict arises, care, services, or discharge (including transfer) decisions must be made in response to the care required by the patient, and not solely in response to the recommendation made by the external agency. Home health agency administrators and staff must be aware that accreditation standards require that a process exists and is implemented for resolving internal and external denial issues, when appropriate, to meet ongoing care and/or discharge (including transfer) needs of the patient."[10] Written documentation of the verbal process of informing the patient of changes in the plan of care and obtaining the patient's consent to the plan must be included in the clinical record.

As part of the communication network, it is important to keep the payers informed of what types of computer linkages are currently available or planned for the future. In this time of instant communication and need for up-to-date patient and billing information, discussions should be ongoing to determine the compatibilities between the automated systems used by the home health agency and the managed care company. Some home health agencies have installed a computer terminal in the managed care company's office that provides "view-only" access to the plan subscriber's patient care information. Current patient data and visit statistics can be retrieved at the convenience of the PCM. All home health agencies need to strive to meet the computer-age need for instant information.

Written communication is the third strategy for success. Verbal communications must be supplemented with written documentation that is readily available to the clinical and billing personnel. At the VNA, a standardized form—Service Authorization Progress Note (Exhibit 19-1)—is used to document contacts with the PCMs. This form records the patient's name, identification number, and designated PCM. Authorized services are listed with visit frequency, duration, and total visits. Space is provided for authorization codes if needed. If there are denials of payment for bills, the supervisor can use this form to substantiate that a certain number of visits was approved, by whom, and on what date. Often, the PCM will adjust the payer's records and pay the bill if the error was on their part. Without this type of documentation, the home health agency has no grounds to substantiate that telephone approvals were obtained.

Clinical documentation in the form of clinical notes and medical orders are contained in the patients' records. These essential written communications among the PCM, HCCM, and physician are readily available to meet myriad standards such as professional, legal, agency, certification, and accreditation.

Exhibit 19-1 Service Authorization Progress Note

Patient #: _____ Patient Name: _____

Telephone call to: _____ at _____
                                  Contact person   Insurance Co. Name

Services	Frequency and Duration	# of Visits	From–Thru Dates	Authorization Number	MA Alpha Modifier

Treatment Plan: ____ Initial POT ____ Interim Update ____ Recertification
                       ____ Service Addition or Modification

To call for additional approval on: _____

Comments: _____

_____

_____

Signature: _____ Date: _____

Source: Courtesy of Visiting Nurse Association of Eastern Montgomery County/A Department of Abington Memorial Hospital, Willow Grove, Pennsylvania.

QUALITY ASSESSMENT/PERFORMANCE IMPROVEMENT (QA/PI) ISSUES

The National Committee for Quality Assurance, located in Washington, D.C., evaluates health plans' internal quality processes through accreditation reviews and develops measures to gauge health plan performance. Quality improvement, physician credentialing, member rights and responsibilities, utilization management, and medical records are evaluated for each plan. Plans may receive full, one-year, or provisional accreditation.[11] This same reference listed the status of Pennsylvania HMOs as of January 31, 1995. "Managed care plans are eager to develop comparable data because they increasingly see quality of care as a sales tool. Employers want quality data for use in choosing plans. Those that offer more than one plan also want employees to be able to compare them before choosing one."[12] The value that is placed on the public release of this type of status report is evident from an article that describes a Florida HMO's lawsuit to block release of a negative report.[13]

As one aspect of attaining and maintaining an individual plan's accreditation, a plan may require a home health agency with which it contracts to submit to one or more of the relevant reviews mentioned above. It is important that a home health agency have and be able to sort its internal quality outcome data related to patients who subscribe to a specific plan to report back to that plan. For example, one plan that contracts with the VNA requests that the VNA submit the results of its QA/PI reports for patient satisfaction for the subscribers of the plan as compared with the agency's patient satisfaction report for its total population (Figure 19-1). The plan also carries out its own patient satisfaction survey. Another plan sends a representative to the agency, where selected records of the plan's subscribers are pulled on site and reviewed to determine that standards of care are met. A written summary report is sent to the VNA director after the site visit that compares the VNA results with the standards established by the plan and the average for all other agencies.

It is imperative that the home health agency administration and staff have the written standards that the managed care company uses in reviewing uti-

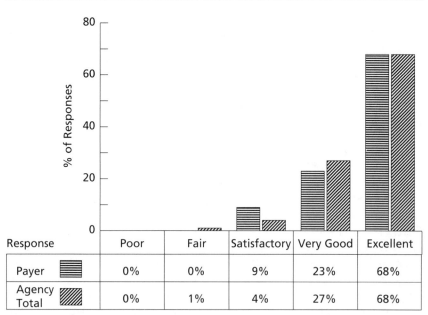

Response		Poor	Fair	Satisfactory	Very Good	Excellent
Payer		0%	0%	9%	23%	68%
Agency Total		0%	1%	4%	27%	68%

Questionnaires from 8/1/94 through 2/28/95.

Figure 19-1 Visiting Nurse Association Home Care Discharge Patient Questionnaire. *Source:* Courtesy of Visiting Nurse Association of Eastern Montgomery County/A Department of Abington Memorial Hospital, Willow Grove, Pennsylvania.

lization and quality of care. These standards need to be incorporated into the home health agency's policies, procedures, and QA/PI plan. It is not adequate, however, to be paper compliant. These standards, and expectations that they will be met, need to be communicated to the staff. Specific requirements of each plan are shared with staff by the supervisors in formal conferences and in-service programs. The sharing of new and supplemental information is accomplished through written and verbal memoranda from administration and clinical supervisors. When requirements are included that the administrative staff know are not currently met (e.g., cardiopulmonary resuscitation training for all staff and contracted home health aides) or will not be met based on current practice, the administrator must communicate these concerns to the contract manager so that contract-related issues can be addressed and resolved before they become a noncompliance issue. From our experience, the representatives from the plans have been willing to discuss specific issues or requirements and make revisions when there is candid communication and rationales are expressed.

A home health agency must have systems in place to identify, collect, track, analyze, and present information on the outcomes of patient care for the patients it serves. One reason is to share this information with the managed care company. Another reason is to compare the agency's data with published national data based on studies that compare fee-for-service patient outcomes with HMOs and other managed care plans' patient outcomes.[14]

Only 21 percent of 314 home care executives who responded to an informal poll stated they used a management information system (MIS) to calculate outcomes for either Medicare or private insurers.[15] A manual or computerized MIS is essential for a home health agency administrator who is interested in survival in the age of managed care. This is necessary to identify patient outcomes by myriad methods including payer source, disease categories, and costs.

Quality standards also need to address the qualifications of the home care staff. This is extremely important when new services are added to the agency. Information must be communicated to the managed care company's PCM and the person responsible for modifications or additions to the existing contract to make them aware of new patient care programs and services and assure them that staff meet professional licensure and/or certification standards. It is important both to provide care and be paid for the services rendered. Most times, the contract, or addendum, must identify the covered disciplines before billing.

Opportunities should be accepted to participate on a professional advisory committee or clinical committees that enable the agency's representative to have input into the plan's QA/PI process. The home care administrator, although often the person to whom the invitation is extended, may not be the appropriate person to serve on these committees. Another member of the administrative team, possibly the director of professional services or director of QA/PI, is more familiar with the clinical operations and can provide the needed input and expertise on a committee.

The role of advocate is another administrative responsibility. This includes being an advocate for quality patient care for individuals who do not know what services they are being denied. Staff also need an advocate as they seek to provide quality patient care while meeting the home care agency's expectations. Therefore, establishing smooth working relations that are efficient and effective will convey administration's commitment. Sometimes, this may mean running interference by scheduling a face-to-face meeting with personnel from the managed care company.

Home care administrators also need to be aware of the many opportunities to be on the cutting edge of technology. This includes availability to monitor a patient's status via computerization (e.g., daily check-ups of expectant mothers with high-risk pregnancies and other electronic "visits" in the home).[16,17] Administrators must also be aware of special clinical programs that are promoted by insurers (e.g., cardiac care, asthma, back pain). Your home health agency may provide the same type of service under generic names such as skilled nursing or physical therapy. The managed care company needs to be aware of this information.

Current managed care enrollment represents less than 10 percent of the Medicare population.[18,19] According to a 1995 Health Care Financing Administration publication, the percentage of Medicaid enrollees in managed care plans has increased from 9.5 percent in 1991 to 23.2 percent in 1994.[20] A survey of 547 managed care organizations showed that a little more than 18 percent of the population of the United States is enrolled in HMOs.[20] As of April 1995, 21 percent of the VNA's discharged Medicare patients' services were paid by a managed care plan. Twenty-nine percent of the VNA's total patients are currently enrolled in some managed care plan (Figure 19-2). In Pennsylvania, all individuals who are on the Medical Assistance Program are covered by a managed care plan, either through the department of health or a private HMO. It is anticipated that the percentage of individuals who choose to enroll in managed care plans will continue to increase.

A recent article states that "HMOs want your nurses and therapists to show up on time and look presentable. They want you to respond to their calls for a nurse at 5 p.m. on a Friday. They want you to provide specialty home care services if you claim to be a full-service provider. And if you want to contract with them, managed care companies want you to fill out their forms completely, follow their rules, and not be an administrative nuisance for

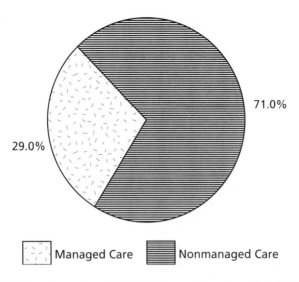

71.0%

29.0%

Managed Care   Nonmanaged Care

Figure 19-2 Visiting Nurse Association Homecare Payer Type (April 1995). *Source:* Courtesy of the Visiting Nurse Association of Eastern Montgomery County/A Department of Abington Memorial Hospital, Willow Grove, Pennsylvania.

them."[21] The article lists the following criteria for a successful experience with a managed care company:

- professionalism
- punctuality
- reputability
- availability
- complete the job in the fewest number of visits
- be your own utilization reviewer
- understand how HMOs work
- be persistent
- follow through on provider credentialing
- do not demand too much
- do not make waves

In addition to these criteria, home health agency administrators and staff must be aware of the recently published home care and case management guidelines.[22] Previously published guidelines for inpatient and surgical care

are widely used by CMs across the country. The new home care-oriented guidelines, published in June 1994, are for use with both commercial and Medicare populations, with straightforward cases. The issue of multiple diagnoses patients is not addressed.[23] These guidelines, which do not appear to be as widely used as yet, could give home health agencies a preview of CMs' future expectations of home care services.[24]

CONCLUSION

Home health care agencies are experiencing rapid changes in this era of health care and insurance reform and cost containment. Working with managed care companies brings new opportunities, challenges, and stress. The key is to be flexible, cooperative, and cost effective while continuing to provide high-quality care to clients in their homes. Emphasis must be placed on administrative and clinical communications. Continuous QA/PI efforts must receive high priority, with the goal of attaining positive outcomes for patients and families while at the same time keeping the home health agency financially viable. "How home care providers respond to the reforms and opportunities will determine the future fate of many agencies. Limited thinkers will be left behind."[24] These are the challenges of the 1990s as health care reform progresses into the twenty-first century.

REFERENCES

1. Millahy CM. *The Case Manager's Handbook.* Gaithersburg, Md: Aspen Publishers, Inc.; 1995:3–13.
2. Billows LA. Case management. In: Harris MD, ed. *Handbook of Home Health Care Administration.* Gaithersburg, Md: Aspen Publishers, Inc.; 1994:411–415.
3. Cline B. Case management: organizational models and administrative methods. *Caring.* 1990;9(7):14–18.
4. Faherty B. Case management—the latest buzzword: what it is, and what it isn't. *Caring.* 1990;9(7):20–22.
5. Sampson E. Offensive case management vs. defensive case management. *Pennington Rep.* 1994;8:17–19.
6. Wolfe G. Cooperation or competition? Collaboration between home care and case management. *Caring.* 1993;12(10):52–60.
7. Halamandaris V. Case management: blessing or curse? *Caring.* 1990;9(7):50, 52.
8. Halamandaris V. Cooperation in competition: e pluribus unum. *Caring.* 1993;12(10):4–6.
9. Smeltzer CH. The art of negotiation: an everyday experience. In: Hein E, Nicholson M, eds. *Contemporary Leadership Behavior.* Philadelphia, Penn: JB Lippincott; 1994:351–356.

10. Joint Commission on Accreditation of Healthcare Organizations. *1995 Accreditation Manual for Home Care.* Vol. I and II. Oakbrook Terrace, Ill: Joint Commission; 1994.

11. The Hospital Association of Pennsylvania. National accrediting agency evaluates Pennsylvania HMOs. *Penn Hosp Nineties.* 1995;6:2.

12. Knox A. HMOs' quality of care reviewed. *Philadelphia Inquirer.* February 25, 1995: D:1,5.

13. Bell C, ed. Florida HMO sues to block release of negative report. *Mod Healthcare.* 1995;25:56.

14. Shaughnessy P, Schlenker R. Medicare home health reimbursement alternatives; access, quality and cost incentives. *Home Health Care Services Q.* 1992;13:91–115.

15. Rak K. Only 21% of home care companies track outcomes and costs electronically. *Homehealthline.* 1995;20(5):7.

16. Joyce M. HMOs turn to home health firms to monitor patients. *Philadelphia Bus J.* 1994;13:5B–13B.

17. Mahmud K, LeSage K. Telemedicine—a new idea for home care. *Caring.* 1995;14(5):48–50.

18. Kertesz L. Medicare: the final frontier for HMOs. *Mod Healthcare.* 1995;25:76–84.

19. Cerne F. Rehabbing Medicare—is managed care a cure-all or just a crutch? *Hosp Health Networks.* 1995;69(8):23–26.

20. American Hospital Association. *AHA News.* 1995;32(17):2.

21. Friend A. Wake-up call for home care providers: managed care decision-makers tell what they want and what they're willing to pay. *Homehealthline.* 1995;25(special report):1–4.

22. Doyle R, Pinney M, Spong F. *Healthcare Management Guidelines. IV. Home Care and Case Management.* Radnor, Penn: Milliman & Robertson, Inc.; 1994.

23. Mann L. Milliman & Robertson home care management guidelines expect a lot from both nurses & patients. *Homehealthline.* 1995;20(5):4–7.

24. Coleman JR, Algie BA. Health care reform: reinventing health care provides new opportunities for ancillary and alternate site providers. *Remington Rep.* 1994;8(6):36–39.

■ 20 ■

Cost Savings and Financial Analysis of Case Management Models

▓▓▓▓▓▓▓

Sandra Pelfrey, MBA, CPA
Mary Lou Wesley, MSN, RN

One issue in managed care that is becoming increasingly important is continuity of care, defined as the extent to which services are received as part of a coordinated and uninterrupted succession of events consistent with the needs of the patient. Continuity of care encompasses events across the continuum, including primary care, acute care, subacute care, home care, and long-term care. Coordinated care is viewed as a methodology for providing a patient with the best efforts to reach and maintain a state of wellness.

Case management is an effective methodology for developing patient care strategies. A commonly used tool in case management is critical pathways, which are defined by one hospital as follows:

> A critical pathway is a tool that helps practitioners manage an episode of care for a patient population or condition by providing a timeline of the expected course of care with expected patient outcomes. The critical pathway is designed to improve quality of patient care and promote efficient utilization of resources.[1]

Because case management and critical pathway use requires active participation of a patient care team comprised of physicians, nurses, and medical and other support personnel, one outcome is a standardized medical treatment plan with scheduled assessment intervals and expected patient outcomes. Comparisons of planned care and expected outcomes to actual treatment and resulting patient conditions furnish timely feedback to the patient care team. The overall result is improved patient care through collaborative practice and coordinated care.

One side benefit to case management's standardized clinical outcomes is the ability to value and quantify a standard in terms of expected costs or reimbursement and length of stay. A comparison of the standard for these measurement bases to the actual data on a patient-by-patient basis affords the patient care team a means of quantifying the changes that have taken place over time. Periodic summaries of these data with the variances isolated and their respective reasons identified will enable nurse case managers and, ultimately, patient care team members to evaluate the potential cost impact from their actions. Streamlining operations and closing the feedback loop can lead to modifications of the standard, the goal of continuous quality improvement being met. This chapter identifies a methodology and an orientation that can enable nurse case managers and patient care teams to establish standards of care, identify variances, and analyze the financial results effected by implementing a case management regiment.

STANDARDS

A standard can be used as a gauge against which actual activities are measured needs to be established. As a general treatment plan, the standard is comparable with a recipe that states the number of individual treatment components that are needed, when they should be performed, and the expected (patient) outcomes at stated time intervals. The goal is to arrive at a quality product (i.e., quality patient care).

The standard becomes not only the means to an end but also a tool to be used to evaluate current operations. Standards can be established based on perfect activity or best-case scenarios. Taking an instance of lowest cost and length of stay (LOS) and using it as a standard by which all other cases will be compared and analyzed will, by definition, yield many variances. Although it may be desirable for the institution to strive constantly for perfection, it is impossible to maintain that level of activity and outcomes, especially in the health care setting. The number and degree of variances may, in fact, reduce the motivation and level of active participation on the part of patient care team members.

It is better to provide a standard based on realistic expectations, even though it may include inefficiencies initially. Because a standard is intended to be a guideline for action, it should be reviewed at regular intervals, and modified or adjusted depending on consensus of the patient care team. For example, the current patient LOS for a specific diagnosis-related group (DRG) may average 4.5 days. Once the standard is set initially, the target patient LOS may be 4.2 days. After some time using this target LOS, the patient care team may refine its treatment plan so that a better target LOS is 3.8 days. As better information becomes available, the patient care team should include these data in the standard.

Where To Begin: Find a Sponsor

Before you attempt to implement a case management program, it will be necessary to find an organizational sponsor who will support project efforts at all levels of the organization. To be effective, the sponsor should be an individual who is respected by the medical staff as well as administration. The chief medical officer would be a good choice for the role of sponsor.

It may be necessary to convince your sponsor that case management is a worthwhile effort. A review of the literature will furnish examples of how case management tools such as critical pathways have improved patient outcomes, assisted in achieving expected clinical outcomes, promoted collaborative practice and coordinated care, ensured the use of appropriate (and often reduced) resources, and promoted professional development and satisfaction.[2-5]

Create a Steering Committee

Many organizations have begun their case management project by establishing a critical pathway steering committee. This should be an interdisciplinary group that acts as an oversight committee to develop, implement, and evaluate critical pathways within the organization. To gain unilateral support across the organization, the steering committee should draw its members from the directors of pharmacy, nursing, laboratory, radiology, dietary, and any other key stakeholders who might support this activity.

The steering committee must decide how critical pathways will be used within the organization. It will need to decide whether critical pathway usage will be mandatory. If critical pathways are mandated, the committee must decide next (1) which practitioners (nurses only or all members of the interdisciplinary team) will be required to use critical pathways, (2) how the steering committee will enforce the mandate, and (3) whether practitioners will be permitted to individualize a critical pathway standard to meet a specific patient's needs.

The steering committee should develop a timeline that has the goals and objectives of the critical pathway project identified, along with their expected date of completion. Once the overall plan is formulated, the steering committee should develop a plan to create the initial critical pathways. The plan should include the means of implementation. The final stage of the plan is to develop an evaluation process and ascertain that a feedback loop is in place to improve the critical pathway continuously.

Gather Data from Other Supporting Departments

Medical Records

Information must be gathered from various service departments of the hospital. The medical records department will need to provide information concerning the medical record coding process for DRG assignments. Each patient is assigned a DRG on discharge, based on the physician's diagnosis, resulting treatment, and the patient's clinical signs, symptoms, and outcomes. The DRG assignment determines reimbursement. Medical records coders review each patient's chart to determine the appropriate DRG assignment. A sampling of these records will then be reviewed by third-party payers to determine if coding was proper. Information that needs to be contained in the record includes the following:

- medical necessity of admission and continued stay
- validation of DRG assignment
- appropriateness of care site (inpatient versus outpatient)
- discharge planning
- appropriateness of surgery if performed

It will be helpful for case managers to be familiar with the medical record coding process to ensure that the necessary documentation is recorded to support the DRG assignment, the need for the LOS, the intensity of services required, and the patient's readiness for discharge.

It is important to remember that the critical pathway assignments and the reimbursement DRG may not match, in part, because one is determined at admission and the other at discharge. Another factor that often provides a mismatch is that medical records coders try to assign DRGs based on the highest reimbursement possible for each case. Medical records staff can be very helpful in developing a system to track data specific to each clinical pathway.

Finance Department

The finance department should provide nurse case managers and their patient care teams with data regarding how they perform the following:

- Identify costs per patient case. Generally, finance personnel apply cost ratio percentages determined on a departmental basis to departmental charges.
- Determine how the organization currently monitors cost per case and LOS data. This includes the identification of the type and frequency of reports generated, as well as the preparers and recipients of these reports.
- Discover if the hospital is currently using benchmarks against which it compares current case data.
- Identify the organization's reimbursement trends, such as the composition of third-party payers, the high-volume DRGs, the current LOS per DRG, as well as reimbursable cost and LOS by payer.

Utilization Review

Generally, the hospital's utilization review department reviews the hospitalization of all patients on a concurrent basis. Personnel review all admissions to determine their appropriateness, and conduct extended stay review to identify problems of overuse, underuse, and efficient scheduling of resources. Utilization review personnel should furnish the following information:

- an overview of the utilization review process, including who performs the reviews and their frequency
- identification of the process for identifying and dealing with physicians who admit patients inappropriately, use resources inappropriately, or fail to discharge patients in a timely manner.

Once the above information has been gathered, case managers can develop their own utilization management process. Utilization management involves a set of activities that ensures patient LOS is within appropriate time frames and that health care resources are used appropriately.

FIRST CRITICAL PATHWAY

The steering committee should decide which critical pathways need to be developed first. Because DRGs are a fact of life, it will be easiest if the DRG becomes the common denominator for developing critical pathways that will become the standard of patient care. It will be impossible to tackle all DRGs at once, so a starting point needs to be selected. For this project, it may be possible to combine DRGs that are similar. For example, one hospital combined DRG 148 and 149 (bowel resection) into one initial critical pathway.

When selecting the starting point, the steering committee should consider that DRG which will provide material benefits to the provider. One possible target could be either a high-volume DRG or a DRG associated with high-risk patient groups. Choosing either of these DRGs would provide sufficient data for establishing the initial standardized medical treatment plan, and because there is already a high level of activity or risk, standardization of treatment and constant monitoring should improve patient care.

An alternative choice of a target DRG could be one that is currently operating at a loss or one in which the possibility of removing inefficiencies is suspected. Concentrating effort here should refine medical care. Many institutions have proved that using good case management techniques yields improved medical care because medical treatment and other care is prescheduled and patient progress is monitored against the established standard.

A second benefit of this improved care is that patients leave the hospital sooner, thus increasing the potential for hospital cost reductions and improved reimbursements. The challenge for the steering committee is to select those DRGs (either high-volume or loss generators) for conversion to critical pathways that will be likely to provide positive institutional feedback on the benefits to be realized. Once these benefits are documented, they will fuel not only the patient team's enthusiasm but also provide the momentum needed to enlist future patient care team members.

PATIENT CARE PROJECT TEAM

The steering committee should identify the interdisciplinary critical pathway project team. The membership of the team depends on which critical pathway is being developed. Even though the critical pathway project team is often temporary, the team should plan to continue meeting even after the critical pathway is implemented as a means of evaluating data and continually improving the system.

The team must plan team meetings and develop a work plan that includes a communication tool, a plan for identifying and dealing with obstacles, and an evaluation plan.

CREATING THE FIRST CRITICAL PATHWAY

Step 1

Once a DRG or DRG grouping has been selected for analysis, its recent historical data should be collected. Medical records and individual patient accounts can serve as the source of this information. Other data and information should be examined. These include requirements of the Joint Commission on Accreditation of Healthcare Organizations, peer review guidelines, "best-practices" information from other facilities, and literature reviews.

Length of stay information should be gathered. This should include (1) DRG LOS by category of patient insurance payer (Medicare, Medicaid, Blue Cross), and (2) the average actual LOS experienced by the organization for a representative prior time interval. Using this information as benchmarks, the patient care team should target a LOS for the DRG under review.

After the targeted LOS is determined, the patient care project team should begin by identifying the time frame (minutes, hours, days, or weeks) for the critical pathway. Then they should identify the actual care a typical patient received according to this time frame, along with actual patient outcomes. The patient care team should focus on critical activities that will ensure that patients receive the care required to allow discharge within the expected time frame. Finally, the group should incorporate best-practice recommendations on which the team agrees into the critical pathway.

If the DRG selected is currently being provided at a loss, then the most prevalent category of patient payer's LOS and reimbursement should be used as the standard's targets. If a high-volume DRG has been selected as the target, then the lower of (1) the hospital's actual average LOS and average total charges and (2) the prevalent provider's reimbursable LOS and rate should be used as the standard.

Step 2

Once the standard LOS to be used has been determined, the nurse case manager should develop a critical pathway that can start with either preadmission testing, if applicable, or admission to the hospital and ends with the expected patient discharge. The time between actual admission and discharge should equal the standard LOS adopted.

Step 3

A review of medical records can then allow nurse case managers to insert the usual prescribed procedures, therapy, and/or tests, as well as the expected patient outcomes on the critical pathway. Physician input can then be sought to determine whether the normal tests, procedures, medication, and/or therapy are considered best practices. Next, physicians can be asked whether the order and timing are correct and whether any of these planned treatments can and should be initiated earlier.

Crucial outcomes can be identified. For example, if the results of a specific test are positive or the patient becomes ambulatory, then with advance physician approval, a second course of treatment can be started. Different patient outcomes would trigger different responses. To the extent that the patient follows a normal recuperative process, standing physician orders can be built into the critical pathway. It is not necessary that the critical pathways of all physicians participating in the program agree. Tentative standards of treatment along the critical pathway may be physician specific. Although the long-term goal is to develop just one standard medical treatment plan, that may not be possible in the short term. Because physician acceptance is crucial, any initial concessions needed to guarantee positive attitudes should be made. However, LOS should not be compromised. If the number of physicians participating in the pilot program is limited, these differences will be manageable. The institution should look ahead. It may be necessary to develop a decision support system on the computer to maintain the details of the various treatment plans.

The level of nursing care can also be built into the case management plan. For this step to occur, nursing must identify the levels of care provided from acute patient care requiring highly skilled registered nurses to the use of nursing aides to administer medication and monitor vital signs. The nursing staff can identify as many levels as they believe to be operable and cost effective. These levels of nursing care can then be built into the critical pathway yielding a valuable system for planning and scheduling nursing staff on the various units. For example, if DRG 148 requires 2.5 hours of registered nurse contact hours and 3 hours of practical nurse contact hours per 24-hour period, these data can be accumulated and added to the nursing hour requirements of other patients on the unit to determine the work schedule.

Once the initial critical pathway standard has been developed for a specific patient, the patient care team may identify extenuating factors that could affect the prescribed items and/or the timing and frequency of prescribed items scheduled along the critical pathway. Factors such as patient age, history of smoking, chronic conditions, and general well-being can have an effect on the patient's response to treatment. A modified critical pathway may be adopted to adjust for these factors or the original standard can be used and the cited conditions used to explain the variances in LOS and total charges.

The alternative selected should be chosen based on cost-effectiveness. There is a cost associated with creating new standards for the various pre-existing patient conditions. However, there is benefit to be had in comparing a patient's actual critical pathway with one that best projects what should take place at stated intervals. The patient care team must decide at what point the benefits of the added information exceed the costs of providing it.

EVALUATING CRITICAL PATHWAY RESULTS

To determine the financial impact of case management techniques, it will be necessary to identify patient critical pathway information on a case-by-case basis and then summarize the relevant information for all patients with the same critical pathway for a designated time period. This is generally performed at one-month intervals. To facilitate this process, it will be helpful to develop pre-case management data to be used as benchmarks if they have not been developed previously by finance or nursing personnel.

Most providers using critical pathways identify two statistics for comparison: LOS and average cost per case. Length of stay is the easiest statistic to track. Lengths of stay for all patients using a specific critical pathway are averaged. This average can then be compared with the pre-case management statistic obtained from finance personnel to track the trend over time. It can also be compared with the targeted LOS, which may differ from the original benchmark.

Next, the average cost per patient case for post-case management patients is compared with the average cost per case statistic calculated for the pre-case management period. It is important to note that cost data are used. Deriving these costs can be difficult and requires the assistance of the finance department. The process necessitates converting patient charges as recorded on the patient account to an appropriate cost component.

The finance department prepares a cost allocation grid annually for inclusion in its Medicare cost report. That report uses the step allocation method, the purpose of which is to allocate the costs of all service or non-revenue-producing departments to the patient service or revenue-generating departments. Exhibit 20-1 provides a simplified example for review.

Accountants use the cost allocation data to determine the total cost, both direct and indirect, of the revenue-generating departments. Direct departmental costs are the salaries, supplies, and expense that are charged to and used by the department. Indirect costs are the direct costs of other supporting departments such as maintenance and administration, which are charged to departments that do not provide patient treatment and are then allocated to the patient service departments using a rational activity basis.

Accountants then compare total costs with the total service revenue generated and develop a ratio of cost to charges. This ratio can then be applied to any patient department charge to derive the approximate cost of the service. For example, using the information in Exhibit 20-1, if the total revenue generated by the laboratory is $100,000 and its total costs, both direct and indirect, amount to $92,000, the cost-to-billed charges ratio is 92 percent (92,000/100,000). This approach is an averaging exercise and presupposes that there is a constant markup on cost to arrive at treatment fees. It also presupposes that the impact of charity care and contractual adjustments are

---

Exhibit 20-1 Cost Allocation Spreadsheet

		Local Hospital				
	Administration	Maintenance	Laundry	Nursing	Lab	Total
Direct Costs	$51,600	$28,000	$12,000	$100,302	$60,098	$252,000
Administration	($51,600)	$5,160	$5,160	$25,800	$15,480	$0
Maintenance		($33,160)	$9,948	$14,922	$8,290	$0
Laundry			($27,108)	$18,976	$8,132	$0
Total Costs				$160,000	$92,000	$252,000
Total Revenue				$200,000	$100,000	
Ratio of Costs to Revenue				0.8	0.92	

shared equally by all departments. Although these assumptions may be somewhat flawed, the cost of perfecting the cost data currently outweighs the benefits associated with better data. For this reason, the ratio of costs to charges has been adopted by most health care institutions as the basis for arriving at the cost of services rendered.

Some finance departments realize the relative merits of determining cost data and tracking it over time. As a result, many have refined the Medicare cost allocation spreadsheet. For example, the Medicare cost report lumps all laboratory work into one revenue-producing department. The finance department may subdivide the department further into specialities such as microbiology and tissue typing to trace cost further. Use of computer software can facilitate the speed and frequency with which the cost data can be generated.

Once cost/charge ratios are determined, it becomes a simple matter to convert a patient's billed charges to cost (Exhibit 20-2). One need only apply the appropriate cost/charge ratio to the departmental total of billed charges to determine cost. Again, using the computer can streamline this process. Decision support systems can be designed to convert charges to cost and then accumulate the costs per case by DRG, further identifying and tracking changes in cost over time.

Exhibit 20-2 Patient Charges Converted to Costs Sample for DRG 123

	Charges	Cost Ratio	Cost
Room Rate Level 1	$200		
Room Rate Level 1	$200		
Room Rate Level 1	$200		
Room Rate Level 2	$100		
Total	$700	0.8	$560
Test XXY	$545		
Test YYX	$266		
Test YYX	$266		
Text YYZ	$378		
	$1,582	0.92	$1,455
Total	$2,282		$2,015

A similarly constructed decision support system can be designed to apply the process of converting billed charges to cost to the standard procedures and treatments identified by the patient care team for the critical pathway (Exhibit 20-3). Now, not only the treatment details but the expected cost of service can be determined for each critical pathway. In this way, actual costs per case can be compared with standard costs on both a per case and total DRG basis. These data can then be tracked over time to note changes. A review of the literature shows that most hospitals that have adopted case management techniques report cost reductions on a per case basis as well as for the specific DRG.[3-5]

The primary reason for cost reductions is the reduced length of stay.[6] Because hospital resources are being focused on patient care, all unnecessary time delays are either reduced or eliminated. Reduced LOSs use nursing care to the fullest and permit hospitals to use fully one of its scarcest resources.

VARIANCE ANALYSIS

Variance analysis takes place in two time frames. It can occur concurrently as service is rendered and retrospectively, summarizing the activity for a specific time interval. It is the case manager's responsibility to identify and ana-

Exhibit 20-3 Sample of Standard for DRG 123

		Charges	Cost Ratio	Cost
Nursing Service	Room Rate Level 1	$200		
	Room Rate Level 1	$200		
	Room Rate Level 2	$100		
	Room Rate Level 2	$100		
	Total	$600	0.8	$480
	Test XXY	$545		
	Test XXZ	$315		
	Test YYX	$266		
	Text WWR	$423		
		$1,549	0.92	$1,425
	Total			$1,905

lyze variances as they occur. Individual case variances are generally analyzed concurrently, comparing actual LOS with targeted LOS and standard prescribed treatment plans with actual treatment rendered and results experienced.

Overall LOS and cost variances should be summarized for each DRG or critical pathway monthly and compared retrospectively with similar data from prior periods to determine operating trends. Both statistics should be incorporated into periodic operational reports prepared for the steering committee and other relevant committees, such as quality assurance and utilization review.

Three types of variances can be identified and monitored under this general framework: clinical variances, operational variances, and system variances. A clinical variance occurs when a change occurs in the patient's clinical status. For example, a patient is admitted under one DRG and the appropriate critical pathway is selected. Complications may arise during treatment or tests disclose additional medical problems, either of which can change the patient's DRG and its attendant critical pathway. Clinical variances should be noted in the patient's medical record. A summary of clinical variances should be reported to the original patient care team, as well as the steering committee, for review to determine whether any interim action could have affected the outcome.

System variances occur when tests and procedures as outlined on the critical pathway are not performed within the appropriate time frame. Reasons for noncompliance with the critical pathway stem from either communication failures or an inability of an ancillary, patient support department to provide the requisite resources at the time needed. These variances should be logged on a separate variance report and reviewed. Variance data may provide information for adjusting staff assignments or other resource allocations.

Operational variances occur when tests or treatments occur within the DRG that can be attributed to alternative medical practices or unique patient conditions. These situations may cause modifications to the established treatment plan.

POTENTIAL VARIANCE ANALYSIS MODELS

There is definite room for improvement in the area of variance analysis. Again cost/benefit models must be reviewed to determine whether the improved information is worth the cost of gathering it.

Once a critical pathway has been developed, it is possible to determine what the standard cost should be. Again, the services of accounting should be enlisted. The critical pathway components can be divided into two general sets of components: nursing and other patient chargeable treatments. The LOS can be equated with nursing care. Billed room charges can be converted to cost using the cost-to-charges ratio. This would provide an average nursing cost per patient day, without reference to level of nursing care provided.

Because total cost per nursing unit is available, along with patient day information, it is possible to refine LOS cost based on patient acuity and level of nursing care needed. To do this, it will be necessary to identify the different levels of nursing care provided and then gather information regarding hours of care provided by the different levels of care. An average cost per patient care day can be calculated and used for simple variance analysis similar to that provided above. To identify nursing costs further by level of care provided, it will be necessary to develop a relationship of costs to the base unit provided (either hours or days), as well as the number of hours of each level of care provided to patients during the period under review. For example, assume the monthly cost data for the nursing unit under review are:

- Total nursing costs (both direct and indirect) $160,000
- Total patient care days provided   1,000
- Number of level 1 care days   600
- Number of level 2 care days   400
- Ratio of level 1 cost to level 2 cost   2 to 1

Then, it would be possible to calculate the cost of one day of each level of care. Level 2 care costs average $100 a day, whereas level 1s are twice that, or $200.

The next step of the process is to calculate the expected charges for providing the tests, procedures, and treatments prescribed by the critical pathway. See Exhibit 20-3 for a simplified example of a costed critical pathway. These charges can then be converted to cost by applying the appropriate departmental ratio. Once this information is calculated, it can be added to the standard cost of providing nursing services to arrive at the standard cost of the critical pathway associated with the DRG.

Again, prescribed treatment modifications can be identified and converted to cost to arrive at unique standards for specific physicians or patient conditions. This is another instance in which decision support systems can be used to facilitate operations.

Once these data have been calculated, variance analysis can be generated. The LOS can be adjusted to reflect the various levels of nursing care provided. Exhibit 20-3 depicts the standard treatment and costs for DRG 123. The patient's actual bill is shown in Exhibit 20-2.

Analysis

Actual LOS level 1	3 days
Less standard LOS level 1	2 days
Difference in LOS for level 1	+1 day
Multiplied by the standard cost of level 1 nursing care	× $200
Yields level 1 variance	+$200
Actual LOS level 2	1 day
Less standard LOS level 2	2 days
Difference in LOS for level 2	−1 day
Multiplied by the standard cost of level 2 nursing care	× $100
Yields level 2 variance	−$100
Total personnel variances = levels 1 + 2 variances or +$100	

The personnel variance identifies the cost associated with experiencing a LOS for the different nursing care levels that are at variance with the standard.

A similar analysis can be performed for the costs of each ancillary area.

Analysis for Lab

Actual costs	$1,455
Less standard costs per critical pathway	$1,425
Usage difference	$30 unfavorable

Once variances have been identified, they should be explained. Not only is there the fact that a variation in treatment has occurred, but the cost implications of that change are available.

Explanations can include the additional tests and procedures prescribed or the substitution of an alternative test other than that listed on the critical pathway. Once identified, the reasons can be reviewed by the patient care team. Although this information appears to create additional work, the use of decision support systems to provide data can reduce the nurse case manager's time involvement. By valuing the impact of the variance, alternative courses of treatment and their cost impact can be quantified. Although it may be impractical to implement a sophisticated variance analysis system at this time, it is often beneficial to identify the possibilities that loom on the horizon and can be used once their benefits are determined.

DATA RETRIEVAL

As previously mentioned, data must be accessible to provide for the smooth operation of a case management system. These data must be updated regularly. Decision support systems or comparable systems should be designed to create and store critical pathways by DRGs. A similar system should also be created to accumulate and monitor cost changes over time, first on a case-by-case basis and then for the DRG.

Case manager data needs to include the following for the patient population on a monthly basis:

- patient volume by DRG
- patient volume by critical pathway
- LOS by DRG
- LOS by critical pathway
- cost per case by DRG
- cost per case by critical pathway
- reimbursement received on a per case basis

The case manager should identify and analyze ongoing trends in financial outcomes. This information should be formalized regularly and reported to administration and other members of the patient care team.

MAXIMIZING REIMBURSEMENT

The major challenge facing hospitals today is how to maximize revenue in an environment where reimbursement for care does not keep pace with the cost of its delivery. More and more, hospital revenues are fixed payment reimbursement plans, such as Medicare, and managed care plans (health maintenance organizations and preferred provider organizations). These plans typically pay less on a case-by-case basis than the actual cost of the care provided. This puts tremendous pressure on hospitals as they try to keep pace with medical technology, improve aging facilities, recruit physicians and other medical and nursing staff, and provide quality care for patients. Such financial challenges have provided the incentive for many hospitals to develop case management programs.

Case management encourages patient-focused care, emphasizing appropriate LOS, careful monitoring of resources based on specific case types, and integration and coordination of clinical services. Many organizations think this emphasis is exactly what they need to harness runaway costs, reduce the negative impact of reimbursement decreases, and improve patient care across the continuum.

Reimbursement limitations have forced organizations to focus on cost-effectiveness and efficiency of their operation. Hospitals have been struggling for decades to identify the costs of the various components of patient care. By associating costs with specific areas such as nursing, radiology, pharmacy, and laboratory, to name a few, financial managers hope to determine the organization's fixed and variable costs. Once these costs are identified, it is hoped that they can be controlled and, in some instances, even eliminated.

Despite continuous efforts to control costs, health care costs continue to grow faster than any other sector of the economy. Because of this growth, the health care industry remains a major public concern. In an attempt to control industry cost increases, managed care plans have been developed and are being adopted throughout the country.

Managed care plans are prepaid coordinated health plans designed to control costs by limiting unnecessary service, physician, and hospital fees. They often include comprehensive insurance plans, such as HMOs and PPOs. These plans contract with a group of hospitals, physicians, and other health care providers to provide care to individuals enrolled in the plan. The individual usually pays a predetermined monthly fee, and this fee is expected to cover all the individual's health care needs, including hospitalizations, treatments, and physician visits.

Because most of a hospital's costs are fixed in nature, they do not change with the number of services provided. To keep costs in line, it becomes necessary to increase the number of patients treated so that the unchanging fixed cost can be divided among more people, thus reducing the per patient cost. The continuing trend to treat patients at alternative sites that use minimal hospital facilities has also had a detrimental effect on patient charges. To increase the dollars needed to offset fixed costs, health care providers often agree to provide their services at discounted fees in exchange for patient referrals, and individuals are given strong incentives to use only those providers covered by their plan.

Once providers have entered into these insurance-type arrangements, their incentives change. They will receive the premium regardless of whether the individual uses the facilities. The fewer resources used on the individual, the better. The health care emphasis changes to one of promoting wellness and keeping patients out of the hospitals. Should group members require admittance, the emphasis should be on reducing LOS while ensuring that discharged patients have received the best care and are not expected to return in the near future. As the managed care percentage of hospitals' payer base increases, with the associated increase in discounted payments and the necessary decrease in usage of inpatient services, the efficiency and effectiveness of hospital services becomes essential for survival.

CONCLUSION

As hospitals continue to concentrate on being cost efficient and cost effective while providing high-quality health care, it becomes vitally important for institutions to adopt case management techniques. Because many practitioners prefer to focus on the clinical aspects of patient care, the case manager must remember the financial implications of actions taken for the patient. Patient care teams must be made aware of the impact that extended LOS, inflated costs, and appropriate use of resources will have on the hospital. The case manager serves the pivotal role of keeping the patient care team focused on the patient's care while reviewing the other financial areas of concern.

REFERENCES

1. Zander K. Managed care within acute care settings: design and implementation via nursing case management. *Health Care Supervisor.* 1988;6(2):27–43.
2. Del Togno-Armanasco V, Olivas GS, Harter S. Developing an integrated nursing case management model. *Nurs Manage.* 1989;20(10):26–29.
3. McKenzie CB, Torkelson NG, Holt MA. Care and cost: nursing case management improves both. *Nurs Manage.* 1989;20(10):30–38.
4. Wesley ML, Easterling A. On the scene: restructuring nursing services in the Mercy Health Services Consortium—the St. Joseph Mercy Hospital, Pontiac Project. *Nurs Adm Q.* 1991;15:50–54.
5. Ethridge P, Lamb G. Professional nursing case management improves quality, access, and costs. *Nurs Manage.* 1989;20(3):30–35.
6. Jacobs S, Pelfrey S. Applying just-in-time philosophy to healthcare. *J Nurs Adm.* 1995;24(1):47–52.

■ 21 ■

Data Management through Information Systems

Catherine Noone, MS, BSN, RN, CNA
Cathy A.R. McKillip, MPA, BA

Management of information is crucial for health care systems of the future. Managed care organizations (MCOs) demand access to a comprehensive patient clinical data base to evaluate the results of clinical interventions and to make a financial justification for providing patient care in any setting. This cost-driven climate requires a single point-of-entry information system for patient data that allows sophisticated access to all types of data regarding patients and their care. A single point-of-entry integrated system facilitates patients' access to health care; however, today's data management environment has frequently been described as containing "islands of information." This environment is characterized by the presence of multiple core and specialty systems with little or no linkage among them.[1]

INCREASED NEED FOR ACCESS TO INFORMATION

Existing decentralized information systems create a need for integration to case manage effectively. In most organizations, managers must go to several sources to obtain management information, which is often incomplete or must be analyzed manually. The lack of computerized decision support systems to monitor critical path variances and patient outcome measurements severely hampers the case manager's decision-making ability. Capitated health plans require access to patient care data to manage patient care effectively among the many different levels and sites of care. For example, case managers need quick, accurate, and easy access to data on patients as they move from the hospital to outpatient clinics, day surgery, home care, or their physician's office (Figure 21-1).

Case management is now part of everyday health care operations. Emphasis on case management by MCOs will supersede the nurse's recommenda-

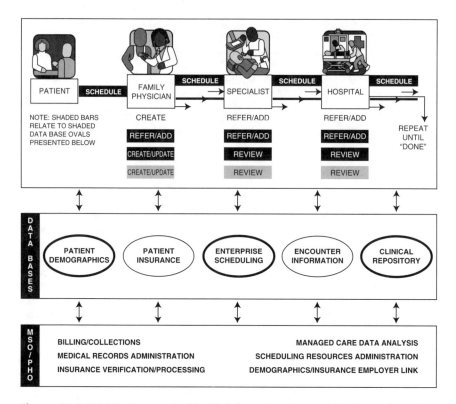

Figure 21-1 N.M.H. Community Health Information Network: Patient Information Flow Diagram. *Source:* Adapted with permission of Wilson, Joel, *Information Systems Strategic Issues: Paper,* Presentation, Newton Memorial Hospital, August 1995.

tions for patient care unless providers have access to their clinical data bases immediately so that an organization can show the cost-effectiveness of their recommendations through objective well-presented data. For example, when a case manager is negotiating with an organization for the care and services that patients need, the providers should have their profile for the diagnosis and outcomes at their fingertips. In many cases, higher rates can be negotiated based on the data compiled and the actual clinical outcomes experienced by the local population.

SYSTEM READINESS

In 1995, the most pressing information system needs were identified by a national consulting group (Exhibit 21-1). An enterprisewide information sys-

Exhibit 21-1 Information System Needs

- Implement user-friendly system interface.
- Access information remotely from all locations.
- Acquire specialized managed care software.
- Use enterprisewide master patient index.
- Implement interface engine to facilitate system communications.
- Develop systems for data comparisons.
- Install conflict resolution resource scheduling.
- Standardize a "limited" number of application vendors.
- Acquire software for longitudinal patient record.
- Use data repository to facilitate data sharing.
- Move toward distributed computing environment.

Source: Adapted from the Fifth Annual Healthcare Computing Conference and Expo, June 25–28, 1995.[1]

tem or community health information network (CHIN) that is user friendly across provider types is needed but does not currently exist in many areas of the country. A CHIN is a fundamental information systems model that encourages the sharing of patient information as a patient travels through a local community health network.[2] The CHIN should include the ability to access information remotely from different provider locations and MCOs (Figure 21-1). An enterprisewide master patient index is needed to transfer patient-specific data easily among the different users of the system. In addition, the ability to store and retrieve longitudinal patient clinical and financial data is essential. The storage of a longitudinal patient record in a data repository is needed to provide data to case managers across provider sources. Standardized clinical systems allow retrieval and statistical analysis of the patient data base, especially as patient services grow.

As traditional indemnity payers and Medicare shift to capitated payment plans, MCOs will require providers to concentrate on proving their high-quality performance through clinical data that can be compared with the performance of other providers. Capitated health plans require access to patient care data to manage patient care effectively across many different levels and sites of care.

Technology, such as an interface engine, to interface different software applications ultimately to obtain a longitudinal patient record is readily available. However, there are currently very few CHINs because the cost of the technology is prohibitive for many providers. In addition, because many providers and payers want access to the CHIN, the allocation of the expense of establishing and maintaining the CHIN is very difficult. Because the cost has been prohibitive for many providers, there has been a lack of patient outcome measurements, which severely hampers the case manager's decision-making ability. For example, without information about the ability of a provider to accomplish a desired clinical outcome, the case manager cannot determine the appropriate level of care for a patient. Computerization of longitudinal financial and clinical data is mandatory to move successfully into the twenty-first century where the technology will be more sophisticated. The ability to retrieve data across a variety of health care settings through data interfaces such as the interface engine will become crucial. The interface engine provides a means for data and information from disparate systems in a health care environment to be connected through a single hub mechanism to share and exchange data. Inpatient and multiple outpatient settings must be linked to provide the case manager with the necessary data to make effective decisions regarding patient care. Accurate tracking of patient visits, outcomes, and costs enable the case manager to manage each case using the optimum resources for each patient.

CONSUMER IMPACT

Patient satisfaction is greatly improved by centralized information systems that allow patient information to be captured and updated at the point of encounter. With centralized information systems, patients provide demographic information at their initial encounter with a provider. Each subsequent provider along the continuum of care has access to the information system to retrieve the patient's information without asking the patient repetitive questions, such as name, birth date, and Social Security number. One example of improved patient satisfaction is that as patients move along the health care continuum they will not be asked to provide their medical history to a number of different providers because the information is online and accessible. As clinical information is added to the demographic data base, each provider verifies and updates patient information at each encounter. The data base or CHIN demonstrates to patients an operational efficiency that has been lacking in many health care settings.

Increased access to medical information has raised many concerns regarding patient confidentiality. Secure systems that protect and restrict information on a need-to-know basis must be developed to give the public trust in their providers. Providers must educate the consumer on the benefits of a data repository to overcome the confidentiality issue. Managers of CHINs must develop procedures to ensure that access to the information system is limited to only those providers who have the patient's authorization to access data.

BENEFITS OF DATA MANAGEMENT THROUGH INFORMATION SYSTEMS

Computerized clinical and financial management information systems are basic for economy and efficiency and must be contracted out if not done internally. Nursing organizations often have to reduce costs to compete in the managed care marketplace. Comprehensive data management enables the organization to submit bills in a timely manner and reduce the average number of days that accounts are outstanding. Without comprehensive data management, organizations are at risk of increasing costs due to lack of the necessary authorizations, certificates of medical necessity, duplicative paperwork, etc. As costs increase, the organization will lose managed care contracts because the organization is not efficiently managing its data. Administrative costs of care are significantly higher with a manual system than with a computerized system.

Financial outcomes and client-specific variables are required in managed care contracts. Comparing charges with real costs and actual reimbursement is necessary to know the true cost of one kind of service compared with another. For example, at a minimum, an organization's information system must track costs by diagnosis and patient outcomes. To negotiate managed care contracts effectively, the information system must have the capability of generating patient-specific differences in response to treatment. The ability to aggregate data for all members of a system or network is an important advantage in the managed care arena.

Providers must use standardized information data sets to capture information to compare the data from one provider with another. The data set is essential to ensure that MCOs are evaluating providers based on the same criteria. Computerized clinical records used for tracking variances from established care plans can boost cash flow through close utilization monitoring from the provider. Electronic approvals from MCOs based on data from the provider will eliminate time-consuming telephone contact between the provider and the MCO. The on-line availability of basic demographic data such as eligibility, geographic location, and insurance plan limitations eliminates the need for duplicative telephone calls from the provider, the patient, and the case manager. Whole packages of health care services can be offered to individuals and families based on the information gleaned from outcome-based data.

Fiscal viability is inevitably linked to the ability to provide quality services in a cost-effective competent manner. Quality controls based on variations from critical pathways are needed because case loads will be smaller but the complexity of patient needs are greater. In the managed care environment, the patient's increasingly complex needs must be met with fewer dollars and resources. Therefore, communication at point of entry regarding the patient's care plan to all members of the service team is logical and cost effective. Instead of saying staffing pattern changes are necessary, hard data will back up this statement so that when redesign of the workplace is implemented, it is not as costly as constantly updating and playing catch-up.

More and more, the business plan for the organization will drive the information systems plan. Following the patient through the health care paper maze is an excellent way to evaluate the need for point-of-entry automation to enhance system efficiency. Forms required by regulatory bodies are standardized and thus lend themselves to easy automation. The managed care environment uses more complex data collection systems (Exhibit 21-2).

IMPACT ON NURSING MANAGEMENT

The interest in computerization as a tool for nursing goes back to the President's Commission on the Nursing Shortage in 1988.[3] One of the 16 recommendations made by the commission was to enhance the nursing work environment using computers to assist nurses with voluminous documentation. Community health settings were known for the amount of redundant manual record keeping they did to meet state and federal reimbursement guidelines.

With the growing interest and demand for products to computerize manual functions, software was developed specifically for health care providers by the leading vendors of health care software products. The array of functions that was adaptable to automation increased from registration, billing, and accounting systems to the nursing process elements. Clinical data, including assessment, problem lists, care plans, and evaluations of care, appeared on the market in growing numbers. The vision of an integrated system with a single point of entry for the patient became a reality for the 1990s.

Exhibit 21-2 Traditional versus Managed Care

Traditional Data Need	Managed Care
Standard formats	Point-of-entry integration
Input/output	Interface engines
Islands of data	Consolidation
Fragmentation	CHIN
Laundry lists	"Convergence"
Encounters of care entry	Permanent lifetime record
Process oriented	Standardization emphasis
Departmental storage of data	Repository storage of data

MCOs have sophisticated integrated systems and demand that providers be capable of retrieval of specific data from their systems that may have interface with other members in the networks. The data available include not only basic demographic information but outcomes, patient profiles, length of stay statistics, information by physician utilization, and specific diagnosis for case managers to track.

Nurses in all settings are affected by this trend because they will need to be computer literate to practice in settings that incorporate entry and retrieval of clinical data in addition to basic census data. Nursing organizations and institutional providers are trying to remain current in a constantly changing environment and often are part of changing organizational structures within the areas of practice. To survive in the new environment, providers need solid information systems that are integrated and contain all the elements needed.

Nurse case managers need computer fluency to communicate with management information staff at all levels and to plan the best interface among departments. They have to be educated in the use of these systems from how to do staffing assignments and determine eligibility for service to tracking important patient outcome data (Exhibit 21-3).

STEPS IN PLANNING AND IMPLEMENTING AN INFORMATION SYSTEM

The case management process is the framework for the Standards of Practice[4] published by the Case Management Society of America. When applied to information systems for case management, the process involves the following steps:

1. *Assessment/case identification*—The case manager must have the ability to identify basic demographic and clinical data about patients in the system.
2. *Problem identification*—The case manager needs longitudinal data about individual physicians, providers, and outcomes by disease category, patient outcomes and payer liability, and insurance variations.
3. *Planning*—The information systems plan must meet the needs of the team in its ability to retrieve information by patient, family, and treatment team, often for multiple sites.
4. *Monitoring*—Case managers need built-in quality indicators to compare goals that were planned for the patient initially to assess appropriate services and products that may need revision or updating.
5. *Evaluating*—Retrieval of individual client responses to the care plan and management that are relevant to other similar cases can be used by the case manager for evaluation steps in process.

Exhibit 21-3 Data Required for Managed Care Communications

- Name of Patient
- Address
- City and Zip
- Age, Sex
- Significant Other
- Occupation
- Company
- Date of Birth
- Social Security Number
- Insurance
- Plan
- Type
- Coverage Exclusions

- Services Requested
- Services Delivered
- Settings for Care
- Charges

- Primary Diagnosis
- Secondary Diagnosis
- Length of Stay
- Number of Visits/Encounters

- Outcome
- Time Elapsed to Goal/Resolution
- Comparison to Region
- Readmission
- Hospitalizations

6. *Outcomes*—The ability to determine whether client outcomes and practice patterns in treatment compare with similar cases and regional providers will demonstrate optimal case management in a cost-effective manner.

CONCLUSION

We have come a long way since the early 1980s when most health care agencies did not have clinical data computerized. The days of "islands of lost slips" and "black holes" where papers disappeared can no longer exist. This has enabled a decrease in redundant paperwork, allowing agencies to focus on the clinical outcome data that are accumulated in an automated system.

There is still a long way to go to integrate different information systems to enable providers with access to all the available data for a patient and then make decisions regarding the optimal setting for the patient. Establishing levels of care based on clear outcomes of nursing interventions makes sense. We can model our delivery of services to patients using systems that fit our needs. Nursing's business is meeting the needs of individual recipients of nursing, and most of those individuals will be in a managed care environment. To connect our clients and other care providers, as well as the new players and payers, we need to link data across new boundaries.

REFERENCES

1. Lafarance S. *Open systems, closed to intruders: how to secure an enterprise-wide system.* Presented at the Fifth Annual Healthcare Computing Conference and Expo. June 1995.
2. Wilson J. *Information systems strategic issues: paper.* Presented at Newton Memorial Hospital. 1995.
3. U.S. Department of Health and Human Services. *Secretary's Commission on Nursing: Final Report.* Washington, D.C.: U.S. Department of Health and Human Services; 1988.
4. Case Management Society of America. *Standards of Practice for Case Management.* Little Rock, Ark: Case Management Society of America; 1995.

BIBLIOGRAPHY

Chu S, Thom J. Information technology as a proactive strategic weapon in healthcare. *JONA.* 1994;24(4):5–7.

■ 22 ■

Case Management As a Service Economy Job Design: Toward a Theoretical Model

Mary Crabtree Tonges, MBA, MSN, RN

The nature of American business is undergoing a dramatic transformation from manufacturing to service, and health care is a growth industry within the burgeoning service sector. Yet the development of job design theory has not kept pace with changes in the economy. Existing theories of job design are based primarily on the industrial model used by manufacturing and may thus be less applicable to service jobs.

Some individuals may regard theory as too abstract or "academic" to be useful and fail to see lack of theory as an important issue; however, the purpose of theory is to provide an explanation, and theory that successfully explains how something important works is highly practical to individuals interested in influencing those outcomes. Job design theory explains the mechanisms that produce intrinsically motivating work and suggests approaches to designing jobs that enhance motivation, satisfaction, and performance. Given the current economic trends, there is a pressing need for theory development to guide the design of service jobs.

Within the context of the transition to a service economy, existing jobs are also being changed as firms reengineer their business processes. Case management is emerging as a new job design in a variety of different types of businesses interested in improving continuity in their service relationships with clients.[1,2] This new approach focuses on process redesign at the customer interface[1] and is characterized by the creation of a quintessential service role in which case managers buffer clients from the difficulties of dealing with complex organizational structures and processes.[2] In health care, case

Acknowledgment: The author thanks Professors Hannah Rothstein and Abraham Korman, Baruch College of the City University of New York, for their feedback, suggestions, and guidance through the ongoing development of this model.

manager jobs are frequently performed by nurses, who coordinate patients' care among providers and across settings to bridge gaps in fragmented delivery systems and facilitate the attainment of desired outcomes.

This is a hyperturbulent time in health care, and many changes are being made in the organization and delivery of patient care. To guide this restructuring toward positive outcomes, explanatory job design theory is needed for nursing as a service profession, and more specifically, for nursing case management as an emerging, highly service-oriented role.

The purpose of this chapter is to extend the limits of job design theory through an analysis of (1) the characteristics of service work and nurses' jobs, (2) the effects of these characteristics on satisfaction and performance, and (3) the influence of dispositional difference moderators on the strength of these relationships. The chapter presents a review of the job design literature, which focuses on nursing job design and available research on the characteristics of the nurse case manager role. Building on this background, a theoretical model for the design of nursing jobs is proposed and potential research opportunities are identified.

JOB DESIGN FOR A SERVICE ECONOMY

Our current understanding of job design is based primarily on the study of industrial, goods-related jobs;[3-5] however, the nature of business activity in the United States has undergone a dramatic transformation, resulting in the creation of a postindustrial, service-based economy. Service and manufacturing organizations are thought to differ on several important dimensions.[6] For example, criteria commonly cited as the distinguishing characteristics of service organizations include (1) intangible output, (2) indispensable personal interaction between the producer and consumer, and (3) information processing properties.[7] These characteristics appear to have important implications for job design theory and application in the service sector.

Among the defining attributes of service work, the nature of client–firm interaction is thought to be the seminal element.[7] Because the essence of this type of work is so interpersonal, relationships with others would seem to have important motivational consequences. Yet the job characteristics model,[8] which is considered the most influential paradigm in contemporary job design research,[9-11] places little importance on the interpersonal aspects of work, relegating required interaction with others to a supplemental element that is not included in the motivational theory itself.

The interactional nature of service work also underlies the information processing properties of service organizations. Because the work focuses on people rather than things, the technologies of service delivery must incorporate communication, knowledge, and energy.[7] Information from clients is the raw material input to the transformation process of service systems, which prevents these organizations from sealing off their technical cores and shielding service workers from customer-induced uncertainties.[12]

Finally, consider the issue of intangible output and its effects on job characteristics. It is likely that the nature and sources of feedback from work are different in a job that generates intangible services as compared with a job that produces physical goods. For example, the evaluation of intangible output may necessarily be more subjective and, therefore, more strongly influenced by personal differences and/or social views.

Mills and Moberg[12(p.467)] provide a succinct description of the change to a service economy and its potential implications:

> The growth of the service sector in the U.S. economy is well documented. Approximately 70 percent of the employable work force is engaged in service activities and predictions of further increases are common. Yet, the growth of knowledge specifically pertinent to the operations of services has not kept pace with these developments. What is known is that caution should be exercised in applying models derived from and for manufacturing to service operations.

Although the industrialization of service was widely advocated in the 1970s,[13,14] service organizations' adoption of the assembly-line approach to organizing work has rarely worked as well as it did in manufacturing and appears to exemplify the misapplication of manufacturing solutions in service situations.[1]

In addition to changes in job design attributable to the creation of new jobs in the growing service sector, the structure of existing jobs is also being altered as competition intensifies and the quest for productivity improvement generates waves of business process reengineering. Based on a growing recognition of the need to focus on business processes rather than functional activities, many firms are reorganizing to enable one individual to ensure continuity in the performance of a series of tasks from beginning to end.[1,2] This new approach is known as case management.

Reintegration of fragmented tasks and processes is a hallmark characteristic of case management, which may explain why it has been described as one of the most radical changes in job design since the division of labor.[1] Given that the case manager job has been created for the express purpose of facilitating clients' interactions with complex service organizations, this role may represent an archetypal service job within the movement toward a service economy.

Changing Structure of Nursing Jobs

Nursing is a service profession in transition, and there have been many changes in nurses' jobs in recent years.[15,16] The impetus for these changes can be found in the combined effects of economic, political, and professional forces affecting the cost and quality of American health care.

The two major factors driving and influencing the development of new nursing roles are the ongoing changes in health care financing and nursing leaders' desire to enrich the staff nurse job.[17-19] The interaction of these forces has resulted in the creation of the nurse case manager (NCM) position to manage a case load of patients with the objective of achieving desired clinical outcomes as quickly and inexpensively as possible. Because hospitals are now paid a predetermined amount for many cases, regardless of length of stay or actual expense, there is great interest in nurses managing patients' care through the hospitalization, and sometimes beyond, across a wider continuum of services.[19,20]

Due to the recurrent nursing shortages of the past several decades, considerable attention has been devoted to the study of job satisfaction and turnover among staff nurses (SNs).[21,22] Research suggests that inadequate working conditions and counterproductive attitudes within employing organizations are the most serious sources of dissatisfaction.[23] Specifically, role stressors, limited autonomy, and inadequate communication and feedback have been identified as major sources of dissatisfaction among nurses.[24,25] In response to these concerns, nursing leaders have used the opportunity created by health care economics to design the NCM role as an enriched job.

Fueled by the pressure to control health care costs, implementation of nursing case management is expanding rapidly across the country.[17,26] Despite the growing popularity and rapid expansion of nursing case management, there is a lack of research concerning its effects.[27] Of the limited number of studies that have been conducted, most focus on patient and organizational outcomes rather than effects on nurses. Given its intended function as an enriched job and the growing popularity of this role, there is a clear need for research concerning the NCM job and its effects on nurses' work experience.

Progress in studying these issues is hampered by a lack of theory. As Loevinger[28] notes:

At least since Thomas Kuhn published *The Structure of Scientific Revolutions* (1962), it has been recognized that observations are the result of theories (called paradigms by Kuhn and other philosophers), for without theories of relevance and irrelevance there would be no basis for determining what observations to make.

Thus, a theory that is applicable to the design of nursing jobs is needed as basis for research.

The framework for the model proposed to meet this need is drawn from several different bodies of theoretical and empirical literature. Specific elements from the domains of work redesign, role theory, need theories of motivation, and nursing practice are central issues and thus provide the basis for explaining the constructs and interrelationships of interest. Key elements from each domain include the following:

1. *Work redesign*—job design and the influence of organizations as social systems on the design and management of work[8]
2. *Role theory*—relationships and interactions between and among role senders and role occupants and effects on occupants' affective and behavioral outcomes[29]
3. *Need theories of motivation*—individual needs, or internal states of disequilibrium, as motivational forces driving behavior;[30] specifically, needs for achievement and affiliation,[31] and influence[32]
4. *Nursing practice*—the professional nature of nursing as viewed from a larger perspective, as well as the specific defining components of this work

These concepts are complementary, and a theoretical model resulting from their synthesis facilitates the development of a better understanding of nurses' work experiences and reactions than any smaller subset of ideas. Specifically, nursing practice is the work performed by nurses in their jobs and is a primary antecedent of perceived job characteristics. Job and work redesign focus on the dimensions characterizing the work experience and employees' affective and behavioral responses, as mediated by a critical set of psychological states. Role theory augments the narrower consideration of task characteristics and design with a more global perspective, which encompasses interpersonal interactions in the work setting, thereby creating an avenue for the extension of job characteristics theory. Finally, need theories of motivation focus on the unique qualities individual workers bring to a job and highlight the importance of examining the dynamics of working from the perspective of person–job interaction. The review of literature that follows begins with a discussion of work redesign as the foundation on which the model is built.

JOB DESIGN THEORY AND RESEARCH

Work redesign can be defined broadly as altering "the design of the work itself—that is, changing the actual structure of the jobs that people perform."[8] Hackman[33] expands this definition by specifying that such changes are intended to increase both the quality of employees' work experience and their job productivity. He also suggests that the term *work redesign* subsumes other related terms including *job rotation, job enrichment,* and *sociotechnical systems design,* which refer to specific methods for changing the design of work.[33]

There are several different approaches to designing jobs. Hackman and Oldham[8] group these approaches into three categories: (1) traditional approaches derived from classical organizational theory and industrial engineering; (2) behavioral approaches that focus on the impact of jobs on the people performing them; and (3) systems approaches that consider interrelationships among networks of jobs in large organizational units. The theoretical model described in this chapter is drawn from the behavioral and systems perspectives and focuses on the motivational characteristics of the work entailed in performing a job, both independently and in the context of interactions with others.

Job Enrichment and the Job Characteristics Model

Most job design theory and research in the past 40 years have been philosophically based in the human resources school of management. This perspective assumes that a combination of increased opportunities for self-direction and more meaningful work leads to higher levels of job satisfaction.[34]

The human resources philosophy may represent a corrective response to earlier approaches to job design, specifically scientific management,[35] or Taylorism, and the human relations movement resulting from Mayo's well-known Hawthorne studies.[36] Although scientific management recommends that jobs be designed as simply as possible, requiring minimal skill and initiative to achieve maximum efficiency, the human relations perspective emphasizes social aspects of the work situation and shifted the focus of research from workers' relations with machines to interpersonal and group relationships. Thus, scientific management focused too narrowly on the technical aspects of the work to the exclusion of workers' needs as people, and the human relations approach emphasized the importance of social and interpersonal issues without sufficient consideration of the work itself. Because the human resources perspective considers good performance in a meaningful job to be causally related to satisfaction, this management philosophy views the design of work as important and encourages the development of enriched jobs.

Behavioral Approach to Work Redesign

The roots of the behavioral approach to job design lie in the work of Frederick Herzberg. Based on a survey of 200 engineers and accountants in the late 1950s, Herzberg and associates[37] developed the two-factor or motivator-hygiene theory of work motivation. This theory posits that job satisfaction and dissatisfaction have different antecedents: motivators (i.e., the work itself, achievement, promotions, recognition, and responsibility) lead to satisfaction, whereas dissatisfaction is caused by hygiene factors (i.e., supervisors, interpersonal relations, working conditions, company policies, and salary). Jobs that are designed to include motivator factors are expected to be intrinsically motivating and satisfying and are therefore described as "enriched."[38]

A major contribution of the two-factor theory is that it has stimulated a large body of research that examines the effects of job design on motivation; however, it also has several limitations, including a lack of empirical support for its major tenets[39,40] and insufficient attention to individual differences in predicting the effects of enriched jobs.[8,40,41]

Job characteristics theory is a behavioral approach to the design of work that focuses on objective attributes or characteristics of jobs.[8] This theoretical perspective is grounded in the work of Turner and Lawrence[5] and the requisite task attributes model that they proposed. These researchers identified six requisite task attributes considered to be required by the intrinsic nature of the job: variety and autonomy in activities, required and optional interactions, and the mental states of knowledge or skill and responsibility. They also developed an instrument to measure these attributes and a summary index of overall job complexity.

Turner and Lawrence[5] hypothesized that workers express a more favorable response (in terms of job satisfaction and attendance) to "more complex or involving tasks than to more highly programmed, less demanding work." Findings from their study of industrial jobs supported the hypothesized positive relationship between challenging work and positive outcomes for employees who worked in factories in small towns; however, for urban employees satisfaction was negatively related and attendance was unrelated to the index. The researchers concluded that subcultural differences moderated the relationship between job complexity and employee response. Turner and Lawrence laid the groundwork for the development of job characteristics theory by initiating the development of an approach to classifying and measuring characteristics of jobs across different types of work and by identifying the need to consider the moderating effects of individual and situational differences.

Lawler,[42] a major contributor to job characteristics theory, provides an explanation for the relationship between job design and employee performance. Briefly, he suggests that "job design changes can have a positive effect on motivation because they can change an individual's beliefs about the probability that certain rewards will result from putting forth high levels of effort." Specifically, good performance in a job that has the potential to satisfy higher-order needs (e.g., self-esteem and self-actualization) is intrinsically rewarding because the employee experiences positive valued outcomes such as feelings of accomplishment, achievement, and use of skills and abilities.

Job Characteristics Model

The job characteristics model (JCM) developed by Hackman and colleagues[3,4,8] is regarded as the dominant paradigm in task design research.[43,44] This model has provided the framework for hundreds of studies, and the evidence generated by this research has been the subject of many qualitative and quantitative reviews.[9,11,44]

The first version of the JCM was described and tested by Hackman and Lawler.[3] In developing the JCM, Hackman and Lawler reconceptualized the individual difference issue and changed its focus from the sociological to the psychological level of analysis. Although Turner and Lawrence[5] suggested that McClelland's need for achievement motive might be one of the most relevant individual motivational predispositions to consider, Hackman and Lawler chose to incorporate higher-order need strength from Alderfer's[45] modification of Maslow's[46] hierarchy of needs theory.

Hackman and Lawler developed measures for the job characteristics, higher-order need strength, experienced work motivation, general and specific types of satisfaction, and performance. Their test of the model with telephone company personnel suggested that employees working in complex jobs who desire higher need satisfaction tend to have high motivation, satisfaction, quality performance, and attendance.[3] Although the two interpersonal dimensions related to required and optional interaction were positively and significantly related to general satisfaction, they were negatively associated with performance. Hackman and Lawler concluded that the consequences of having jobs with high interpersonal components are primarily social in nature.

Hackman and Oldham[47] refined the measures used by Turner and Lawrence[5] and Hackman and Lawler[3] to create the job diagnostic survey (JDS), which assesses employees' perceptions of the characteristics of their jobs. They used these tools to evaluate an extension of Hackman and Lawler's[3] conceptual framework, which they called the JCM.[4]

The JCM identifies five core job dimensions (skill variety, task identity, task significance, autonomy, and feedback) that evoke three critical psychological states (experienced meaningfulness of the work, experienced responsibility for outcomes of the work, and knowledge of the actual results of the work activities), which in turn lead to five desirable personal and work outcomes (high internal work motivation, high-quality work performance, high satisfaction with the work, and low absenteeism and turnover). The first three core dimensions (variety, identity, and significance) relate to experienced meaningfulness, autonomy is linked to experienced responsibility, and feedback influences knowledge of results. The five core dimensions can be combined in a summary measure called the motivating potential score (MPS) by multiplying the overall mean score for variety, identity, and significance times autonomy times feedback. All three of the psychological states are seen as antecedents of the affective and behavioral outcomes. Finally, the relationships between the core dimensions and the psychological states and between the states and the outcomes are moderated by employee growth need strength (GNS).[4] A test of the JCM with 658 employees on 62 different jobs in seven organizations supported its general validity.[4]

Evaluation of the Cumulative Evidence. Hackman and Oldham provide an enlightening critique of the JCM that makes the following key points:

1. Evidence for the proposed moderating effects is mixed, and there is a need to explore different conceptualizations and measurements of relevant individual differences, such as need for achievement or intrinsic versus extrinsic work values.

2. The feedback concept used in the model is flawed in its failure to consider the effects of feedback from other sources besides the work itself.[8]

Its developers conclude that although the validity of the JCM is generally supported by empiric evidence, it has not been demonstrated to be a completely accurate or comprehensive explanation of the motivational effects of job characteristics. Thus, it is best viewed as a guide to further research in this area.

The most comprehensive recent review of JCM research is reported by Fried and Ferris.[9] These authors conducted a meta-analysis of correlational data from 76 studies and a narrative review of additional studies for a total of nearly 200. The purpose of the study was to evaluate the extent to which empiric evidence supports the JCM. Their overall conclusion is that some elements of the model were supported, but corrections or modifications are needed in other aspects. Specifically, their main findings can be summarized as follows:

1. Although job characteristics relate more strongly to psychological than behavioral outcomes, relationships between job characteristics and behavioral outcomes (performance and absenteeism) are more meaningful and consistent than has been suggested. Task identity has the strongest relationship to performance.

2. Effects of job characteristics on performance are moderated by individual and situational differences.

3. The multidimensionality of job characteristics is supported, but the exact number of dimensions is not clear.

Reviews of the cumulative evidence informed the development of the theoretical model presented here, as follows:

- Support for the relationship between job characteristics and behavioral effects[9] provides a basis for the inclusion of performance as an outcome.

- Evidence supporting the multidimensionality of job characteristics and suggesting the need for further exploration of additional dimensions[9,44] is addressed in the development of a more comprehensive set of characteristics.

- Findings concerning the questionable role of GNS as a moderator[8] suggest the inclusion of several alternative dispositional difference constructs.

Although all the controversies concerning the JCM have not been resolved, the weight of the evidence appears to provide reasonable support for the general validity of the model. Thus, although not perfect, the JCM does provide a useful foundation for the development of further research in this area.

Many authors have suggested the need for modification and extension of the JCM.[8,44,48–50] Recommendations have included both the identification of potential additional dimensions[44,48–50] and the consideration of different moderators.[8,44] Johns and colleagues[10] report strong support for the mediating role of the psychosocial states, which leads them to recommend using the states as "more sensitive criteria in job design efforts and as preliminary criteria in studies of job characteristics other than those specified by the JCM." The model developed in this chapter responds to these recommendations and builds on previous studies of job characteristics and job enrichment in nursing and other professional jobs.

Job Characteristics and Enrichment in Nursing

The JCM approach has been used to assess nurses' perceptions of the motivational characteristics of their jobs and associated outcomes by several researchers.[51–54] In response to cyclical shortages, many job enrichment interventions have been initiated in nursing.[55–56] The JCM has been used as a framework to evaluate the effects of several past approaches to enriching nurses' jobs;[57] however, the NCM job has not yet been systematically evaluated.

Assessment of Characteristics and Effects

A consistent pattern of findings emerges from research focusing on the identification of SN job content characteristics.[51,52] In comparison to JDS norms for professional and technical jobs reported by Hackman and Oldham,[8] SNs perceive higher levels of significance and variety, about the same levels of autonomy and feedback, and lower task identity.

Depending on the composition of the sample, the overall MPS for SNs can be higher[52] or lower[51] than the professional/technical norm of 154 reported by Hackman and Oldham.[8] Roedel and Nystrom's[52] sample included a small percentage of nurse managers, which may have increased the mean MPS. The results of Joiner and colleagues[51] suggest differences in the motivational characteristics of SN jobs in different clinical areas. Although they report an overall MPS of 155, the mean for medical/surgical nurses was 139 versus 188 for nurses in coronary care.[51] Subgroups of Joiner et al., however, were quite small (i.e., 14 coronary care nurses and 47 medical/surgical nurses). A similar pattern of findings is reported by Wulff,[54] who found that critical care nurses scored their jobs as significantly higher for skill variety, experienced meaningfulness, and meeting individual growth needs than medical/surgical nurses. However, Roedel and Nystrom[52] found that medical/surgical nurses perceive significantly more task identity than critical care nurses, but MPSs are not available for comparison.

What are the effects of these characteristics on nurses' outcomes? In their sample of 135 nurses, Roedel and Nystrom[52] report significant relationships, albeit at several different significance levels, between all five job characteristics and general job satisfaction (feedback, $r = .30$, autonomy, $r = .24$, and identity, $r = .22$ [$P < .01$]; variety, $r = .14$, and significance, $r = .12$ [$P < .10$]). Four characteristics were significantly correlated with the work satisfaction facet of general satisfaction. Autonomy and feedback had the strongest relationships ($r = .30$, $P < .01$), followed by task identity ($r = .24$, $P < .01$), and skill variety ($r = .14$, $P < .10$). Correlations for task significance and variety may be attenuated by range restriction as nurses consistently report high scores for these characteristics.

The pattern observed suggests that task identity, autonomy, and feedback are important to nurses' psychological states and affective outcomes, but nurses report lower levels of these characteristics in their jobs. These studies focused on satisfaction versus performance, which is a general pattern in nursing research, but may also be related to the inclusion of scales for affective variables in the JDS.

Seybolt[53] examined the effect of nurses' hospital career stage on the relationships between job characteristics and satisfaction and turnover intentions. The most relevant findings to this discussion are that nurses in the first few years of their careers focus on performance feedback and supervisory expectations, but the emphasis shifts to the work itself during the three- to six-year period, and after six years, interactions at work are seen as the major sources of career satisfaction.

Harrison[58] reports a study of the effect of GNS as a moderator of the job characteristic-affective outcome relationship for nurses. The author compared reported job characteristics, GNS, and growth and general satisfaction for nurses in three different types of positions: SNs, head nurses, and specialized roles, such as clinical nurse specialist or patient educator. Key findings included significantly higher MPSs for nurses in specialized roles than those reported by either SNs ($t_{76} = 3.62, p < .01$) or head nurses ($t_{50} = 2.04, p < .05$). Nurses in specialized roles perceived their jobs as significantly higher in task identity than SNs ($t_{76} = 4.02, p < .01$) and head nurses ($t_{50} = 2.16, p < .05$). Both nurses in specialized roles ($t_{76} = 3.77, p < .01$) and head nurses ($t_{94} = 2.52, p < .05$) reported significantly higher autonomy than SNs.

Head nurses ($t_{94} = 4.02, p < .01$) and nurses in specialized roles ($t_{76} = 2.64, p < .01$) also reported significantly higher growth satisfaction than SNs. Characteristics with the strongest relationships with growth satisfaction were autonomy ($r = .64, p < .001$) and skill variety ($r = .59, p < .001$). Head nurses' scores for overall job satisfaction were significantly higher than those reported by SNs ($t_{94} = 3.33, p < .01$), but there was no significant difference between nurses in specialized roles and SNs.

It is interesting to note that although nurses in specialized roles report higher levels of perceived job characteristics than either head nurses or SNs, head nurses have the highest satisfaction scores. The author unfortunately does not report an analysis of the demographic homogeneity of the three groups because it would be interesting to see if perhaps the head nurses have more experience or the nurses in specialized roles have more education. Although experience has been shown to be positively associated with job satisfaction, education appears to be negatively related,[59] which may be a factor in these findings. It is also possible that the nurse managers are the highest paid group, and they may experience different types of control other than autonomy.

There were no significant differences among the different functional groups in level of GNS. A subgroup analysis based on high versus low GNS revealed that all correlations between job characteristics and growth satisfaction were stronger in the high GNS group. Harrison's findings are congruent with other studies reporting low levels of task identity and autonomy in SN positions.[51,52] Moreover, this study demonstrates that nurses in other types of positions perceive higher levels of these motivational characteristics. It is also important to note, however, that dispositional and individual differences will influence how nurses respond to and evaluate a more complex job.

Evaluation of Job Enrichment in Nursing

In their book on job enrichment in nursing, Joiner and van Servellen[57] present a comprehensive literature review intended to "describe in some detail the phenomenon of job enrichment as it applies to job design, in theory and in practice, and to the work world of the nurse, particularly in the hospital setting." Their discussion focuses on several job enrichment strategies that were popular in nursing at the time.[55,56] Interventions of particular relevance to this discussion include primary nursing and collaborative practice.

Joiner and van Servellen[57] speculate that primary nursing should lead to higher levels of autonomy, direct feedback, identification with the whole, and task variability. Their explanation is as follows:

1. Autonomy, authority, and accountability are warranted on the basis of the nurse's in-depth knowledge of the patient—a byproduct not only of the RN's skills, but also of the continuous relationship of the nurse with the patient and family from admission to discharge.
2. Feedback in all cases—from patient, physician, associate nurses, and head nurses—is direct.
3. Identification with the whole patient is encouraged by several concepts [including a patient-centered versus task-oriented approach, comprehensive care, continuous nurse-patient relationship, and increased attention to outcomes].
4. Task and skill variety . . . is greatly enhanced, because the nature of the primary nurse's interventions with assigned patients is comprehensive.

No study that explicitly tested these predictions has been located.

The qualitative review of Joiner and van Servellen suggests that primary nursing has a positive effect on recruitment and retention; however, the impact on job satisfaction is less clear. The relationship between primary nursing and satisfaction appears to be influenced by other factors, including motivation to accept change, the quality of care provided, recognition and rewards inherent in the enriched role, and organizational context, particularly availability of resources and consistency of expectations.

Development of collaborative nurse-physician practice programs was stimulated by a grant from the W.K. Kellogg Foundation in 1978.[60] In addition to primary nursing, collaborative practice initiatives included these elements: (1) encouragement of nurses' clinical decision making, (2) integration of nurses' and physicians' notes in the medical record, (3) participation in joint review of patient records, and (4) joint practice committees to address issues arising in relationships between the two disciplines.[57] Case study reports indicate that nurses perceive benefits and find some satisfaction in collaborative practice, but it is frequently difficult to engage physicians in meaningful collaboration with nurses.[61,62] The writer is reminded of a physician's comment that he is willing to collaborate with anybody as long as he has control.

An empirical test of the effects of primary nursing and collaborative practice on nurses' perceptions of the characteristics of their jobs has not been located. Of the research reviewed, investigations of the effects of primary nursing, and results suggest that this intervention has a positive effect on recruitment and retention; however, findings concerning the relationship between primary nursing and job satisfaction are mixed.[57] Collaborative practice programs report positive effects on nurses' satisfaction, but physician resistance is a common obstacle to meaningful collaboration.[61,62] In summary, findings from studies of these job enrichment efforts in nursing suggest that further intervention is necessary.

Nurse Case Manager As an Enriched Job

Case management is gaining popularity as a work redesign technique among companies striving to streamline their business processes.[1,2] Within hospitals, nursing case management has been introduced both to improve the coordination of patient care and create enriched jobs for nurses. The concluding section of this review presents an overview of case management as a job design in business in general and health care specifically. The section ends with a summary and discussion of available findings on the design and characteristics of the NCM job.

Reintegrating Labor through Case Management Job Design

Several authors have described a business trend toward combination, not division, of labor.[1,2] Based on a growing recognition of the need to focus on business process, which originated in the quality movement,[63] firms are reorganizing to enable one individual to perform a series of tasks, such as fulfillment of a customer order from beginning to end. This "radical new work design" is called a case management approach, possibly in reference to social work case managers who help clients to deal with multiple agencies.[1]

Davenport and Nohria[1] make several relevant points about case management in general business. They identify the following as components of a successful case manager's role: (1) completes or manages a "closed loop" work process to deliver an entire service; (2) mediates between customers and complex organizations at a point where customers and other functions intersect; and (3) has an expanded role to make decisions about customer issues.

These elements suggest that a case manager's job can be described as a boundary-spanning function, high in job identity, autonomy, and influence. Davenport and Nohria[1] point out that the case manager job includes several elements that theorists of work motivation identify as desirable, yet they caution that the potential for job satisfaction in these jobs may be paradoxically low. Because the job is frequently mediated through a telephone or computer workstation, a loss of face-to-face social interaction can radically reduce case managers' work life quality.[1]

From a macro perspective, these authors observe that case management generally leads to strains within an organization. Specifically, they state, "Because it is a role based on a process view of the organization, some aspects of case management will frequently conflict with functional or divisional structures and with existing policies and procedures."[1(p.21)] This suggests that the case manager may also experience high levels of role stressors.

Interestingly, Davenport and Nohria identify the case manager role as a potential bellwether of a new organizational form. They report that case management is being widely adopted across multiple industries and conclude that "it has the potential to become the future of all business organizations, and it has already become the present for some."[1(p.22)] Clearly, there is a need to increase our understanding of this important new role and its effects on employees.

Nursing Case Management

Organizations with complex processes for bringing their products and services to market are identified as the best candidates for case management.[1] For example, case management is highly suited to service organizations in which "the service cannot be performed simply and straightforwardly in assembly line fashion . . . because multiple types of services are offered to one customer, perhaps even simultaneously (e.g., as in a health care institution)."[1(p.16)]

Health care organizations have, in fact, been ahead of this trend. Pioneering hospitals began to implement case management in the mid-1980s.[64,65] Case management in health care is defined as:

> A clinical system that focuses on the accountability of an identified individual or group for coordinating a patient's care (or a group of patients) across a continuum of care; insuring and facilitating the achievement of quality, clinical, and cost outcomes; negotiating, procuring, and coordinating services and resources needed by the patient/family; intervening at key points (and/or at significant variances) for individual patients; addressing and resolving patterns in aggregate variances that have a negative quality-cost impact; and creating opportunities and systems to enhance outcomes.[66(p.1)]

There are many different types of case management models in health care. Nursing case management, the model of interest in this discussion, is defined by the American Nurses Association as a process of care that includes assess-

ing, delivering, coordinating, and monitoring services and resources to ensure service needs are met.[66] Nursing case management is provided by registered professional nurses, frequently through a department of nursing within
a hospital or another type of health care organization. NCMs may use clinical
management tools known as CareMaps® that organize, sequence, and time
the major interventions of the various health professionals who care for a
particular case type and identify expected patient responses and outcomes.[67]
These tools provide a framework for managing care and assessing patients'
progress.

Nursing Case Management Research

My review of the nursing case management literature suggests two general conclusions, which are supported by the findings of other reviewers:
(1) most of this literature is largely anecdotal,[68] and (2) the research that exists
focuses primarily on patient and institutional outcomes, rather than nurses'
outcomes.[69]

A few relevant studies were located, however, including two recently completed, unpublished nursing masters theses. Several studies that used qualitative approaches to explore and describe the NCM experience were reviewed,
and two studies that reported quantitative findings concerning nurses' outcomes were identified.

Van Dongen and Jambunathan[70] report a small pilot study that examined
the role of the NCM. These researchers used survey data from 24 psychiatric
outpatients, 5 NCMs, and 2 psychiatrists to develop a composite description
of the nature of NCM practice and care. They found that the psychiatrists and
NCMs both described the NCM role as autonomous, yet collaborative with
the psychiatrist.

Carondelet St. Mary's Hospital in Tucson, Arizona, developed one of the earliest nursing case management models.[64] Carondelet has had an active evaluation research program in place to evaluate quality and cost outcomes, and researchers there have recently begun to turn their attention to studying the
process of nursing case management practice.[71] Key findings from the study
of Newman et al.[71(pp.405,407)] of NCM roles at Carondelet include the following:
(1) "NCMs are not bound by space or time; they establish ongoing partnerships with people and move across the spectrum of health care settings";
(2) NCMs are "organizationally empowered to carry out professional service";
and (3) relationships between NCMs and hospital nursing staff were "sensitive" initially but improved with time. The investigators concluded that nurses
were experiencing something different when practicing as case managers.

Rheaume and colleagues[72] also studied the effects of community-oriented
nursing case management on practice, specifically, its effects on nurse-client

and nurse-colleague relationships. Regarding the nurse-client relationship, they report that case management has the potential to shift the usual roles of community health nurses: the care coordination role may expand, and the direct care provider role may decrease. Thus, "the development of a therapeutic relationship with clients may be more difficult to achieve," and "the caring relationship described in the literature that bonds nurse and client may be replaced under case management by a more formal relationship that may also benefit the client, but in a different way."[72(p.32)]

Findings concerning nurse-colleague relationships can be summarized as follows: (1) "case management has the potential to alter fundamentally the usual lines of authority between nurses and physicians"; (2) occasional difficulties are encountered between NCMs and hospital discharge planners who think that case management is duplicative; and (3) "relationships with other healthcare workers can be troublesome if the case manager's role is not understood clearly. This is even a potential problem in relationships with other nurses."[72(p.33)] Despite the potential difficulties, the authors conclude that case management appears to improve the quality of working relationships with other health care workers in that it makes collaborative relationships feasible.

McGill's[73] thesis is a qualitative evaluation of the impact of the role of the hospital-based NCM on leadership development. Content analysis of the data revealed three major themes: changing relationships, changing self, and changing support systems. McGill concluded that NCM's relationships with physicians and other disciplines changed positively, but relationships with SNs changed negatively.

McGill's research report is a rich source of information about how NCMs experience their jobs. She provides direct quotes from focus group transcripts, and many of them are very telling. The following are among the most pertinent.

Regarding changes in self

I think you are focused more on the total picture of the patient rather than maybe just your shift. You are looking at the overview of the whole patient stay and the outcomes that you are trying to work toward.[73(p.47)]

We are pioneers in the hospital for how we are delivering care to patients. You have to be able to take a lot of criticism and a lot of questions about what exactly are you doing, from peer to doctors. Part of that is being in a new role, and just that for a long time the role is not clearly defined . . . you are being repeatedly asked to verify what your role is.[73(p.49)]

Regarding changes in relationships

With physicians. On pulmonary, trying to get the pulmonary rehab ordered. The doctor will say, "No, they don't need it." Now you can say, "Why not? I think they do." Not a feeling of being threatening, a challenge. Just you know you can make it better.[73(p.50)]

With other disciplines. From my standpoint, I think there is more collaborating going on. There is more communication. The dietitians are looking for us now. The social workers are looking for us.[73(p.41)]

With staff nurses. My peers don't understand the full scope of my practice. They only see that you get the same patients on the unit every day that you work. I think that is what is upsetting to them because I think there is a feeling of envy when you get the same patients that you get more continuity with assignments.[73(p.43)]

I have really felt a separation that I'm not one of these normal bedside care givers, there's a little more scope to my practice. I'm also not into a management position either, so I'm kind of in this No Man's Land, and because there are not a lot of other people joining me, I'm kind of alone.[73(p.43)]

Two studies that contain relevant quantitative findings are worthy of note. Ethridge's[64] report of initial efforts to evaluate the outcomes of the Carondelet model is the only study found that contrasts NCMs' outcomes with those of other nurses. Findings from this study indicate that NCMs ($N = 7$) report significantly higher levels of autonomy, enjoyment of their work, and professional status than SNs ($N = 72$).

Lancero's[74] thesis examines differences in perceived control over nursing practice, job stress, and work satisfaction among 30 NCMs practicing in two different case management models and evaluates relationships between control over nursing practice and job stress and satisfaction. NCMs who participated in the study worked in two different types of models, a system with a strong community focus and a more hospital-oriented program. Lancero's main findings were that work satisfaction was positively correlated with control over nursing practice ($r = .65$, $p = .01$) and negatively correlated with job stress ($r = -.43$, $p = .01$). Control over nursing practice had a stronger impact ($B = .59$) on work satisfaction than job stress ($B = -.33$), and together they explained 53 percent of the variance in NCM work satisfaction.[74]

Lancero developed an instrument to measure job stress in the NCM role. Among the items that NCMs reported to be most unique to nursing case management practice were:[74]

- focusing on a continuum of care rather than on an episode of care
- wanting to focus on illness prevention and wellness while serving a primarily ill population
- having independence and autonomy
- maintaining long-term relationships with clients and families.

Other interesting findings include that the second-highest scoring item on the time-task requirement subscale of the work satisfaction instrument was "I think I could do a better job if I did not have so much to do all the time."[74(p.88)]

In summary, job characteristics and job enrichment research in nursing suggests that the core job dimensions of the JCM reflect important aspects of nurses' practice and that SN jobs may be deficient in job identity, autonomy, and feedback. This is a valuable starting point; however, the JCM may not include the full range of dimensions inherent in nurses' jobs, and all nurses cannot be expected to respond equally well to enriched jobs. A more comprehensive theoretical framework may be needed to enhance our understanding of the relationship between characteristics of nurses' work and their personal and work outcomes.

THEORETICAL EXTENSIONS: SITUATIONAL CONSTRUCTS

Beyond characteristics of the work itself, there are at least three additional broad situational constructs that are relevant to nurses' jobs: control, social integration, and role stressors. Control can also be conceptualized with increased specificity. Two types of control or influence that are particularly relevant to nurses' work are collaboration with physicians and influence with other disciplines. Similarly, role stressors include a number of applicable role dysfunctions, specifically role conflict, overload, and ambiguity.

Control

Control is an important motivational construct,[75,76] particularly in nursing,[77] a field that has been described as a subordinate, helping profession.[78] Personal control has been shown to significantly predict satisfaction and performance among nursing employees.[75]

Autonomy can be defined as control or self-direction in the work itself,[4] and research has consistently shown that autonomy is a critical factor in nurses' job satisfaction.[79–81] Yet autonomy represents only one aspect of situational control. What about the degree of control nurses experience in their interactions with physicians and other disciplines? Due to the interdependent nature of nursing practice, it appears that these relationships may be an important potential source of experienced control.

Nurse/Physician Collaboration

From a control or influence perspective, nurses' relationships with physicians are particularly important and troublesome. Interdependence with physicians is a central feature of nursing, and physicians are, therefore, key players in nurses' work lives. Because of the nature of the nurse-physician relationship, the quality of nurses' interactions with physicians affects their job satisfaction and may affect performance. Weisman and colleagues[81] found that nurses are more satisfied if they perceive that physicians do not delegate inappropriately.

Physicians hold a position of professional dominance in many hospitals and frequently resist decision-making discretion by nurses. As one physician expressed, "There are nurses and there are doctors and . . . the highest ranking nurse is lower than the lowest ranking doctor, and that system will not change."[82(p.2)] Fagin[60] suggests that collaboration is a relationship of interdependence involving complementary roles. Describing a nurse's relationship with physicians as collaborative suggests that the nurse has more influence than is typical in most nurse-physician relationships.

Evaluations of collaborative practice projects have shown increases in nurses' satisfaction.[83] Findings from other research indicates that patients cared for in intensive care units characterized by collaborative physician-nurse relationships have better outcomes, which suggests that collaboration makes a positive performance difference.[84]

Influence with Other Professional Coworkers

Nurses also interact with many other health professionals. They routinely work with social workers, physical therapists, dieticians, pharmacists, and other disciplines in relation to patient care issues and decisions. Yet the nature of these relationships and their effects on nurses' workplace well-being and productivity have not been well-researched.

Studies have shown that poor support services can impair nursing productivity and lead to frustration,[85] but I was unable to locate research that directly examined nurses' relationships with other disciplines. These relationships may not be as charged with gender and status issues as nurses' dealings with physicians, but such interactions do appear to represent a legitimate source of feelings of influence in clinical decision making.

Social Integration

The effects of nurses' interactions with other nurses have been studied by several investigators. McCloskey[80] examined the impact of autonomy and social integration on several outcomes, including job satisfaction. Social integration was defined in this study in terms of supportive relationships with nurse colleagues. Findings suggest that nurses with low scores for social integration and autonomy experienced lower levels of job satisfaction. McCloskey also reported that higher than average amounts of social integration can effectively buffer the negative effects of low autonomy. This author concluded that women, including nurses, want a combination of autonomy and connectedness.[80]

Price and Mueller[21,22] also include social integration in the job satisfaction model imbedded within their causal model of nursing turnover. These authors define social integration as the degree to which an individual has close friends among organizational members within the immediate work unit[22] but do not explicitly restrict the set to just fellow nurses. Price and Mueller's broader conceptualization is used in the model proposed here.

Price and Mueller[22] found that friendly interactions in the work setting are an antecedent of satisfaction and turnover for nurses. Similarly, Pincus[86] reports that communication with peers explained 13 percent of the variance in nurses' job satisfaction, and Everly and Falcione[87] found that a factor related to relationships with fellow workers and supervisors accounted for close to 24 percent of the total variance in satisfaction.

To summarize, the tasks and activities of the work itself comprise the content of nursing jobs captured by the core dimensions of the JCM; however, relationships with physicians, other health care professionals, and fellow nurses are also important features of nurses' work lives. Development of a more comprehensive model of the motivational characteristics of nurses' jobs should, therefore, include constructs related to these coworker relationships. Given the interactional nature of nurses' work with both clients and coworkers, it appears that it would also be useful to give consideration to the integration of role theory to explain additional aspects of both sets of relationships.

Role Stressors

Several researchers have identified the need to integrate narrower considerations of task design with more global aspects of role design to gain a better understanding of employees' reactions to their work.[53,88,89] Abdel-Halim's[88] research suggests that employees working in complex, high-scope jobs in service organizations are most vulnerable to negative effects of role stressors, which supports Tumulty's[89] assertion that role dynamics may overshadow specific tasks in jobs of enlarged scope.

Drawing on the work of sociological theorists, Kahn and colleagues[29] developed a conceptual framework for the study of role stressors in organizations in 1964 that has shaped much of the ensuing research on this topic. Interested readers are referred to this seminal work, as space restrictions limit this discussion to selected basic concepts and definitions.

Kahn et al.[29] identify two broad types of potential role dysfunction: role conflict and role ambiguity. Role conflict occurs when different members of a role set communicate disparate expectations, which arouse motivational forces within the individual toward different behaviors. Role ambiguity stems from a lack of information required to perform the job. Within the role conflict category, they delineate several specific forms of sent role conflict, such as intersender conflict in which pressures from one sender oppose pressures from others. Kahn and colleagues also describe other types of conflict created by a combination of sent pressures and internal forces, such as person-role conflict, which involves a conflict between the needs and values of the person and the demands of the role set. The classic study by Rizzo et al.[90] of role stressors in complex organizations found that role conflict and ambiguity are negatively related to employee satisfaction and positively related to anxiety and propensity to leave.

Role Conflict

Role conflict and ambiguity are frequently studied together. Vredenburgh and Trinkaus[91] report a study of role conflict, uncertainty about acceptance of one's behavior, and role ambiguity among hospital nurses. These authors suggest that nurses are a particularly suitable sample for studying role stressors because they are professionals who work for bureaucratic organizations. Their findings indicate that complexity of patient conditions is significantly associated with the three role stressors evaluated, whereas task specialization is negatively related to uncertainty and ambiguity.

Within the general category of role conflict, Kahn et al.[29] identify even more specific types of conflict. Role overload is defined as a complex combination of intersender and person-role conflict, in which various role senders hold legitimate expectations that are compatible in the abstract but impossible for the individual to fulfill completely because of time constraints.

Role Overload. Findings from the evaluation of Dear et al.[92] of a contract professional practice model suggest that role overload may be a greater problem for nurses than role conflict or ambiguity. Nurses on both the contract and the control units reported higher levels of role overload than either of the other two types of role stressors. This is not surprising considering that staffing levels are a critical issue in nursing, and work overload has been identified as a significant negative factor through meta-analysis of job satisfaction research in nursing.[25] Price and Mueller[22] added role overload to their revised model of nursing turnover based on their observations and feedback from nurses and found that it had a significant negative relationship with satisfaction.

Role Ambiguity

A study of human service workers reported by Glisson and Durick[93] analyzed the simultaneous effects of multiple predictors on satisfaction and commitment. Predictors included job, organizational, and worker characteristics. Results indicated that the two best predictors of job satisfaction are role ambiguity and skill variety, which supports the importance of situational factors in the development of satisfaction.

In summary, environmental pressures have destabilized the hospital industry. Factors identified as role stressor antecedents, such as frequent reorganizations and changes in personnel,[29] are prevalent in hospitals as they struggle to anticipate and adapt to impending reforms. At the nexus of these organizational stresses, nurses function in a liaison role linking patients to their physicians and to the organization. Nurses' boundary-spanning roles make them particularly vulnerable to the negative effects of role stressors, and a strong case can be made for the extension of the job characteristics model through the integration of role theory constructs.

THEORETICAL EXTENSIONS: DISPOSITIONAL DIFFERENCES

As previously described, the job characteristics model proposes that GNS moderates relationships between the core job dimensions and the critical psychological states and between these states and the personal and work outcomes. Hackman and Lawler[3(p.262,269)] define individual need strength as the "desire for higher order need satisfaction." They offer "needs for personal growth and development or for feelings of worthwhile accomplishment" as examples of higher-order needs and refer to Maslow and Alderfer as sources of more information concerning the nature of higher needs and their motivational implications.

There appears to be some inconsistency and confusion in the literature regarding exactly what the term *higher-order need strength* encompasses.[40,94] Maslow is credited with drawing attention to the role of positive, as opposed to deficit needs in human motivation;[31] however, substantive problems have also been identified in his work.[31,40] For example, Locke[40] notes that Maslow's term *self-actualization* has no coherent meaning and cannot be used to explain anything. In view of evidence that GNS may be a broad construct encompassing several more specific needs that are not strongly related,[95] it may not be surprising that the moderating role of GNS remains unclear.

Several potential alternatives to GNS have been identified, including the Protestant work ethic, need for achievement, intrinsic versus extrinsic work values, and need for autonomy or independence.[8,94,96–98] Among these, need for achievement has been repeatedly suggested, with supportive empirical evidence.[97–99]

Need for Achievement

McClelland[31] states that "doing something better" is the natural incentive for the achievement motive. He indicates that individuals high in need for achievement are characterized by the tendency to seek out and do better at moderately difficult tasks, take personal responsibility for their performance, seek performance feedback on how well they are doing, and try new and more efficient ways of doing things.

Orpen[97] reports an investigation of need for achievement as a moderator of relationships between perceptions of the five core dimensions and job satisfaction and performance in a sample of middle managers from manufacturing firms. Findings suggested that individual differences in the managers' needs for achievement did affect the relationship between their perceived job characteristics and affective and behavioral responses.

The authors of a study of the effects of drive for achievement and task characteristics on satisfaction and performance outcomes also report a significant interaction between motivational characteristics of the job and drive for achievement.[99] Employees with high personal drive for goal achievement who described their jobs as highly intrinsically motivating were more satisfied.

A critical question that requires careful examination is whether need for achievement is a construct different from GNS. The study of Stone and colleagues[98] comparing the relationships between the JDS growth need scales and other measures of higher-order needs supports the position that need for achievement and GNS share some overlap but are also relatively independent. Specifically, the correlation between a JDS GNS scale and Jackson's[100] need for achievement scale was $r = .34$, which indicates that these two measures share only 11.6 percent common variance. Thus, it appears that it would be useful to include need for achievement as a potential alternative to GNS.

Need for Influence

Because interpersonal interactions are not central to the basic JCM, need for power and need for affiliation are not commonly examined in relation to task characteristics. With the extension of the JCM to include characteristics of nurses' relationships with coworkers, however, these needs become more salient. Stahl[101] found that SNs report need for affiliation and need for power percentiles, which are both above the norm. He concludes that SNs are characterized by concern for others, interpersonal relationships, and friendships. They are also concerned with influencing others and expect that their help and advice will be accepted.

Need for power is related to impact, control, or influence over others.[31] Control and power are interrelated constructs in that power provides the basis for the exercise of control. Bacharach and Lawler[102] delineate two distinct dimensions of the power construct: authority and influence. Authority is a formal power that implies involuntary submission to the direction of a superior office, but influence is more informal, deriving primarily from an individual's ability to persuade or convince others of one's position. Given that nurses do not have formal authority in relation to physicians and other disciplines, influence appears to be the more appropriate focus for this discussion.

Bennett[32] identifies a construct he labels need for influence, rather than power. He defines the need for influence as the desire to persuade and affect others, as opposed to his description of need for power as an egoistic striving for position, and reports the development of an instrument to measure the two constructs separately. Factor analysis from several different samples was used to demonstrate the construct validity of the separate scales, and additional analyses supported their discriminant validity.

Bennett's[32] findings suggest that the need for influence may be more prevalent in women than the need for power. McClelland[103] also indicates that because women's values differ from men's values, women are more sociocentric than men. Given that the vast majority of nurses are female, need for influence may be a more appropriate construct than need for power to include as a potential moderator of nurses' responses to collaboration with physicians and influence with other disciplines.

Need for Affiliation

McClelland[31] describes the need for affiliation as the need to be with and interact with other people. Affiliative imagery is defined as the concern for establishing, maintaining, or restoring a positive, affective relationship with another person or persons. The research of Steers and Braunstein[104] indicates that a preference for working together and helping coworkers is significantly related to the need for affiliation. As noted earlier, Stahl[101] found that SNs report a higher-than-average need for affiliation, which is not surprising given the nurturing, interpersonal nature of their work. Thus, need for affiliation may moderate the nurses' response to the degree of social integration they experience at work.

THEORETICAL MODEL: ANTECEDENT CONDITIONS RELATED TO NURSES' SATISFACTION AND PERFORMANCE

The proposed theoretical model is broadly depicted in Figure 22-1. This diagram indicates that tasks, activities, and relationships with clients and co-workers lead to both perceived characteristics of work and coworker relationships and role stressors. It also suggests that the relationships between objective job characteristics and related perceptions are moderated by dispositional differences. For example, McClelland[31] reports that individuals high in the need for achievement are more sensitive to achievement-related cues, such as those related to performance improvement.

As in the JCM, the five core dimensions of job content are expected to be related to satisfaction and performance through mediating relationships with the three critical psychological states.[4] These relationships are moderated at two points in the model. Interactional effects of dispositional differences are predicted to moderate the relationships between perceived characteristics and psychological states and between psychological states and outcomes. Instead of the effects of GNS, however, it is proposed that the needs for achievement, influence, and affiliation moderate these relationships.

The JCM is further extended through the inclusion of three characteristics of nurses' relationships with coworkers: collaboration with physicians, influence with other disciplines, and social integration. These characteristics are also expected to influence satisfaction and performance through mediating relationships with the psychological states, with moderating effects at the previously specified points. To capture more fully the interpersonal nature of nurses' work, the three role stressor variables of role conflict, overload, and ambiguity are predicted to affect satisfaction directly and indirectly affect both satisfaction and performance through the psychological states.

Although constructs included in the model and their primary interrelationships are discussed in the preceding review of literature, it may be helpful to provide specific definitions of the constructs used to extend the JCM and some additional explanation of their underlying mechanisms.

Characteristics of Coworker Relationships

Nurse/physician collaboration is defined as "interactions between nurse and physician that enable the knowledge and skill of both professionals to synergistically influence the patient care being provided."[105] It is suggested that nurses who perceive that they can influence physicians' decisions will feel a stronger sense of responsibility for patient outcomes. It is also predicted that nurses will find their work more meaningful because they perceive that they are influencing important events.

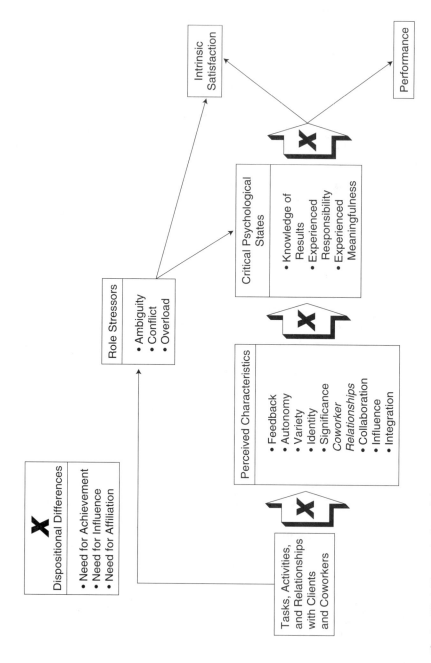

Figure 22-1 Theoretical Model

Influence with other professional coworkers is defined as the extent to which the nurse perceives that professional coworkers from other disciplines, besides physicians, ask nurses' opinions about patient care problems and are inclined to take nurses' opinions and suggestions into account. It is proposed that the effects of this variable will be similar to collaboration in increasing nurses' experienced responsibility for outcomes and enhancing the meaningfulness of their work.

Social integration is considered "the extent to which members of an organization have close friends in their immediate work units."[22] It is suggested that close friendships with others in the immediate work unit will contribute to the meaningfulness of nurses' work experience.

Role Stressors

"Role conflict is defined in terms of the dimensions of congruency-incongruency or compatibility-incompatibility in the requirements of a role, where congruency or compatibility is judged relative to a set of standards or conditions which impinge upon role performance."[90(p.155)] In a study of the correlates of role indices, Brief and Aldag[106] found significant negative relationships between role conflict and task identity ($r = -.29$, $p < .01$) and autonomy ($r = -.31$, $p < .01$). Findings concerning the relationships between role stressors and core dimensions may provide some insight into patterns of relationships with the psychological states.

Role conflict is predicted to have a negative effect on experienced meaningfulness and responsibility for outcomes. It is expected that nurses who feel torn between contradictory expectations will find it more difficult to feel their work is meaningful because success in meeting one set of expectations is likely to be offset by the inability to simultaneously meet others. It is also proposed that nurses who perceive conflicting expectations will feel less personal responsibility for outcomes as they may be juggling their time between competing demands and feel that they are not making a substantive contribution anywhere.

Role overload is defined as the experience of trying to satisfy multiple role expectations that are virtually impossible to meet due to time constraints.[29] It is suggested that nurses who feel that they do not have time to accomplish all that is expected of them are likely to experience their work as less meaningful because, in this form of role conflict, positive feelings associated with successfully meeting some expectations may be negated by the frustration of being unable to accomplish all that is expected, specifically because of time pressures.

Role ambiguity is defined in terms of "the predictability of outcomes or responses to one's behavior and the existence or clarity of behavioral requirements."[90(p.155-156)] Brief and Aldag[106] report a significant negative relationship between role ambiguity and feedback from work ($r = -.27$, $p < .05$).

It is proposed that nurses who are unclear about what is expected of them will experience difficulty in determining their level of performance. Similarly, a lack of knowledge concerning the standards against which they are to be judged will make it difficult to discern the meaning of what has been accomplished. It is predicted that role ambiguity is negatively related to knowledge of results and meaningfulness.

Moderating Variables: Dispositional Need Strength Differences

Three different dispositional needs are proposed to moderate relationships between characteristics of the work and experienced psychological states and between psychological states and satisfaction and performance outcomes.

The need for achievement is the desire to do something better for its own sake or to show that one is more capable of doing something.[31] As Orpen[97(p.208)] explains:

> The n-Ach model suggests that high need achievers are stimulated by tasks that are inherently meaningful . . . and also provide both ample knowledge of results and opportunities for independent action and thought. Hence, when they perceive their jobs to possess these attributes to a larger degree, we would expect high achievers not only to be very satisfied with their jobs but also to respond with high-level performance.

Individuals who have a high need for achievement respond positively to situations in which they can assume personal responsibility for work and receive individual feedback and recognition.[31] Thus, it is predicted that need for achievement moderates the relationships of job identity, autonomy, and feedback with the specified psychological states and between each of the critical psychological states and satisfaction and performance. The opportunity to exercise discretion in the performance of a substantive piece of work should lead to feelings of ownership for the outcomes, and feedback provides a basis for determining how well one is doing. The underlying motivational mechanisms are similar to those described by Lawler.[42]

Defined as a "desire to persuade and affect others,"[32] the need for influence is expected to moderate an individual's response to perceived interpersonal effects on coworkers. It is proposed that individuals with high needs for influence will react favorably if they perceive that their interactions with others lead to desired psychological or behavioral responses from coworkers.

The need for influence is expected to moderate the relationship between a nurse's perceptions of collaboration with physicians and influence with other disciplines and the specified psychological states, as these characteristics represent the attainment of desired effects in one's interpersonal dealings. Similarly, it is predicted that the need for influence moderates the relationship between experienced responsibility for outcomes and satisfaction and performance because a nurse with a high need to persuade and affect others is expected to respond strongly to the experience of feeling responsible for outcomes attained. Need for influence is also predicted to moderate the relationship between experienced meaningfulness and outcomes on the basis that nurses who have a strong desire to affect others will be strongly responsive to the feeling that they have contributed to meaningful work.

The need for affiliation is defined as the wish to enjoy positive, affective relationships with others.[31] It is expected that individuals with a high need for affiliation will respond positively to opportunities for close friendships with coworkers.

A moderating effect of need for affiliation on the relationships between social integration and experienced meaningfulness and between experienced meaningfulness and outcomes is proposed. Individuals with a high need for affiliation generally have a strong desire for approval and reassurance from others. This suggests that positive relationships with others may play a role in meeting highly affiliative individuals' needs for self-esteem and respect. Thus, in situations in which personal support and approval are tied to performance, people with strong affiliative needs tend to perform better.[34] It is predicted that nurses who want very much to have positive affective relationships with others should find the experience of working in a cooperative, supportive work environment to be meaningful. In turn, it is expected that they will find this satisfying and strive to perform well to receive peer approval.

In summary, 11 constructs have been identified as important motivational characteristics of nurses' jobs. This model's unique potential contribution to increased understanding of the effects of these characteristics may lie in its combination of increased specificity and comprehensiveness. The model delineates three different types or sources of perceived control: autonomy in nurses' own work and influence in relationships with physicians and other disciplines. It is comprehensive in including the potentially important contextual factor of social integration and in integrating role dimensions that transcend the task domain to capture key aspects of nurses' relationships with clients and coworkers and their experiences as professional employees in bureaucratic organizations.

RESEARCH OPPORTUNITIES AND NEEDS

A test of the proposed model may help to answer the following research questions:

1. From the job characteristics and other theoretical perspectives, what are the important motivational characteristics of nurses' jobs?

- In what ways are current theories of job design inadequate to capture the important motivational characteristics of nurses' jobs?
2. Do specific characteristics have the predicted effects on nurses' job satisfaction and performance?
3. What are the combined effects of multiple characteristics on job satisfaction and performance?
4. Do dispositional differences other than the traditional GNS construct moderate the relationships between characteristics of the work and satisfaction and performance outcomes?

Some additional areas that would provide rich research opportunities include:

1. perceived characteristics of the NCM job
2. relationship of these characteristics to affective and behavioral outcomes
3. similarities and differences between the characteristics of the NCM and other nursing jobs, such as SN, nurse manager, clinical nurse specialist, and other advanced practice roles
4. effects of introducing NCM on job characteristics reported by SNs and related outcomes
5. effects of introducing NCM on job characteristics reported by other health professionals and related outcomes

These ideas represent examples rather than an exhaustive list. Clearly, the design of nursing and other service jobs is a fruitful avenue for further research. With a better understanding of the key dimensions and their motivational effects, jobs can be designed to strengthen positive and minimize negative characteristics, resulting in enhanced job satisfaction and performance. Moreover, the suggestion that case management may be the bellwether of a new organizational form[1] highlights the need to evaluate the effects of this potentially important new role on employees. There appears to be a dearth of research on this topic and a compelling case for the development of job design theory to reflect twenty-first century jobs.

REFERENCES

1. Davenport TH, Nohria N. Case management and the integration of labor. *Sloan Manage Rev.* 1994;35:11–23.
2. Hammer M, Champy J. *Reengineering the Corporation: A Manifesto for Business Revolution.* New York, NY: HarperCollins; 1983.

3. Hackman JR, Lawler EE. Employee reactions to job characteristics. *J Appl Psychol.* 1971;55:259–286.

4. Hackman JR, Oldham GR. Motivation through the design of work: test of a theory. *Organizational Behavior Hum Performance.* 1976;16:250–279.

5. Turner AN, Lawrence PR. *Industrial Jobs and the Worker.* Boston, Mass: Harvard University Graduate School of Business Administration; 1965.

6. Schneider B, Bowen DE. Employee and customer perceptions of service in banks: replication and extension. *J Appl Psychol.* 1985;70:423–433.

7. Mills PK, Hall JL, Leidecker JK, Marguiles N. Flexiform: a model for professional service organizations. *Acad Manage Rev.* 1983;8:118–131.

8. Hackman JR, Oldham GR. *Work Redesign.* Menlo Park, Calif: Addison-Wesley; 1980.

9. Fried Y, Ferris GR. The validity of the job characteristics model: a review and meta-analysis. *Personnel Psychol.* 1987;40:287–322.

10. Johns G, Xie JL, Fang Y. Mediating and moderating effects in job design. *J Manage.* 1992;18:657–676.

11. Taber T, Taylor E. A review and evaluation of the psychometric properties of the Job Diagnostic Survey. *Personnel Psychol.* 1990;43:467–500.

12. Mills PK, Moberg DJ. Perspectives on the technology of service operations. *Acad Manage Rev.* 1982;7:467–478.

13. Levitt T. Production-line approach to service. *Harvard Business Rev.* 1972;50:41–52.

14. Levitt T. Industrialization of service. *Harvard Business Rev.* 1976;54:63–74.

15. Mayer GG, Madden MJ, Lawrenz E. *Patient Care Delivery Model.* Gaithersburg, Md: Aspen Publishers, Inc.; 1990.

16. Sherer JL. Health care reform: nursing's vision of change. *Hospitals.* 1993;67(8):20–26.

17. Sherer JL. Next steps for nursing. *Hosp Health Networks.* 1993;67(16):26–28.

18. Tonges MC. Redesigning hospital nursing practice: the Professionally Advanced Care Team (ProACT™) Model, part 2. *J Nurs Adm.* 1989;19(8):19–22.

19. Zander K. Nursing case management: strategic management of cost and quality outcomes. *J Nurs Adm.* 1988;18(5):23–30.

20. Bower KA. Case management: work redesign with patient outcomes in mind. In: McDonagh KJ, ed. *Patient-Centered Hospital Care: Reform from Within.* Ann Arbor, Mich: Health Administration Press; 1993: 47–65.

21. Price JL, Mueller CW. *Professional Turnover: The Case of Nurses.* New York, NY: Spectrum; 1981.

22. Price JL, Mueller CW. *Absenteeism and Turnover of Hospital Employees.* Greenwich, Conn: JAI Press; 1986.

23. Seymour E, Buscherhof JR. Sources and consequences of satisfaction and dissatisfaction in nursing: findings from a national sample. *Int J Nurs Stud.* 1991;28:109–124.

24. Blegen MA. Nurses' job satisfaction: a meta-analysis of related variables. *Nurs Res.* 1993;42(1):36–41.

25. Irvine D, Evans M. Job satisfaction and turnover among nurses: a review and meta-analysis. *Quality Nurs Worklife Res Monogr.* Toronto, Canada: Faculty of Nursing University of Toronto; 1992.

26. Wake MM. Nursing care delivery systems: status and vision. *J Nurs. Adm.* 1990;20(5):47–51.

27. Lamb GS. Conceptual and methodological issues in nurse case management research. *Adv Nurs Sci.* 1992;15(2):16–24.

28. Loevinger L. The paradox of knowledge. *Skeptical Inquirer.* 1995;19(5):18–21.

29. Kahn RL, Wolfe DM, Quinn RP, Snoek JD. *Organizational Stress: Studies in Role Conflict and Ambiguity.* Reprint ed. Malabar, Fla: Krieger; 1981.

30. Cherrington DJ. Need theories of motivation. In: Steers RM, Porter LM, eds. *Motivation and Work Behavior.* 5th ed. New York, NY: McGraw-Hill; 1991:31–44.

31. McClelland DC. *Human Motivation.* Cambridge: Cambridge University Press; 1987.

32. Bennett JB. Power and influence as distinct personality traits: development and validation of a psychometric measure. *J Res Personality.* 1988;22:361–394.

33. Hackman JR. Work design. In: Steers RM, Porter LM, ed. *Motivation and Work Behavior.* 5th ed. New York, NY: McGraw-Hill; 1991: 418–444.

34. Steers RM, Porter LW. *Motivation and Work Behavior.* New York, NY: McGraw-Hill; 1991.

35. Taylor FW. *The Principles of Scientific Management.* New York, NY: Harper; 1911.

36. Mayo E. *The Human Problems of an Industrial Civilization.* New York, NY: Macmillan; 1933.

37. Herzberg F, Mausner B, Synderman BB. *The Motivation To Work.* New York, NY: Wiley; 1959.

38. Paul WH, Robertson KB, Herzberg F. Job enrichment pays off. *Harvard Business Rev.* 1969;47(2):61–78.

39. House RJ, Wigdor LA. Herzberg's dual factor theory of job satisfaction and motivation. *Personnel Psychol.* 1967;20:369–390.

40. Locke EA. The nature and causes of job satisfaction. In: Dunnette M, ed. *Handbook of Industrial and Organizational Psychology.* 2nd ed. New York, NY: Wiley; 1976: 1297–1350.

41. Steers RM, Mowday RT. The motivational properties of tasks. *Acad Manage Rev.* 1977;2:645–658.

42. Lawler EE. Job design and employee motivation. *Personnel Psychol.* 1969;22:426–435.

43. Griffin RW. Moderation of the effects of job enrichment by participation: a longitudinal field experiment. *Organizational Behavior Hum Decision Processes.* 1985;35:73–93.

44. Roberts K, Glick W. The job characteristics approach to task design: a critical review. *J Appl Psychol.* 1981;66:193–218.

45. Alderfer CP. An empirical test of a new theory of human needs. *Organizational Behavior Hum Performance.* 1969;4:142–175.

46. Maslow AH. *Motivation and Personality.* New York, NY: Harper & Row; 1954.

47. Hackman JR, Oldham GR. Development of the Job Diagnostic Survey. *J Appl Psychol.* 1975;60:159–170.

48. Griffin RW. Objective and social sources of information in task redesign: a field experiment. *Adm Sci Q.* 1983;28:184–200.

49. Sims HP, Szligayi AD, Keller RT. The measurement of job characteristics. *Acad Manage J.* 1976;19:195–212.

50. Stone E, Gueutal HG. An empirical derivation of the dimensions along which characteristics of jobs are perceived. *Acad Manage J.* 1985;28:376–396.

51. Joiner C, Johnson V, Chapman JG, Corkrean M. The motivating potential of nursing specialties. *J Nurs Adm.* 1982;12(2):26–30.

52. Roedel RR, Nystrom PC. Nursing jobs and satisfaction. *Nurs Manage.* 1988;19(2):34–38.

53. Seybolt JW. The impact of work role design on the career satisfaction of registered nurses. *Proc Acad Manage.* 1980;40:42–46.

54. Wulff KS. *Nurse Participation in Unit Decisions.* Seattle, Wash.: Seattle University. 1991. Dissertation.

55. McClure ML. Managing the professional nurse: part I: the organizational theories. *J Nurs Adm.* 1984;14:15–21.

56. McClure ML. Managing the professional nurse: part II: applying management theory to the challenges. *J Nurs Adm.* 1984;14:11–17.

57. Joiner C, van Servellen GW. *Job Enrichment in Nursing.* Gaithersburg, Md: Aspen Publishers, Inc.; 1984.

58. Harrison JK. Tuning into the growth needs of registered nurses. *Nurs Econ.* 1987;5: 297–303.

59. Grunberg NN. *Understanding Job Satisfaction.* New York, NY: Wiley; 1979.

60. Fagin CM. Collaboration between nurses and physicians. *Acad Med.* 1992;67:295–303.

61. Browning G, Marino P. Joint practice: a rural hospital can make it work. *Nurs Manage.* 1983;14(3):22–25.

62. Vaughn RA. Collaborative practice. *Nurs Manage.* 1982;13(3):33–35.

63. Davenport TH, Short JE. The new industrial engineering: information technology and business process redesign. *Sloan Manage Rev.* 1990;31:11–27.

64. Ethridge P. Nurse accountability improves satisfaction, turnover. *Health Progress.* 1987;5:44–49.

65. Zander K, Etheredge ML, Bower KA. *Nursing Case Management: Blueprints for Transformation.* Boston, Mass: New England Medical Center; 1987.

66. Bower KA. *Case Management by Nurses.* Kansas City, Mo: American Nurses Association; 1992.

67. Zander K. Critical pathways. In: Melum M, Sinioris M, eds. *Total Quality Management.* Chicago, Ill: American Hospital Association; 1992.

68. Marschke P, Nolan MT. Research related to case management. *Nurs Adm Q.* 1993;17:16–21.

69. Erkel EA. The impact of case management in preventive services. *J Nurs Adm.* 1993;23: 17–32.

70. Van Dongen CJ, Jambunathan J. Pilot study results: the psychiatric RN case manager. *J Psychosoc Nurs.* 1992;30:11–14.

71. Newman M, Lamb GS, Michaels C. Nurse case management: the coming together of theory and practice. *Nurs Health Care.* 1991;12:404–408.

72. Rheaume A, Frische S, Smith A, Kennedy C. Case management and nursing practice. *J Nurs Adm.* 1994;24:31–36.

73. McGill RL. *Nursing Case Management: Developing Clinical Leaders.* St. Paul, Minn.: College of St. Catherine; 1994. Thesis.

74. Lancero AW. *Work Satisfaction among Nurse Case Managers: A Comparison of Two Practice Models.* Tucson, AZ: University of Arizona; 1994. Thesis.

75. Greenberger DB, Strasser S, Cummings LL, Dunham RB. The impact of personal control on performance and satisfaction. *Organizational Behavior Hum Decision Processes.* 1989;43:29–51.

76. Seligman MEP. *Learned Optimism.* New York, NY: Knopf; 1991.

77. Fox ML, Dwyer DJ, Ganster DC. Effects of stressful job demands and control on physiological and attitudinal outcomes in a hospital setting. *Acad Manage J.* 1993;36:289–318.

78. Korman AK. Seminar in organizational behavior: work motivation and performance. New York, NY: Baruch College of the City University of New York. 1993.

79. Dwyer DJ, Schwartz RH, Fox ML. Decision-making autonomy in nursing. *J Nurs Adm.* 1992;22:177–183.

80. McCloskey JC. Two requirements for job contentment: autonomy and social integration. *Image.* 1990;22:140–143.

81. Weisman CS, Alexander CS, Chase GA. Job satisfaction among hospital nurses: a longitudinal study. *Health Serv Res.* 1980;15:341–364.

82. Prescott PA, Dennis KE, Jacox AK. Clinical decision making of staff nurses. *Image.* 1987;19:56–62.

83. Kellog to Fund. *Am J Nurs.* 1981;12:2134–2135.

84. Knaus WA, Draper EA, Wagner DP, Zimmerman JE. An evaluation of outcomes from intensive care in major medical centers. *Ann Intern Med.* 1986;104:401–408.

85. Swenson B, Wolfe H, Shroeder R. Effectively employing support services: the key for increasing nursing personnel productivity. *Mod Health Care.* 1984;14:101–102.

86. Pincus J. Communication: key contributor to effectiveness. *J Nurs Adm.* 1986;16(9):19–25.

87. Everly GS, Falcione RL. Perceived dimensions of job satisfaction for staff registered nurses. *Nurs Res.* 1976;25:346–348.

88. Abdel-Halim AA. Effects of role stress–job design interaction on employee work satisfaction. *Acad Manage J.* 1981;24:269–273.

89. Tumulty G. A model for nursing role redesign. In: Henry B, ed. *Practice and Inquiry for Nursing Administration.* Washington, DC: American Academy of Nursing; 1992: 67–71.

90. Rizzo J, House R, Lirtzman S. Role conflict and ambiguity in complex organizations. *Adm Sci Q.* 1970;13:150–163.

91. Vredenburgh DJ, Trinkaus RJ. An analysis of role stress among hospital nurses. *J Vocational Behavior.* 1983;23:82–95.

92. Dear MR, Weisman CS, O'Keefe S. Evaluation of a contract professional practice model. *Health Care Manage Rev.* 1985;10:65–77.

93. Glisson C, Durick M. Predictors of job satisfaction and organizational commitment in human service organizations. *Adm Sci Q.* 1988;33:61–81.

94. Stone E, Mowday RT, Porter LW. Higher order need strengths as moderators of job scope-satisfaction relationships. *J Appl Psychol.* 1977;62:466–471.

95. Steers RM, Spencer DG. The role of achievement motivation in job design. *J Appl Psychol.* 1977;62:472–479.

96. Morris JH, Snyder RA. A second look at need for achievement and need for autonomy as moderators of role perception-outcomes relationships. *J Appl Psychol.* 1979;64:173–178.

97. Orpen C. The effects of need for achievement and for independence on the relationship between perceived job attributes and managerial satisfaction and performance. *Int J Psychol.* 1985;20:207–219.

98. Stone E, Ganser DC, Woodman RW, Fusilier MR. Relationships between growth need strength and selected individual differences measures employed in job design research. *J Vocational Behavior.* 1979;14:329–340.

99. Joyce W, Slocum JW, Von Glinow MA, Hellriegel D. The interaction effects of achievement-oriented climates on employee attitudes and behaviors. *Acad Manage Proc.* 1976;36:228–232.

100. Jackson DN. *Personality Research Form Manual.* 3rd ed. Port Huron, Mich: Research Psychologists Press; 1967.

101. Stahl MJ. *Managerial and Technical Motivation.* New York, NY: Praeger; 1986.

102. Bacharach SB, Lawler E. *Power and Politics in Organizations.* San Francisco, Calif: Jossey-Bass; 1980.

103. McClelland DC. *Power: The Inner Experience.* New York, NY: Irvington; 1975.

104. Steers RM, Braunstein DN. A behaviorally-based measure of manifest needs in work settings. *J Vocational Behavior.* 1976;9:251–266.

105. Weiss SJ, Davis HP. Validity and reliability of the Collaborative Practice Scales. *Nurs Res.* 1982;34:299–305.

106. Brief AP, Aldag RJ. Correlates of role indices. *J Appl Psychol.* 1976;61:468–472.

■ 23 ■

Legal Liabilities in Case Management

Deborah J. Nichols, JD, MBA, RN

The case manager has a professional obligation to participate actively in the management of the medical case file to ensure quality health care in the most cost-effective manner. Shocking words! Just five years ago, these would be fighting words, igniting a hostile response among physicians, administrators, the public, and yes, even nurses.

Today, nursing case managers can take pride in all they have achieved. Unthought of just a few years ago, case managers are increasingly recognized as well-educated, independent, autonomous, and respected professionals. No longer the handmaidens of physicians and hospitals, case managers stand alongside physicians and other health care providers in formulating, implementing, and managing the care of patients in all aspects of the health care and insurance industries.

However, as case managers become the gatekeepers of the once exclusive province of the physician and patient, they find themselves increasingly involved in the complex and vague world of legal liability. As responsibility and autonomy expand, legal accountability heightens.

Increasingly, in the past decade, nurses have been named as defendants in lawsuits. Although there are yet few cases finding a particular case manager directly liable for his or her involvement in a case, it must be remembered that case management is in its infancy. Case manager liability is surely to follow.

As more case managers involve themselves in the integration of the diagnosis and treatment decisions of health care with the financial and cost control considerations, existing tort doctrine is likely to expand to include case manager liability when the case manager's decision making is shown to result in harm to the patient, denial of an essential diagnostic procedure or treatment, or interference with or corruption of acceptable medical judgment. In addition to these new legal theories, case managers, like all health care professionals, face all the historical legal liabilities including malpractice and negligence.

Unfortunately, there is no map available to help case managers navigate the murky legal waters. But the case manager can significantly reduce the risk of liability by understanding the basic premises of legal responsibility.

Case management liability should be thought of as a model. When case managers normally describe their professional duties and the interplay with law, the model that appears is global in form. There are multiple components in this model, each existing and acting independently while interacting with every other component. The typical model involves physicians, nurses, hospitals, insurers, governments, allied health professionals, and of course, patients. Adding to the mix are conflicting theories including the duty to advocate for the patient, the physician-patient relationship, rising health care costs, and the public demand to contain medical costs. Then there are the obligations of the professionals including licensure, education, one's duty to the employer, and ethics, to name a few. Overshadowing all these elements is the risk of exposure to legal liability.

The conflicting theories, lack of cohesiveness, and the absence of integration of the various elements result in a failure to provide direction to the case manager on precisely how he or she should proceed in any given situation. The consequence is that most case managers and providers engage in defensive practice, always reacting to the unknown, to what might happen.

This is the case management model that most practitioners learn, so it is little wonder that case managers are so often unclear about their professional risks and responsibilities. The global model breeds confusion. Changing the way you think about legal liability can alter the way you practice and ultimately your legal risks.

The simpler model is to think of case management liability as a pyramid structure. Without a foundation, there can be no structure. Without a strong foundation, the structure is always at risk of collapse.

The foundation of the pyramid model is the basic legal principles and guidelines that should guide every practitioner in *every* decision. It encompasses a sound understanding of professional responsibility, patient rights issues, malpractice, negligence, and ethics. It is not necessary to understand every nuance or to remember every case. Legal liability is a dynamic process. It is, however, imperative that the case manager have a firm grasp on the basic principles of the law and be able to incorporate them into daily practice. As the various elements are discussed, keep in mind the model and build your case management practice on top of this foundation.

PROFESSIONAL RESPONSIBILITY

Professional responsibility—We are all familiar with the phrase. It is tossed about, often carelessly, to defend a position or win a point: "But I have a professional responsibility" to act this or that way. Professional responsibility should not be taken or treated lightly. It is the sum and substance of the case management profession. It is the heart of the case manager's credibility and liability. It is the primary and most important building block in the pyramid model.

It sounds simple and is certainly important. So surely there must be a book of rules, a definition, something? Sadly, there is no book of rules and no clear definition of professional responsibility.

Professional responsibility is a broad concept that encompasses many ideas and is in a constant state of flux. It includes:

- The code of conduct or ethics that govern how members of the profession should or must behave
- The case manager-client relationship
- The competence of the individual case manager
- The duty of the case manager to keep abreast of changes in the field
- Conflicts of interest
- The quality of practitioners in general
- The case manager's reputation
- The relationship between the case manager and society at large

When the case manager finds him- or herself at the center of a legal issue, all these concepts will come into play in evaluating the reliability and credibility of the case manager. Only a few of these issues are discussed at length. It is important to note that ethics is an integral part of legal liability and should always be considered in evaluating your obligations and risks. Ethics is discussed briefly throughout this chapter and in more detail in other parts of this book. The discussion that follows should serve to raise the awareness of the practitioner to be vigilant in pursuit of excellence in the profession and in clinical practice.

Every case manager has a duty to be reasonably competent. There is no nationally recognized standard of competence. There are acceptable avenues for achieving "reasonable" competence. At the lowest level, the case manager must obtain a basic nursing education and be licensed at all times and in good standing in accordance with his or her state's law.

It is not enough, however, for a case manager to complete a basic education, obtain a license, get a job as a case manager, and then sit back. Case management is more than a job, it is a profession. As with any profession, there are responsibilities and expectations. Failure to accept these responsibilities can result in grave moral, ethical, and legal consequences. All case managers have an ethically charged duty to reach beyond the basics to achieve a level of knowledge and education that results in the safe delivery of quality health care in a manner that meets the needs of the individual client while meeting society's demand for cost-effective medical care.

Case managers have a professional responsibility to continue their education formally or informally throughout their professional life. Education includes knowing the particular legal doctrines in your field of practice that potentially may affect a patient's outcome. It may include Medicare/Medicaid rules and regulations, the Americans With Disabilities Act, worker's compensation laws, general tort principles, patient rights bills, child and elder abuse laws, which generally require mandatory reporting, patient confidentiality laws, etc.

A case manager's professional responsibility does not require that he or she become an expert in any of these areas. It does require he or she to become generally aware of the applicable laws so as not to harm a patient or inadvertently abrogate a patient's legal rights.

It is advisable for case managers to become actively involved in one or more professional associations and regularly read one or more professional journals. The best defense against legal liability is education, knowledge, and credibility.

The case manager also has a professional obligation to act within the scope of practice. The scope of practice is defined by state law and standards of practice that are discussed in detail. Failure of the case manager to understand the scope of practice can result in a lengthy and costly suit in negligence.

STANDARDS OF PRACTICE

Every case manager worries about being sued for negligence or malpractice by a patient or patient's family. But before negligence is discussed, there must be a full comprehension of the relationship between negligence and the standard of practice. The standard of practice is the measuring stick against which a case manager may be found legally liable for negligence.

Because case managers are presumed to have both the skills and knowledge that are beyond the scope of the general public, they must then act in a manner consistent with those superior skills and knowledge. This is known as the standard of care or the standard of practice.

Case law has traditionally defined a nurse's duty to include the "ordinary or reasonable care to see that no unnecessary harm comes to a patient."[1(p.353)] The standard of care is then "predicated upon the degree of care ordinarily exercised by other nurses in the locality involved, or similar localities."[1(p.353)] Extrapolating that definition to case management, the case manager would be held to the standard of conduct or practice of an ordinary, prudent case manager in the same or similar situation in the same or similar locality. To prove negligence, the plaintiff would have to show the case manager deviated from or acted in some manner that was inconsistent with the standard.

If the case manager is held accountable to the standard of practice, then the logical question that follows is how the courts determine the standard of the "ordinary and prudent case manager." Like most issues in law, the answer is complex. The most common approach to the establishment of a standard is through the standards of care that have been written, reviewed, and formally adopted by recognized organizations and governments.

On the government side, every state has some form of a nurse practice act. The nurse practice acts delineate the scope and authority under which a nurse can function, including the requirements to be licensed in that state. In some instances, the act will recognize a specialty area such as the nurse practitioner and will then further set out the special duties and functions that can be performed by the specialist. Case managers need to be familiar with their states' practice act. These acts are generally written in broad language, and the courts are likely to hold all nursing practitioners to these more generalized standards.

The case management field has brought life to a virtual cottage industry of national and state associations and certification programs designed to meet the needs of case managers in various fields from rehabilitation to insurance to geriatrics. They are too many to list and beyond the scope of this chapter. It is advisable for the case manager to identify a respected state or national organization that is closely aligned with the practitioner specialty area and then become familiar with the association's standards of practice. It is generally not necessary to join an organization to receive a copy of the standards of practice. Ignorance of the standards or failure to investigate the standards of practice will generally not be held by the courts to be an excuse for negligence.

If the case manager is working for a company, hospital, insurer, or other institution, they will generally be held to the policies and procedures set forth in the company manuals. The accountability of the case manager to meet those standards becomes even greater if the negligence he or she is accused of has been specifically set out in the policy and procedure manual.

Less often used standards, although still valid, are standards that may be found in professional journals and textbooks and through the use of expert professionals to testify as to the recognized standard of practice. Therefore, it becomes critical that the case manager communicate and interact with other professionals within their field and community, attend continuing education classes, and in general, keep up on changing theories of practice.

Last, the courts generally follow the principles of common law. That is the law that develops from case law precedent. Even if the state practice act or a recognized association does not specifically recognize an act as negligent, if a higher court has determined that a case manager was negligent in the performance of a duty then that finding might be used in a similar case as the standard of practice. Courts will generally follow precedent established within their own states or circuits (several surrounding states). Although case managers are usually not lawyers, it is prudent advice to keep up with current legal precedent through professional journals and associations.

PATIENT CONFIDENTIALITY

Case managers, like all health care professionals, have an affirmative legal and ethical duty to safeguard the confidentiality of a patient's heath care information. Unauthorized disclosure is generally considered the highest breach of professional ethics and even reprehensible. The principle of confidentiality arises from the privileged communication presumed to exist between the physician and patient. The communication between the physician and patient must be swathed in trust so the patient will feel confident in disclosing all the information necessary to ensure appropriate diagnosis and treatment. Therefore, the presumption of confidentiality is grounded in the belief that every individual has an unqualified right to privacy in certain nonpublic matters. The physician is then bound to nondisclosure of a patient's medical information unless the patient specifically grants permission to release the information.

In recent years, the issue of confidentiality has become anything but clear. If the patient is hospitalized or institutionalized, then the facility owns the record and is responsible for the dissemination of information. With HMOs, preferred provider organizations (PPOs), managed care, government agencies, third-party payers, and case managers all on the health care scene, it has become difficult to protect the confidentiality of medical information. In addition, the technology boom has placed confidentiality in jeopardy by computerizing many medical records, although not always addressing safety concerns on who is granted access to those records.

In response to these growing concerns, *The Case Management Advisor*[2] cites model legislation by Computer-Based Patient Record Institute, Inc., that establishes three levels of clinical data and the consent necessary to access the information:

Nonprivileged Information: Includes the patient's name, address, the fact that they are hospitalized, and some demographic information. This information is generally considered to be public in nature and does not require consent from the patient for disclosure.

Privileged Information: Includes the diagnoses, symptoms, prognosis, and any information that directly discusses the patient's specific medical history. This information requires the patient's permission for release.

Deniable Information: Includes extremely sensitive data, such as HIV/AIDS status, substance abuse treatment, and psychiatric care. It requires a separate explicit release from the patient. It may also require that only specific named parties access the information.

As a result of the growing concern that a patient's record may not be as safe as we all presume, many states have enacted specific legislation that extends the obligation to protect a patient's confidentiality to all providers and institutions. Disclosure of or access to medical records generally must be gained through a specific written authorization from the patient.

That, of course, does not include patients themselves. Patients in general have the right to access medical information about themselves unless it would prove harmful to them. Unauthorized disclosure of private medical records can result in a suit for violation of the state or federal statute demanding confidentiality, invasion of privacy, and in some instances, defamation.

To prevail on a theory of invasion of privacy, the plaintiff would have to demonstrate that the details released were "truly private ones, which are not contained anywhere on the public record."[3(p.330)] In addition, the plaintiff would have to prove the material released is "not of any legitimate concern to the public" and the details were, in fact, "publicized" in a tangible form to more than just a few people.[3(p.331)]

Defamation is a more difficult theory to prove. Plaintiffs must prove that the defamatory statement exposed them to hatred, contempt, or ridicule. They must show a tendency to harm but not necessarily an actual harm to their reputation.[4] Further, it must be demonstrated that a "significant and respectable minority of persons would draw an adverse opinion of the plaintiff from it."[4(p.308,309)]

There are defenses, even obligations, to disclosure of certain confidential information. The case manager may not, in some instances, be held liable for disclosure of medical information if there is shown to be overriding competing interests in which the law will provide greater protection for the person disclosing the information than the interest of the patient.[5] Such information may include health reasons, public policy, or if the individual is required to release the information by law.[6] For instance, most states have mandatory reporting requirements for child or elder abuse, sexually communicable diseases, drug reactions, infectious diseases, violent crimes, and so forth. Case managers should make every effort to become familiar with these reporting statutes as they may be held accountable to the state for failure to report this information. In these instances, patient consent is not necessary.

The case manager should bear in mind some simple questions that should be asked any time a patient's medical record is at stake:

1. Is the information contained in the record public, private, or extremely sensitive in nature?
2. What information may I disclose?
3. What information requires express authorization to disclose?
4. Do I have a signed, dated, written authorization to disclose private information?
5. Is the date on the authorization within a reasonable time frame of the date I am seeking the information?
6. Does the written authorization contain a clause to allow disclosure of deniable information?
7. Are there any defenses or obligations to disclosure?

MALPRACTICE/NEGLIGENCE

When case managers speak of legal liability, they are generally referring to suits in malpractice. Malpractice suits are suits against professional persons who generally have a level of skill or knowledge that is greater than the general public while commonly shared by members of the same profession. In other words, these are suits against professionals who practice under a similar standard of practice in the same or like profession.

Malpractice suits are, for the most part, based on a theory of fault or negligence on the part of the practitioner. In a malpractice suit against a case manager, the plaintiff would have to prove the case manager's conduct fell below the minimal skill or competence of the ordinary prudent case manager under a similar situation in a like environment.

These are unintentional torts. The plaintiff does not have to prove the case manager *intended* to act in a certain way, only that the *conduct* of the case manager fell below an acceptable standard of practice.

To understand the current case law and how it applies to case managers and to specific situations in which case managers might find themselves, it is necessary to understand all the elements of negligence and the burden of proof. If a plaintiff sues a case manager for malpractice on a theory of negligence, three distinct elements must be proved. In negligence, there must be a duty owed, a breach of that duty, and an injury or actual damages. Each and every element must be proved by the plaintiff or the case fails. For instance, if the plaintiff proves that the defendant had a duty to the plaintiff to act in a certain way, but fails to show a breach of that duty or a failure to conform his or her conduct to a recognized standard, then he or she loses. If, however, the plaintiff proves all three elements, the burden of proof has been met. It is then incumbent on the defendant to disprove the element or put forth defenses to the charge.

The duty owed by a case manager arises when a client-patient relationship exists. The case manager has a duty to conform his or her conduct in such a manner that the patient is not at an unreasonable risk of harm. The case manager must take reasonable steps to avoid an unreasonable risk of harm to the patient.

The second element is proof that the second duty was breached. The plaintiff must show that the case manager breached the duty to exercise a reasonable standard of practice. The breach of duty must be shown to be sufficiently close in proximity to the harm suffered by the patient. This is the cause-and-effect element of negligence and the most difficult to understand and prove. The act of negligence must be the proximate or legal cause of the injury or harm claimed by the plaintiff. If there is an independent, intervening cause that resulted in the harm to the plaintiff, then the second element fails.

It is the interplay between these first two elements where the relationship between negligence and standards of practice comes into play. The courts will generally look to the standard of practice established by peers in the community, expert witnesses, and written standards of governments and professional associations. The case manager is required to conform his or her conduct to the minimally recognized standard of care for his or her skills, knowledge, and education.

Finally, the plaintiff must show actual damages or injury. The damages may be an injury to the person, property, or rights as a direct result of the defendant's negligence.

All three elements must be proved. The duties of the case manager and the elements of negligence should be kept in mind while reading about specific types of negligence.

BENEFIT DECISION MAKING VERSUS CASE MANAGEMENT

As health care costs skyrocketed and society began demanding a reduction in heath care costs, more and more case managers have become closely involved in managing the health care benefits through or for third-party payers. The third-party payers may include workers compensation insurers, Medicare/Medicaid payers, managed care companies, health insurance companies, liability insurers, and others.

These case managers find themselves in a dichotomy. On the one hand, they are patient advocates. On the other hand, they must see that health care is delivered in a quality but cost-efficient manner. For case managers practicing in these areas, the risk of liability is greatest. There are no national standards of care to fall back on, no national outcome criteria, no clear guidelines to follow.

To reduce the liability risks, it is important for these case managers to understand their role and to practice in a manner that is consistent with their obligations. The case manager is primarily advisory or administrative in function. The role of the case manager is to evaluate the patient or the medical record to determine if the care received is reasonable, cost effective, and efficacious based on the complaints of the patient and in the light of all the information available. That information must then be fairly balanced and weighed against the benefits outlined in the insurer's policy. The case manager can then refer the patient or patient's records to an appropriate and qualified reviewer or provider to make a final determination on whether the care is or was needed. It is critical for the case manager to avoid placing him- or herself in a position of actually making a medical decision, interfering with prescribed care, or prescribing treatment. That role remains exclusively a physician's responsibility.

Benefits decision liability has become more prevalent in the past decade as utilization review and case management programs were instituted to enhance patient care while making insurers and hospitals more competitive in the marketplace. It is this environment in which many case managers find themselves. This liability warrants a review of the utilization review process and the subsequent court cases defining benefits decision making.

Utilization review is an "evaluation based on established clinical criteria that are used by third party payers to evaluate the quality and appropriateness of the medical care at various stages in its delivery."[7(p.883)] To be cost effective, the peer reviewer must have some say or control over the treating physician's decision as to what care is needed.[7] There are three types of utilization review: prospective, concurrent, and retrospective.

Retrospective review is the oldest and, in the past, the most widely used type of utilization review. It occurs after the physician has rendered all the care to a patient. Although the goal of retrospective review is to identify care that was unnecessary and therefore not reimbursable by the insurer, in actuality most claims were rarely denied and the cost of the review process simply added to the growing health care costs.[8] Retrospective reviews have been abandoned by most third-party payers in favor of concurrent or prospective review programs.[8]

Prospective or concurrent utilization review processes were implemented because these types of review take place before the care is rendered in the case of prospective reviews or on an ongoing basis as the care is received in the concurrent review process. It is thought to be a more effective cost-containment system because if the care rendered exceeds the "approved" or "preauthorized scope" of care, the provider is less likely to be reimbursed and may be doing the care for free.[8] It is, however, the prospective and concurrent review systems that offer the greatest legal liability to insurers and case managers because the risk exists that a patient may be harmed or denied an essential treatment or diagnostic procedure if the insurer refuses to pay for it. It is these reviews that recent case law has addressed.

The landmark case linking a third-party utilization review process to negligence liability is *Wickline v. California*.[9] The patient, Lois Wickline, sued Medi-Cal, a third-party insurer, for negligence when the prospective utilization review process resulted in her premature discharge from the hospital and her subsequent readmission and amputation of her leg.

Lois Wickline was hospitalized for complaints of back and leg pain, which ultimately required vascular surgery to correct the problem.[9] Wickline's attending physician submitted a preauthorization request for the surgery. On the date Wickline was to be discharged, the attending physician determined it was medically necessary to keep Wickline an additional eight days. The attending physician completed a request for an extension, which was submitted to Medi-Cal utilization reviewers.

The Medi-Cal reviewers included a nurse and general surgeon. After reviewing the records, the nurse and physician reviewers authorized an additional four days instead of the requested eight days. The attending physician complied without protest, discharging Wickline after four days. Wickline developed a life-threatening infection in one leg, which necessitated an emergency admission and subsequent amputation of the limb.

The trial court jury found in favor of Wickline, holding the third-party insurer liable for negligence resulting from the utilization review process. The court of appeals reversed. The court found third-party liability did not exist given the facts of the case. However, the court identified three key elements that should send a resounding message to case managers and third-party insurers: (1) when a patient is harmed, he or she should be able to recover from all responsible parties, including the third-party insurer; (2) the third-party payer can be held legally accountable for an inappropriate decision resulting from defects in the design or implementation of cost-containment mechanisms; and (3) when a treating physician disagrees but carries out the requests of a third-party reviewer without exhausting all avenues of protest, he or she is liable for any resulting harm to the patient.[9]

The utilization review process came under scrutiny again in *Hughes v. Blue Cross of Northern California*.[10] The third-party payer was found to have acted in bad faith in denying coverage for a psychiatric hospitalization. The court found that the utilization reviewers, a nurse and a physician, used a standard of medical necessity that significantly deviated from the medical standard of the community.

In coming to the decision in *Hughes*, the court found evidence that the reviewers analyzed fragmented medical records and failed to investigate the case thoroughly by accessing complete medical records and talking to providers and that the reviewing physician spent as few as 12 minutes reviewing the records, resulting in a cursory review. The court held a third-party insurer has a good faith obligation to construct a medical necessity standard that is "consistent with community medical standards that will minimize a patient's uncertainty of coverage in accepting his physician's recommendations for treatment."[10(p.856,857)]

More recently, a concurrent utilization program came under attack in *Wilson v. Blue Cross of Southern California*.[11] The patient was admitted to the hospital for major depression. While still hospitalized, the concurrent reviewer determined that additional hospitalization was not justified and denied additional coverage. The patient, unable to bear the costs of hospitalization on his own, was discharged. Shortly after discharge, he committed suicide. The court held the third-party payer could be at least partially liable for negligent conduct resulting in the death of the insured and remanded the case to the lower court for findings.

These cases illustrate the pitfalls for case managers involved in utilization review. Other cases have followed and will continue to follow, further prescribing the limits of utilization review. However, utilization review is unlikely to fade away. In fact, there is significant evidence to the contrary, that as more of the country moves to a managed care environment, utilization review will be the norm.

It is the nature of the beast that liability risk will always be present in case management. The case manager should not shy away from practicing in this area because of the risks involved but rather should make every effort to analyze the issues and participate in developing a utilization review program that reduces potential liability. The following guidelines are offered:

- Investigate, develop, and internalize a strong concept of professional responsibility and ethics.
- Always operate within the scope and standards of your practice.

- Understand that the role of the case manager is always advisory or administrative in function. Never become involved in the actual medical decision-making process. Do not interfere with the physician-patient relationship.
- In every case, conduct a thorough and timely investigation by gathering sufficient clinical data to be able effectively and safely to evaluate the clinical status of a patient.
- When possible, develop a written plan of care. Be flexible. Consider alternative plans of care as the patient's condition or situation changes.
- If a treating physician objects to or disagrees with the findings of a reviewer, give him or her every opportunity to respond. Get the objection in writing if possible. If there is a significant disagreement between the reviewer and the treating physician, consider an independent medical examination.
- If there is sufficient evidence to support the position of the treating physician and the utilization reviewer still disagrees, you are professionally obligated to voice an objection if you have a good faith belief that the patient may be harmed. The patient should get the benefit of the doubt.
- In any case, if you have a doubt on how to proceed, you are obligated to seek the counsel of competent peers or physicians.

NEGLIGENT REFERRAL

Case managers often find themselves in the position of recommending or referring a patient to a physician, hospital, institution, or other provider. In the light of the recent court decisions, the case manager may be at risk of liability if the patient is harmed by the provider or institution as a result of the referral. Moreover, Hyatt[12] notes that the case manager may owe a greater duty of care to the patient because he or she is typically more involved in the care of a patient than the typical utilization reviewer. The case manager may be liable not only for the "referral itself but also for the failure to refer when warranted."[12(p.2)]

In determining which provider or institution to refer a patient, the case manager should consider "investigating the practitioner or facility you refer before making the recommendation."[12(p.2)] The investigation should be thorough, including an inquiry into "licensure, accreditation, staffing components, geographical capabilities, area provider endorsement, patient census, acuity levels"[13(p.217)] and any history of complaints or suits against the provider. Sources of the investigation may include the agencies or providers themselves, the government agency licensing the provider or agency, and references from professional peers in the community.

If it is possible to give the patient a choice in providers or facilities, then by all means do so. Allowing a patient to participate actively in his or her health care decision always reduces your risk of legal liability.

ABANDONMENT AND PATIENT DISCHARGE

The duty not to abandon a patient has been around as long as nursing itself. In simple terms, it is the termination of the patient relationship by the provider without informing the patient and/or failing to provide adequate medical care in the absence of the provider. Typically, this situation arises if a nurse is assigned to take care of a patient and then abruptly leaves the patient before making sure that another competent professional is placed in charge of the patient's care.

For nurses involved in hands-on practice, the duty has not changed. For the case manager, there is still a duty not to abandon a patient, but it may arise in a different context. For example, consider a workers compensation case manager assigned to the case of Mr. Jones. Mr. Jones is 50 years old and suffers a debilitating knee and back injury on the job. He has diabetes and chronic obstructive pulmonary disease from years of smoking, necessitating the need for home oxygen, is required to take many medications, and is generally noncompliant and cantankerous. Despite your best efforts, Mr. Jones repeatedly misses his physician appointments, refuses to comply with his physician's recommendations on treatment and medications, has verbally assaulted you with foul language, and has even threatened to sue you.

This is not an uncommon situation. If the case manager simply closes the case file and does not make further attempts to implement the plan of care, he or she can be liable for abandonment if the patient is harmed, even if the patient was verbally told that if he or she missed one more appointment or failed to take his or her medications, the file would be closed.

So what should the case manager do? Take the abuse? Keep the case file open indefinitely? There are measures the case manager can take to avoid being sued for abandonment. *Documentation is essential!* A paper trail must be created, and all interactions with the patient must be carefully and accurately documented. If you observe noncompliant behavior, the behavior should be documented objectively in the file. If the patient misses appointments, it must be documented in the file. All instances of noncompliance should be followed up with a patient verbally, if possible, and always in writing. The letters should document the incident itself and advise the patient of the necessity to continue and comply with the physician's recommended treatment. A copy of the letters should be placed in the file and a copy sent to the treating physician. The treating physician should be kept advised every step of the way.

If after repeated episodes it is necessary to terminate the professional relationship, then this should also be done verbally, if possible, and by certified letter. The patient should always be given an opportunity to mend his or her ways before the relationship is terminated. Therefore, it is advisable to send more than one certified letter and to offer the patient an opportunity to continue the relationship or to accept references to other case managers. Only after a painstaking effort to encourage compliance and documentation of noncompliance should a case manager close the case without the patient's consent. In the final letter, the patient should be offered a referral to other professionals, and the treating physician must be notified.

VICARIOUS LIABILITY

There are several theories of vicarious liability including corporate negligence, agency, ostensible agency, and respondeat superior. The first three are most likely to apply to managed care companies that have the possibility of exerting influence or control over a physician's decisions. They are not discussed here. However, the doctrine of respondeat superior is applicable to the case manager employed by a company, hospital, or facility and to the case manager who employs other case managers.

Under the doctrine of respondeat superior, "an employer is vicariously liable for the acts of an employee acting within the scope of his employment."[14(p.955)] The employer of the case manager could be sued in negligence if the decision of the case manager brings about an injury to a patient's person, property, or rights.

The key is whether the act was intentional or unintentional and whether the individual was acting within the scope of employment. If the case manager intentionally commits a tortious act on a patient, then the employer will generally not be held liable.

The best defense for case managers employing other case managers is a careful development of policies, procedures, contracts, and other materials that are relevant to the employment and an outline of the expected duties of the employee. In developing these materials, the case manager employer should take care to make sure the expectations are grounded in the scope of practice. There should be sufficient documentation in the employment record that the case manager employee was given the materials to review and, in fact, reviewed them.

INTERFERENCE WITH PHYSICIAN-PATIENT RELATIONSHIP

The tort of interference with the physician-patient relationship has historically been limited to the relationship that exists between a hospital or other facility and a physician.[8] The physician-patient relationship arises when a physician actively or prospectively agrees to "be available and provide reasonable medical services"[8(p.1274)] to a patient and the patient agrees to reimburse the physician for services rendered.[8] The relationship is strictly between the patient and the physician. Each is able to exercise judgment independently about the appropriate delivery and receipt of health care.[8]

When that independent judgment is restrained or the physician-patient relationship is disrupted because of the interference of a third party, then the individual or institution that restrained or limited the physician's judgment or relationship could be liable if the patient is subsequently harmed because of the interference.[8]

Unlike hospitals, HMOs, or PPOs, which can interfere with the physician relationship by terminating the physician's privileges or refusing to allow the physician to perform certain treatments, the third-party payer or case manager "can interfere with the medical decision-making process."[8(p.1275)] The liability arises if the third-party payer or case manager denies payment for certain treatments, causes by their conduct the physician-patient relationship to terminate, defames the provider resulting in the termination of the relationship, or substantially interferes or "imposes limitations on a physician's ability to diagnose and/or treat a medical condition in a timely manner."[8(p.1275)]

The lesson here is simple. Case management is the administrative management of a medical case. It is not medical management. It is not medical decision making. The actual decision about whether a treatment is reasonable and necessary should be left to the physicians. You must operate within your defined scope of practice.

INCOMPETENCE, MALPRACTICE, MISCONDUCT, AND REPORTING

We all know it exists. We do not talk about it enough. But what should the case manager do about incompetence, malpractice, and misconduct of other case managers, physicians, and allied health care providers?

Depending on your state's laws or practice acts, you may have a legal obligation to report any incidents that may lead to the harm of a patient. In any event, you have an ethical obligation to report incompetence, malpractice, and misconduct to the appropriate licensing agency. It is, however, improper to go "directly to a patient with adverse information about the individual's attending physician"[13(p.221)] or other provider.

When faced with these situations, the case manager should first decide if the patient is in immediate danger. If the answer is yes, then you are obligated to bring the matter first to the attention of the provider and try to resolve the matter. If the provider is unwilling to alter his or her behavior, the problem should be taken up with the individual's supervisor, peer review committees, or state licensing agency. Even if the immediate situation has been corrected and the error is of such significant magnitude as to be incompetence or if the provider repeatedly engages in such behavior, then you are obligated to bring it to the attention of the appropriate authorities to ensure that the provider's activities are reviewed and do not jeopardize patients in the future.

CONTRACTING

A few words of advice on contracting. Case managers are not always employed by hospitals or insurers. A growing trend in the case management arena is the independent case manager. In these instances, case managers may find themselves in the position of entering into contracts with third-party payers or even the patient him- or herself for his or her case management services.

Verbal agreements should be avoided. It is important always to get the agreement in writing. Whenever possible, the case manager should consult independent legal counsel before entering into a contract or before constructing a blanket contract. It should be remembered that both parties may be held to the contents of the contract.

In contracting, any information should be included that may arise out of the course of the relationship including, but not limited to, the expected duties of the case manager, the obligations of the patient/payer, any and all restrictions on the part of the case manager or patient/payer, the fee or payment schedules, the expected length of time the contract will be in force, a detailed outline of the services that will and will not be provided, conditions under which the contract may be terminated, including who may terminate and whether notice must be given, and any liability or restrictions to liability that may exist, such as malpractice insurance coverage.

CONCLUSION

The information provided in this chapter in no way covers every aspect of potential liability for the case manager and is not intended to substitute for good common sense and the advice of legal counsel when needed. It is intended to provide an overview of the changing world of legal liability as it applies to the case manager.

Exposure to liability is inescapable. However, case managers can significantly reduce the risks of liability by modifying how they think about liability and its effect on daily practice. Going back to the pyramid model, the foundation of every practice should be based on sound ethics and legal principles. The patient should always be at the forefront of your practice. It is the independence and health of the individual patient that forms that top of the pyramid, the reason for case management.

Every time case managers make a decision in the medical case file, they do so for the benefit of the patient. Case managers should ask themselves if the decision reflects the duty to act in the best interest of the patient, if the decision will place the patient at risk of harm, and if every effort has been made to diminish the risks to the patient. Additionally, the case manager should follow a professional code of conduct in daily practice. These parameters will reduce but not eliminate liability risks.

And a final word on verbiage. Medical management and case management are often used interchangeably. They are not interchangeable. In the field of nursing case managment, medical management is the actual management of the patient's care by a physician. Case management is the management of the case file. The distinction is important. It is not the purview of the case manager to make medical decisions or to interfere with the medical decision-making process. It is the duty of the case manager to manage the medical case file for the optimum delivery of health care.

REFERENCES

1. 61 AMERICAN Jurisprudence 2D 353, §224.
2. Computerized records, claims threaten patient confidentiality. *Case Manage Advisor.* 1993;4:119.
3. Emanuel S. Emanuel Law Outlines: Tort Law, *Miscellaneous Torts: Invasion of Privacy; Misuse of Legal Procedures; Interference with Advantageous Relations: Familial and Political Relations; Torts in the Family.* Larchmont, NY: Emanuel Law Outlines; 1988; 330.
4. *Defamation.* Larchmont, NY: Emanuel Law Outlines; 1988: 308–309.
5. 20 AMERICAN LAW REPORTS 3d 1109, 1113, §2.
6. 61 AMERICAN Jurisprudence 2D 304, §173.
7. Griner DD. *Paying the Piper: Third Party Payor Liability for Medical Treatment Decisions,* 25 Ga. L. Rev. 861, 883 (Spring 1991).
8. Phelan JP. *Law and Medicine Symposium Issue: Two Hot Areas in Medical Malpractice for the 1990s,* 24 CRLR 1261 (June 1991); 1261–1275.

9. *Wickline v. California,* 192 Cal. App. 3d 1630, 239 Cal. Rptr. 810 (Ct. App. 1986), *review dismissed, remanded,* 741 P.2d 613 (Cal. 1987).

10. *Hughes v. Blue Cross of Northern California,* 215 Cal. App. 3d 832, 263 Cal. Rptr. 850 (1984).

11. *Wilson v. Blue Cross of Southern California,* 222 Cal. App. 3d 660, 271 Cal. Rptr. 876 (1990).

12. Hyatt TK. *Negligent Referral.* Washington, DC: Powers, Pyles, Sutter, and Verville, P.C.

13. Blum JD. *An Analysis of Legal Liability in Health Care Utilization Review and Case Management,* 26 Houston L. Rev. 191, 217–221 (1989).

14. Parise HL. *The Proper Extension of Tort Liability Principles in the Managed Care Industry.* 64 Temp. L. Rev. 955, 977 (Winter 1991).

■ 24 ■

Ethical Issues in Case Management

Winifred J. Ellenchild Pinch, EdD, RN

Although major health care reform legislation at the federal level was unsuccessful in the 1994 Congress, the promise (or threat) of such reform motivated many changes in the health care system that will continue to affect the delivery of care. One of the most significant changes continues to be the phenomenon of managed care. A managed care approach to the delivery of health care services primarily targets containment of costs. Nursing case management is a system used by the profession for the delivery of health care services in the age of managed care. In this chapter, the effects of managed care and case management on the ethical obligations and responsibilities of the nurse are discussed.

In the context of ethics, two aspects of the role of the nurse in case management may cause ethical conflict. The mandate of advocacy for the patient can be in tension with the mandate for community justice and fairness. One key nursing value is advocacy for the patient and the provision of the highest possible quality of care, which results in beneficial outcomes for patients and significant others. The American Nurses Association Code for Nurses implicitly supports an advocacy stance for nurses:

> The nurse provides services with respect for human dignity and the uniqueness of the client, unrestricted by considerations of social or economic status, personal attributes, or the nature of health problems.[1(p.2)]

In the association's discussion of this statement, the self-determination of clients is an important concept. Services designed for each client cannot be determined unless the person's opinions and preferences have been ascertained. Patient-defined needs and goals are critical for decision making, which cannot occur without correct, sufficient, and relevant information that the patient understands. Support for the patient's decision may be required as the patient role is a vulnerable one in the health care system, open to discriminatory action and paternalistic practices. For example, health care professionals can decide that information related to possible treatment options is too complex for the patient to understand. To simplify the situation, the professional decides what is best for the patient and then leads the patient to chose that option while discussing future treatment.

Another area that can conflict with individual patient advocacy is the nurse's broader responsibility for groups and communities. This is reflected in statement 11 of the Code for Nurses:

> The nurse collaborates with members of the health professions and other citizens in promoting community and national efforts to meet the health needs of the public.[1(p.16)]

Statement 11 exhibits a justice mandate. What actions by the nurse are necessary to promote the good of the aggregate? How can limited resources be fairly distributed? What is fair for the individual given a broad spectrum of needs in the community and an acknowledgement that all needs cannot be met?

As a case manager, the nurse has an obligation to work within the guidelines, policies, and procedures of the employing agency. These directives are developed in various ways but in this age of managed care, cost containment is of critical concern whether the agency is for profit or nonprofit. The limits of health care and the distribution of available resources are concerns of the ethical nurse. The ethical nurse not only desires to do good, but also wants to be thought of as a good person. For decisions to be ethically acceptable, the case manager needs to know, understand, and accept the rationale for decision making related to the available services. When aggregate needs are adequately assessed and fairly balanced against individual needs, then the case manager can maintain a good conscience while working within the system.

A greater understanding of these ethical issues can be realized by first exploring advocacy and justice separately. The historical framework from which each mandate evolved will provide the setting for their interface.

ADVOCACY

The concept of patient advocacy is not new to either health care or the nursing profession. Advocates, or ombudsmen as they were formally known in the legal sphere, date back to the 1800s.[2] Nursing advocacy was popular in the 1970s when discussions of patient rights created high levels of professional interest paralleling the widespread, general concern for consumer rights in the public arena.[3-7] Patient advocacy continues to be vital to the nurse's professional role as related to the ethical dimension of practice[8-11] and is specifically included in the role of the nurse as case manager.[12-15]

Patient advocacy has two facets. One is the provision of information by the nurse so that the patient can make decisions. The second is supporting the decisions that patients make. The process of patient advocacy is a bridge between legal and ethical practice.[6] Generally, legal mandates prescribe a particular level of information that must be provided to the patient when carrying out the informed consent process, whether this be informally in the routine provision of services or the more formal completion of documents before implementing procedures or research. Ethically, the nurse takes the additional responsibility of supporting the patient in the decision-making process. This may be a simple assurance of the right to receive appropriate information and make decisions or a more action-oriented role, in which the nurse intervenes on behalf of the patient to ensure that rights are protected.

Advocacy is not a simple process. It may involve clarifying one's own and the patient's values, although this is not necessary by most definitions.[8-11] The key features, however, are informing and supporting. Ethically, the nurse is required to believe genuinely that the patient needs to possess the appropriate information before self-determination can occur. Occasionally, the patient's need to know and the nurse's belief about what the patient should know may be in conflict. This must be resolved. There may be individuals on the health care team who have similar conflicts. It is the nurse advocate's responsibility to ensure recognition by all team members of the patient's right to know whatever is necessary for adequate decision making. The patient needs to understand that his or her decision will be respected and that abandonment by the health care team will not be a risk.

In recent years, the patients' rights movement involving patient needs, individual rights, and protection of autonomy/privacy has dominated ethical discussion. The American Hospital Association Patient Bill of Rights, the first statement of the Code for Nurses, and the more recent Patient Self-Determination Act support these rights. In turn, these documents represent a focus on maintaining *individual* liberty and freedom. Individual freedom from interference of others and the liberty to do as one individually determines are often expressed ethically through the principle of autonomy.

The importance of autonomy resides in the democratic political system of our country, whose founding documents guarantee individual liberty and pursuit of happiness. In health care, autonomy is the right to make health care decisions in the context of one's own history, life, goals, and relationships. A respect for patient autonomy encompasses a recognition of the importance of the patients' choices as well as the person's inherent dignity and worth.

Autonomy can be threatened by the misuse of power by health care professionals, often referred to as paternalism. Paternalism bypasses patient decision making and places the selection of choices in the hands of the professional. Paternalism is often presented as a practice to be avoided by the ethical professional. However, professional judgment and paternalistic behavior cannot always be clearly separated.

The health care professional does have a right to interject professional opinion about the best possible option for the patient. Objectivity is relative. The professional brings values and beliefs as well as education to the decision-making process in the information provision stage. Professionals are shaped by their own life histories and professional socialization. Yet, the professionals' role is to assess the patient and the situation, use their expertise to draw correct conclusions, and make recommendations about possible treatments or other interventions. Professionals prioritize these recommendations, and prioritization may not be objective. The line between professional discernment and paternalism may be difficult or impossible to identify. Ethically, an ideal goal for the professional would be an appreciation for the possibility of paternalistic practice and an openness to discussion of its meaning in particular situations.

Several other concerns about the role of autonomy in ethics and health care have surfaced recently. One concern relates to the breadth to which autonomy needs to be respected. Should autonomy mean that persons be allowed to do anything they want to do as long as they abide by the law and do not interfere with others' liberty? Another concern relates to the relationship between autonomy and rights. To what extent are rights inherent in the principle of autonomy? People require freedom to act autonomously. Protection is necessary to guarantee privacy and safety from the coercion and misdeeds of others. Additionally, are people owed any privileges and benefits in our society? What can the individual autonomously demand? These questions lead to a consideration of justice—balancing the needs and demands of the one against the needs and demands of many.

JUSTICE

Although the most current health care reform legislation was not passed, there is a growing movement that supports community *rights*. Along with this social movement are the obvious, realistic economic constraints nurse case managers need to work within: capitated budgets, rationing, provider alliances, and shifting government fiduciary accountability.

The epitome of the stalwart rugged individual of Western democratic society has become somewhat tarnished. Individualism and individual rights, so long championed in our political system and reflectively in other social systems including health care, are developing their own flaws. There is a recognition that in some instances, individualism more or less represents a selfish position rather than a self-sacrificing noble one. There is not only a desire in this version of individualism for a share of the available resources but also in some cases a demand to fulfill personal needs irrespective of others' needs or possible future needs of the community at large. The recipient of multiple liver transplants, especially an individual who contributed to a declining health status by life style choices, is often viewed as one who receives more than a fair share of resources. The cost of several transplants and the lifetime support for a person with a transplant uses health care dollars that could be spent on less costly interventions or preventive care benefiting many people.

In health care ethics, the need to protect and support individual autonomy is an important concept. However, the overemphasis on autonomy and the individual has blindsided many to the corollary need to attend to the aggregate needs and desires of society that must be met within existing and potential resources. How are individual needs to be addressed given the needs of many others?

Past discussions of ethical decision making in most situations focused on the individual decision, the patient in the dilemma with attending health professionals involved in that moment of care. People have been held individually responsible for their health practices and status, both in preventing disease and carrying out treatment plans. Many books of bioethics devoted the bulk of their space to this individual orientation.[16–22] The allocation of scarce resources or rationing of health care was often an afterthought discussed after a series of discussions on reproduction, dying, transplantation, genetics, mental health, and experimentation. The allocation of resources appeared to be the least important issue, something one considered after each person already decided what was best for her- or himself. With the ethical consideration of the distribution of resources systematically discussed last, "first come, first served" often appeared to be the most viable alternative for decision making about the allocation of resources. When conflicting needs occurred simultaneously, a lottery system was posed as a decision-making process. In a lottery, all individuals currently requiring a particular intervention become part of the pool from which the recipients are chosen. Some individual needs would be met in the lottery but without regard for future persons, some of whom might possibly benefit more from the treatment. All these allocation strategies were reactive to clashing needs rather than a proactive solution. The relative importance placed on allocation of resources compared with other ethical issues serves covertly to teach the priority of individual issues as opposed to aggregate needs, especially those related to scarce resources and rationing of health care.

We can no longer afford the luxury of the individual as the most significant focus in ethical decision making. A more robust tradition of social ethics needs to be established.[23] A respect for justice must be more than an extension of individualism whereby fairness is determined based on a group of persons, each one viewed as largely detached from others in society. Decisions at the macro level need to appreciate individuality but place it in a social context, not fashion personal choices before a consideration of the milieu in which these choices exist.

The importance of context and relationships, our connections to others, is recognized and fostered in the psychological work by Gilligan et al.[24,25] and feminists in philosophy, theology, and other disciplines.[26–35] The research of Gilligan et al. heightens our awareness of the roles of context and relationships in ethical decision making, albeit at a personal level. Their thesis has consistently challenged the priority of individualistic autonomous decision making in moral dilemmas whether the decision maker be male or female. The centrality of people's interrelationships in some feminist writing has advanced a perspective of morality more supportive of a communitarian orientation than one in which the principle of autonomy holds preeminence. A communitarian consciousness is necessary for implementing the ethical responsibilities of a justice mandate.

Apart from immediate patient situations, institutions and legislatures will have to make decisions about available resources and their distribution. The ethical goal will be the provision of the best possible services using available resources in a fair manner. These decisions are made at the macro allocation level. The case manager at the bedside should not have to choose between patients if an ethical system is implemented. Limitations and restrictions, when necessary, are effective for all individuals included in the pool of patients comprising the target population of the managed care institution or the government. As different needs arise, or characteristics of the population change, revisions in allocation dispersement can be instituted.

FUNCTIONING AT THE INTERFACE OF ADVOCACY AND JUSTICE

Patient advocacy was linked to the ethical responsibility of nurses and the philosophic foundations of nursing most cogently by Gadow[36] through her theory of existential advocacy. For her, advocacy nursing was different from and more than paternalism or patients' rights advocacy, both described above. Paternalism, or the health professional's resolution of the best decision for the patient, is a violation of the patient's self-determination from Gadow's perspective. Additionally, patients' rights advocacy is a narrow interpretation of advocacy in which, first, information is provided to the patient, especially information about rights. Second, action is taken by the advocate when the health care system prevents a patient from exercising those rights. Gadow[36(p.84)] calls this advocate a "troubleshooter willing to intervene when the system violates an individual's rights."

Gadow posits the ideal in a fuller, richer definition of the advocate as a nurse who assists patients "to *authentically* exercise their freedom of self-determination." She goes on to describe this process more fully.

> [Existential advocacy] is not based on an assumption about what individuals *should want* to do, nor does it consist in protecting individuals' *rights* to do what they want to do. It is the effort to help persons *become clear about what they want* to do, by helping them discern and clarify their values in the situation, and on the basis of that self-examination, to reach decisions which express their reaffirmed, perhaps recreated, complex of values.[36(p.85)]

This mode of interaction is not an automated response to infringements of patients' rights nor the registering of a formal complaint of injustice. Rather, it is involvement in which the entire self of the professional is engaged with the patient. This process assists the patient to identify and express important core values, resulting in the nurse's understanding of the lived experience of the patient, the personal meaning of illness, suffering, or dying for that individual. The nurse, Gadow believes, is the best person for this role as nursing encompasses both care and cure. Nursing is concerned about both scientific treatment and the experience of living: before, during, and after illness and injury.

The nurse case manager would be able to practice ethically while balancing the possibly conflicting demands of justice and autonomy in the role of existential advocate. Gadow[36] does not specifically discuss the nurse's obligations to groups and the aggregate. However, in her description of the nurse's role, this community perspective can be inferred. Gadow specifically includes the need for the nurse's perspective to be shared during the patient's decision-making process. The nurse's role complements and completes the partial perspective of the patient, according to Gadow. Existential advocacy can encompass a cyclical processes whereby the nurse implements different roles at different times, each complementing the other, each succeeding because of the perspective gained in the other role. A closer look at these roles as the nurse case manager sensitizes her- or himself to ethical responsibilities to both individuals and communities will illuminate the practical application of these ideas.

One role for the nurse in managed care is as a general existential advocate for patients in the public arena based on the summation of the nurse's experiences with individual patients in professional practice. These experiences provide the nurse with the expertise to (1) inform public officials and administrators/supervisors about patient needs, (2) lobby for changes in the delivery of health care, and (3) create forces within professional organizations that will monitor the health care system for ethical outcomes. These experiences together will support grassroots decision making associated with the allocation of resources and enable the nurse to accept the stipulations of a managed care environment ethically.

The other role for the nurse is as existential advocate for the individual patient within the context of managed care and the set boundaries given available resources and the most fair and just distribution possible. A major component of this latter role will be education during the decision-making process. Patients will require assistance in understanding the extent of resources available to them and the nurse case manager's role in maximizing their access to these benefits. The more difficult challenge in education will be situations in which limitations for services exist or optimum benefits have been exercised. The idea that resources are not unlimited and community needs must be distributed fairly will be an arduous lesson for patients and nurses alike to learn. It is hoped that knowing that decisions regarding restrictions are not made on an individual basis but rather in balancing many needs across myriad groups may ameliorate any sense of ethical compromise for the nurse related to autonomy or injustice regarding allocation of resources.

ETHICAL ISSUES

The specific ethical issues in managed care encompass the entire spectrum of possible health care dilemmas (e.g., transplantation, human immunodeficiency virus (HIV)/acquired immunodeficiency syndrome (AIDS), nutrition/hydration, abortion, high-risk newborns). Ethical issues represent events across the entire life span from before birth (genetics and reproduction) to death (right to die, assisted suicide, refusal of treatment). These topics are discussed in a variety of resources on bioethics.[17,19,37,38]

The unique ethical issues of case management are just beginning to be explored as case managers juggle multiple roles of advocacy, gatekeeping, and quality control.[39] Until these issues are specifically identified, it is reasonable to anticipate that the case manager will encounter a cluster of concerns relating to end-of-life decisions, advance directives, and assisted suicide, as well as HIV/AIDS, multicultural issues, violence, ethics education, ethics committees, professional integrity, and health reform.*[40] The broad ethical dimensions of health reform and the resulting health care delivery systems, including managed care and the use of case managers, have been identified in the review of advocacy and justice. Other remaining issues warrant some additional remarks.

Note: *These are the top ten topics as reported by each U.S. state published by The American Nurses Association's Center for Ethics and Human Rights. See reference 40.

The end-of-life issues are particularly troublesome as they test competing claims of respect for autonomy, beneficence (do good), and nonmaleficence (do no harm).[41] A great value is placed on doing good by health professionals, sometimes to the point of implementing interventions of marginal benefit. At the opposite end of the spectrum, patients sometimes believe they have a right to any and all treatments regardless of their prognoses and predicted outcomes. Futile treatments need to be identified and outcome data utilized in order to avoid needless prolongation of life. Questions of withholding or withdrawing nutrition—especially the provision or removal of hydration—will undergo much debate in the future. When cost containment is a key element in decision making, the case manager needs to be alert to the potential for budgetary constraints to override other ethical considerations such as optimal treatment and quality of life.[42] Case managers can be instrumental in developing critical clinical pathways that include points of possible ethical distress. These will alert all care givers to potential problematic areas—not necessarily to avoid them, but to be prepared for them when they arise.

End-of-life questions are relevant whether the patient is young (newborn) or old. Advance directives are helpful documents when patients are competent adults and have a life history that contains examples of past decision making based on individual values, beliefs, and traditions.[43] The case manager can promote the preparation of such documents before there is a critical need for their use. Discussions with clients are helpful, and many individuals are acutely aware of their preferences immediately after discharge. It is more difficult in the newborn situation when the best interests of the neonate are determined based on general criteria about all newborns. Although parents would seem to be natural decision makers for these infants, decision making for the neonate has presented some particularly thorny problems related to the locus of decision making.[44,45]

Assisted suicide has created a media circus, but when seriously ill clients are referred to case managers, this issue can develop tangible dimensions. Clients discharged early in their recovery phase, dependent and functioning marginally, and those in terminal conditions may judge their situations intolerable. Assisted suicide is not legal at the present time, but believing themselves to be burdensome, some clients may press their cases cogently and persuasively.[46] Each case manager needs to decide what actions constitute treatment to decrease pain and suffering (although such treatment may shorten the life span) and what crosses the line to unacceptable ethical behavior.

HIV and AIDS focus the case manager on ethical obligations of confidentiality and discrimination.[47] Although strides have been made in relation to the societal attitude toward clients with HIV and AIDS, the stigma and discrimination have not been totally erased. Clients who are HIV positive continue to face compromising and dangerous situations. Clients are at risk for losing jobs, housing, friends, and certain services. Trust is an especially important element in the professional relationship between the case manager and the client with HIV/AIDS. The moral obligation of maintaining confidentiality in cases of HIV/AIDS is singularly strong. Initially, clients must clearly understand the difference between anonymity and confidentiality, particularly in relation to HIV testing. Later, the need to disclose information about the diagnosis may create an ethical dilemma for case managers. Sometimes, greater services are available if the diagnosis is HIV/AIDS. Case managers will need to weigh the client's preferences with the need for the services, counterbalanced with the case managers' responsibility to inform and educate their clients. The ethical danger here, of course, is the problem of how persuasive case managers ought to be. There is often a fine line between persuasion and coercion or manipulation when attempting to have clients understand the full range of options and facilitate a wise choice.

The case manager who confronts multicultural issues is faced with provocative questions of relativity.[48] Traditionally, the nursing profession has fostered respect for various ethnic groups and their differing cultural beliefs. Nurses have been cautioned to withhold judgment and attempt to provide value-free services. Accusations of ethnocentrism are to be avoided. However, are any ethical norms universal? Are there any values and beliefs within our culture and society that become bottom-line ethical measures for standards of practice? For example, female genital mutilation is a practice among some groups who have immigrated to the United States.[49-51] This is not as widespread yet in the United States as in some countries, but it is beginning to make an appearance. Countries such as the United Kingdom, France, and Canada have classified the procedure as child abuse. Some health professionals do perform these procedures to avoid the use of primitive equipment and prevent the risks of infection in girls. How does the case manager respond to the woman who wants to discuss this procedure for her daughter?

Another issue involves cultural perspectives of congenital disorders and handicaps. In certain groups, Vietnamese, for example, disfigured and malformed newborns are not always perceived as acceptable.* In the country of origin, these children would be left to die because it is a disgrace to recognize their existence and care for them. This presents a significant dilemma for the case manager who works with families whose children begin life in the neonatal intensive care unit. Many handicaps are compatible with life, although

---

Note: *This has been a personal experience in ethics consultation involving two cases to date. Each infant had severe anomalies that included the physical appearance. In both cases, the parents did not want to have the infant treated. It was also extremely difficult to communicate in these cases because the parents were unable to use English but also did not want a bilingual Vietnamese person present. In each situation, they wanted to hide the results of the pregnancy from the rest of the Vietnamese community and simply be able to say that the baby died.

they may create a disfiguring appearance. Some of these infants are also candidates for reconstructive surgery where normal or near-normal appearances are possible. How does the professional staff respond to parents who prefer to allow the child to die or abandon the child if it lives—a child that is not culturally acceptable in their community? Are there universal human rights that cross these cultural barriers and declare the specific unacceptability of such selected beliefs? Can we take the position of generally affirming a culture and respecting some beliefs yet disregard others because, in this society, a set standard of care prevails? The case manager's dilemmas and decisions are bound to the community in which the practice is implemented. Although these particular examples of clashes may not exist, others will surely emerge as various mixes of cultures continue to thrive in our melting pot society.

Violence tests the case manager's ability to be accepting and nonjudgmental to establish a therapeutic relationship and provide effective services.[52-54] The case manager will undoubtedly be in contact with traumatized persons, both those who were objects of violent acts as well as those who initiated such activity. It is far easier to develop compassion and understanding for a casualty of domestic violence than it is to understand and withhold judgment for gang members caught in their own violent ventures. When working with various aspects of violence, the case manager is quickly thrust into the public policy sphere. Here the case manager is forced to consider the ethics of the distribution of scarce resources as poverty is significantly linked to incidences of violence. Despair and hopelessness are companions for many caught in the turbulence of this violence. Caring for the traumatized person is the case manager's first responsibility, but the more far-reaching implications of violence for the community at large is also within the case manager's purview.

Ethics education and ethics committees are both tools for the case manager to use while investigating ethical dilemmas and attempting to reach a resolution.*[55,56] The process of education is an ongoing one, beginning with some basic ethical concepts and theories and continuing with in-depth study of topics as they arise in practice. Education can be as simple as reading an article or as complex as a formal university program of study.** Case manag-

---

Note: *See the range of articles in *HEC Forum*, a journal targeting hospital ethics committees but including pieces for other types of ethics committees (see reference 56). These contributions discuss all aspects of ethics committees from getting started to membership, responsibilities, and problems frequently encountered.

Note: **Many basic books are available that can provide a ready resource that includes a basic explanation of the discipline of bioethics and selected material on various topics. In addition, the *Encyclopedia of Bioethics* [Reich WT (ed.). New York, NY: Simon & Schuster Macmillan; 1995] is highly recommended as a more comprehensive treatment of the breadth of topics within bioethics. This is a good place to begin self-education about a subject. Each article also includes a bibliography. This combined with material identified on an index search (Medline, BIOETHICS data base at the National Library of Medicine, CINAHL) can help create valuable resources on a selected topic.

ers, as leaders in the nursing profession, can both educate themselves and plan educational experiences for those with whom they work. Case conferences can routinely include considerations of ethical implications. This will foster the ability of all service providers to identify the ethical dimensions of client care and increase their comfort with ethical issues.

Ethics committees are a good resource for the case manager if they already exist. The committee and its members can provide education and consultation, two common roles for the committee. When a committee does not exist, the case manager can be instrumental in initiating the formation of such a group. A major benefit of case consultation with the ethics committee is the provision of a forum in which all parties can present their perspectives and have an opportunity for dialogue with others involved in the situation. Usually, ethics committees do not provide a decision for the problem but alternative actions are explored, and these may be ranked in some sort of priority. However, more gratitude is often expressed for the experience of the consultation than the actual solutions posed. It is a valuable tool for the case manager in problematic cases.

In addition to the familiar topics of ethics just addressed, other problematic issues require ethical examination. Several less frequently addressed ethical issues for the nurse case manager are presented here, as a reminder of particular ethical responsibilities that cross all those health care dilemmas named above, namely, considerations of gender, race, and class.

Nurse case managers need to remember that patients are potentially a very vulnerable group of people. Someone who is injured or ill has less energy and ability to act autonomously or even express ideas and values central to one's integrity. The poor are a special case and an added responsibility. Those in poverty are more likely to become ill for many reasons.[57] Inadequate food, housing, clothing, and other basic necessities can potentially lead to poor health. The poor who are able to find employment often work in high-risk industries, where they are prone to injury or disease. Additionally, the poor are at greater risk for health problems related to mental instability, addiction, and crime. Lack of health insurance can force individuals to delay seeking treatment. The availability of Medicaid or other welfare benefits do not always alleviate the situation. On a television report entitled "Borderline Medicine," pregnant women in California with MediCal benefits encountered great difficulty in locating obstetricians who would accept this form of payment.[58] When access to health care services is finally accomplished by some poor, the existing condition may be further advanced, requiring more expensive treatment than intervention at an early stage. Illness and poverty can operate in either direction. Illness can financially cripple a stable family's functioning, which in turn lowers the socioeconomic status, making the family more vulnerable to additional compromises as a result of poverty. The poor as research subjects have been abused. Notably, poor women were subjects in the placebo trials of contraceptive medications.[59]

Women are the primary recipients of health care, yet the services they receive are not always in their best interest.[57] Women present an interesting phenomenon involving both overtreatment and undertreatment. On the one hand, women are often overtreated. For example, women tend to have excessive surgeries and are prescribed drugs more frequently.[57] Reconstructive surgery is an inducement for women who do not meet the ideal body form.[60,61] Many natural conditions of women are medicalized: menstruation, pregnancy, birth, and menopause. These conditions have been appropriated by medical practice as treatable maladies. Women are often viewed as anxious, overcomplaining, and unstable, incapable of understanding information necessary for adequate decision making. This results in paternalism and the overtreatment of women with psychosurgery and drugs such as tranquilizers.[57]

In some cases, women are less likely than men to receive medical treatment for the same presenting conditions. Discrepancies have been noted in such areas as AIDS, kidney transplants, cardiac catheterization, coronary bypass surgery, and lung cancer diagnosis.[57,62–64] Research based on the study of certain disease processes in women woefully trails the agenda for men.[65] In some studies of breast and uterine cancer, the research was conducted without the use of female animals or females themselves.[66] Researchers have claimed that women's biological cycles distort the data and therefore have been reluctant to include them.[67] Although the research situation has changed dramatically in very recent years based on mandates from the National Institutes of Health and extensive achievements by the Office of Research on Women's Health, vigilance must be maintained to prevent loss of progress in this area. Often the special needs of women are forgotten when health care programs are developed; poor women lack transportation and child care facilities to attend prenatal care, addiction programs, or mammography appointments.[57]

Race plays another influential role in health care experiences. Women of color are at higher risk under certain circumstances in the health care system.[57] More childbirth deaths occur to black women and more high-risk newborns are delivered by them. Black women have significantly higher rates of hypertension, obesity, and lupus than white women and are more likely to die from hypertension as well as from breast cancer.[57,68] Minority women are more likely to be poor and suffer the burdens described above for the poor. Finally, little research has been conducted to identify the distinct health care needs of minority women.

The organization of health care is dominated by the authority of white middle-class (or above) men who control the administration and delivery of services.[57] Women are primarily responsible for family health yet do not have the knowledge and skills in many cases to take an assertive stance. Cultural, linguistic, and sexual orientation differences also widen the gap between practitioner and patient. The usual reliance on pharmacologic prescriptions and sophisticated technological interventions may not always be the appropriate solution to the problems presented or may only provide a stop-gap measure. Deep social and economic etiologies may ultimately be at the base of many problems for which medical interventions are futile. Noninvasive alternative therapies may be preferred by the patient, but when labor intensive or unfamiliar to the practitioner, they are not likely to be implemented and even less likely to be reimbursed by existing payment plans.

Gender, race, and socioeconomic class separately or together are responsible for discriminatory practices in health care. Prejudice and bias can occur within any one individual case or when considering the health care needs of a specific target population. Negative attitudes and practices create conditions of oppression, suppression, and repression for any disadvantaged group. The ethical case manager needs to be alert to these possible unfair limitations in access to and delivery of health care. Test questions can be posed when solutions have been devised for health care problems. The decision maker needs to ask: Given comparable situations and needs, are possible alternatives the same regardless of gender, race, or class? Are the options basically the same for men and women? Black, Hispanic, American Indian, or white? Poor, middle class, or wealthy?

ETHICAL DECISION MAKING

The case manager has several responsibilities in the decision-making process. First, the nurse is required to implement the decision-making process for her- or himself when dilemmas arise. Second, the existential advocate needs to facilitate the decision-making process with the patient or the agency, depending on the level at which the problem exists. Although the process proceeds through similar steps, the sequence and timing may be somewhat different for each individual involved.

Basically, any decision-making process consists of about six steps: (1) determining a problem exists and defining it, (2) gathering relevant information, (3) reviewing the information to generate possible solutions and their most probable outcomes, (4) prioritizing solutions, (5) making a choice, and (6) acting on the choice. This is not a linear process. For example, after reviewing information the decision makers may realize the problem was not defined clearly. Or, in another situation, prioritizing solutions may lead decision makers to realize that some critical piece of information is missing. Or when action is finally initiated, the decision maker may only then understand that the proposed solution is inadequate.

Some ethicists would say that every problem has an ethical dimension. If ethics is defined as a determination of right or good action in our interactions with other individuals in society, then this broad view suffices. Every problem then requires an examination of its ethical dimension. Information for decision making consists of knowledge available from many sources. Sources include a whole range of ideas: clinical information, opinion, theoretical concepts (including morals, values, ethics, and beliefs), and empirical data. The other steps are self-explanatory.

Each individual, the case manager, other professionals, and the patient, brings a different expertise to the situation. The case manager knows the clinical state, the operation of the health care system, and perhaps has dealt with similar problems in the past. Other professionals will have similar information. However, the case manager is best informed about the pool of patients in that particular nurse's practice, especially in relation to administrators' and executives' perspectives. The patient is the ultimate source of self-understanding, although under certain conditions the patient may be incompetent or unconscious.

CONCLUSION

Grappling with ethical issues in this era of managed care can be an exciting experience for the case manager. The case manager can be seriously challenged to provide services and respond in an ethically acceptable manner. Some outcomes may be discouraging, but others can result in exhilarating experiences and satisfying solutions. The case manager should be proactive. Using the philosophical perspective of existential advocacy, the case manager takes the necessary action to carry out the decision-making process whenever a dilemma is identified. The case manager must be mindful of an ethical responsibility to use wisdom to balance both mandates of advocacy and justice. Justice decisions are made using the case manager's information about aggregate needs and practice experiences with various individuals. Individual autonomous decisions are made by patients, facilitated by the case manager, within the boundaries set for the functioning of the defined community. Both of these are dynamic processes, each one informing the other as needs and situations change.

REFERENCES

1. American Nurses Association. *Code for Nurses with Interpretive Statements*. Washington, DC: American Nurses Association; 1985.
2. Specht J. Nurses as consumer advocates. *Nurs News*. 1985;25(4):6–14.
3. Annas GJ. *The Rights of Hospital Patients*. New York, NY: Avon; 1975.
4. Donahue MP. The nurse: a patient advocate? *Nurs Forum*. 1978;17:143–151.
5. Kelly LY. The patient's right to know. *Nurs Outlook*. 1976;24(1):26–32.
6. Kohnke MF. The nurse as advocate. *Am J Nurs*. 1980;80:2038–2040.
7. Kosck SH. Patient advocacy or fighting the system? *Am J Nurs*. 1972;72:694–698.
8. Kozier B, Erb G. *Fundamentals of Nursing: Concepts and Procedures*. 5th ed. Redwood City, Calif: Addison Wesley; 1995.
9. Potter PA, Perry AB. *Fundamentals of Nursing: Concepts, Process and Practice*. 3rd ed. St. Louis, Mo: CV Mosby-Year Book; 1993.
10. Sundberg MC. *Fundamentals of Nursing*. 2nd ed. Boston, Mass: Jones & Bartlett; 1989.
11. Wolff L, Weitzel MJ, Fuerst EV. *Fundamentals of Nursing*. Philadelphia, Pa: JB Lippincott; 1979.
12. Bower KA. *Case Management by Nurses*. Kansas City, Mo: American Nurses Association; 1992. Pub. NS–32 3M.
13. Cohen EL. *Nursing Case Management: From Concept to Evaluation*. St. Louis, Mo: Mosby-Year Book; 1993.
14. Kane RA. Case management: ethical pitfalls on the road to high quality managed care. *QRB*. 1988;14:161–166.
15. Netting FE, Williams FB. Ethical decision-making in case management programs for the elderly. *Health Values: Achieving High Level Wellness*. 1989;13(3):3–8.
16. Bandman EL, Bandman B. *Bioethics and Human Rights*. Boston, Mass: Little, Brown & Co; 1978.
17. Benjamin M, Curtis J. *Ethics in Nursing*. 3rd ed. New York, NY: Oxford University Press; 1992.
18. Mappes TA, Zembaty JS. *Biomedical Ethics*. New York, NY: McGraw-Hill Publishing Co; 1991.
19. Munson R. *Intervention and Reflection: Basic Issues in Medical Ethics*. Belmont, Calif: Wadsworth Publishing; 1992.
20. Reiser J, Dyck AJ, Curran WJ. *Ethics in Medicine: Historical and Contemporary Concerns*. Cambridge, Mass: MIT; 1977.

21. Thompson JB, Thompson HO. *Bioethical Decision Making for Nurses*. Norwalk, Conn: Appleton-Century-Crofts; 1985.

22. Veatch RM. *Medical Ethics*. Boston, Mass: Jones & Bartlett; 1989.

23. Churchill L. *Rationing Health Care in America*. Notre Dame, Ind.: University of Notre Dame Press; 1987.

24. Gilligan C. *In a Different Voice*. Cambridge, Mass: Harvard University Press; 1982.

25. Gilligan C, Lyons NP, Hanmer TJ, eds. *Making Connections*. Cambridge, Mass: Harvard University Press; 1990.

26. Belenky AF, Clinchy BM, Goldberger NR, Tarule JM. *Women's Ways of Knowing: The Development of Self, Voice, and Mind*. New York, NY: Basic Books; 1986.

27. Card C, ed. *Feminist Ethics*. Lawrence, Kan: University Press of Kansas; 1991.

28. Fox-Genovese E. *Feminism without Illusion*. Chapel Hill, NC: University of North Carolina Press; 1991.

29. Keller EF. *Reflections on Gender and Science*. New Haven, Conn: Yale University Press; 1985.

30. Kittay EF, Meyers DT, eds. *Women and Moral Theory*. Totowa, NJ: Rowman & Littlefield; 1987.

31. Noddings N. *Caring: A Feminine Approach to Ethics and Moral Education*. Berkeley, Calif: University of California Press; 1984.

32. Okin SM. *Women in Western Political Thought*. Princeton, NJ: Princeton University Press; 1979.

33. Reuther RR. *Sexism and God-Talk: Toward a Feminist Theology*. Boston, Mass: Beacon Press; 1983.

34. Stevens MA, ed. *Reconstructing the Christ Symbol*. New York, NY: Paulist Press; 1993.

35. Tong R. *Feminine and Feminist Ethics*. Belmont, Calif: Wadsworth; 1993.

36. Gadow S. Existential advocacy: philosophical foundation of nursing. In: Spicker SF, Gadow S, eds. *Nursing: Images & Ideals*. New York, NY: Springer; 1980:79–101.

37. Beauchamp TL, Childress JF. *Principles of Biomedical Ethics*. 4th ed. New York, NY: Oxford University Press; 1994.

38. Silva MC. *Ethical Decision Making in Nursing Administration*. Norwalk, Conn: Appleton & Lange; 1990.

39. Wetle T. Long-term care: home care. In: Reich WT, ed. *Encyclopedia of Bioethics*. New York, NY: Simon & Schuster Macmillan; 1995:1386–1391.

40. American Nurses Association's Center for Ethics and Human Rights. Ethics and human rights issues identified by states. *Communique*. 1994;3:1.

41. Brock DW. Death and dying: euthanasia and sustaining life. In: Reich WT, ed. *Encyclopedia of Bioethics*. New York, NY: Simon & Schuster Macmillan; 1995:563–572.

42. Wetle T. A taxonomy of ethical issues in case management of the frail older person. *J Case Manage*. 1992;1:71–75.

43. Lynn J, Teno JM. Death and dying: euthanasia and sustaining life: advance directives. In: Reich WT, ed. *Encyclopedia of Bioethics*. New York, NY: Simon & Schuster Macmillan; 1995:572–577.

44. Pinch WJ, Spielman ML. Parental perceptions of ethical decision making post NICU discharge. *West J Nurs Res*. 1993;15:422–440.

45. Harris CH. High risk infants: thirty years of intensive care. *Bioethics Forum*. 1995;11(1): 23–28.

46. Hendin H. Selling death and dignity. *Hastings Cent Rep*. 1995;25(3):19–23.

47. Pinch WJ, Brown K, Dougherty CJ, Allegretti J, McCarthy V. Caregivers' perspectives on confidentiality for mothers and newborns with HIV/AIDS. *Pediatr AIDS HIV Infect: Fetus Adolesc*. 1993;4:123–129.

48. Fluehr-Lobban C. Cultural relativism and universal rights. *Chronicle Higher Educ*. 1995;41(39):B1–B2.

49. Kopelman LM. Female circumcision/genital mutilation and ethical relativism. *Second Opinion*. 1994;20:55–71.

50. Toubia N. Female circumcision as a public health issue. *N Engl J Med*. 1994;331:712–716.

51. Schroeder P. Female genital mutilation—a form of child abuse. *N Engl J Med*. 1994;331:739–740.

52. Bell LA. *Rethinking Ethics in the Midst of Violence: A Feminist Approach to Freedom*. Lanham, Md: Rowman & Littlefield Publishers; 1993.

53. Mondragón D. Clinical assessment of gang violence risk through history and physical exam. *J Health Care Poor Underserved*. 1995;6:209–216.

54. Mondragón D. When the streets enter the emergency department. (Unpublished manuscript.)

55. Grafius LC. *Ethics for Everyone*. Chicago, Ill: American Hospital Publishing Co.; 1995.

56. Pinch WJ, Miya P. Ethics committees in states nurses' associations: a report on the national status. *HEC Forum*. 1989;1:167–173.

57. Sherwin S. *No Longer Patient: Feminist Ethics & Health Care*. Philadelphia, Pa: Temple University Press; 1992.

58. Weisberg R. (Writer, producer, director). *Borderline Medicine*. Urbana, Ill: Carle Medical Communication; 1991.

59. Veatch RM. "Experimental" pregnancy. *Hastings Cent Rep*. 1971;1(1):2–3.

60. Bordo S. *Unbearable Weight*. Berkeley, Calif: University of California Press; 1993.

61. Faludi S. *Backlash: The Undeclared War against American Women*. New York, NY: Crown Publishers, Inc.; 1991.

62. Hawthorne MH. Gender differences in recovery after coronary artery surgery. *Image: Journal Nurs Scholarship*. 1994;26:75–80.

63. Rosser SV. *Women's Health—Missing from U.S. Medicine*. Bloomington, Ind: Indiana University Press; 1994.

64. Smeltzer SC, Whipple B. Women and HIV infection. *Image: J Nurs Scholarship*. 1991;23:249–256.

65. Pinch WJ. Research and nursing: ethical reflections. *Nurs Health Care*. 1996;44(1).

66. Dresser R. Wanted: single, white male for medical research. *Hastings Cent Rep*. 1992;22(1):24–29.

67. Cotton P. Examples abound of gaps in medical knowledge because of groups excluded from scientific study. *JAMA*. 1990;263:1051–1052.

68. Bowen DJ, Tomoyasu N, Cauce AM. The triple threat: a discussion of gender, class, and race differences in weight. *Women Health*. 1991;17:123–143.

■ Epilogue ■

Case Management:
The Shape of Things To Come

Suzanne Smith Blancett, EdD, RN, FAAN
Dominick L. Flarey, PhD, MBA, RN,CS, CNAA, NP-C

Throughout the pages of this book, authors have readily demonstrated the evolutionary nature of case management as a model of care delivery. As our health care system continues to change, so too will case management to meet future mandates and challenges.

This final presentation provides a glimpse into the future of case management as a system of care. These views of the future of case management reflect, in part, answers solicited from subscribers to an Internet health care management list. These contributions from health care managers around the world are invaluable to understand fully the developing nature of case management.

To streamline the contributions and provide a clearer focus of the shape of things to come, content is presented around five major themes: continuity of care, patient issues, reimbursement systems, evolving goals, and evolving roles.

CONTINUITY OF CARE

As case management systems continue to evolve, we will see an increase in the development of seamless models of care delivery. Organizational boundaries will disappear, and case management systems will evolve into one model encompassing the full continuum of care. The following trends are emerging:

- People will be case managed throughout their lives, from birth to death with dignity.

Acknowledgment: The authors thank those who responded to queries over the Internet health care management list. Many of the ideas in this epilogue are based on their contributions.

- Each developmental phase of human existence will be case managed with the goal of wellness and disease prevention.
- A seamless system of continuity will be the norm in the overall delivery of health care services.
- Continuity will be achieved through HMO-based and employer-based case management systems.
- The drivers of continuity of care will be case managers; frontline health care professionals will work within the system but not drive the continuity of care.
- Specialized case management systems will merge to allow for the smooth transition of care delivery based on patients' needs in the overall continuum of care.
- Care will be coordinated across multiple delivery sites.
- Collaborative networks of case managers in defined communities will provide continuity of care throughout the life cycle.
- The focus of case management will shift from managing hospitalizations to managing care in general.
- Clinical protocols will become more refined; they will be developed around a model of continuity whereby patient care can be managed in transition from one episode of illness/wellness to another.

PATIENT ISSUES

Patient needs for holistic and preventive care will drive the evolution of newer case management models and systems. Models of case management will evolve based on collaborative input from patients. Patients will define for health care professionals what they need in terms of health care services. Some emerging trends around patient issues include:

- Protocols will be more individualized around patient needs.
- The focus of case management systems will be on patient outcomes, how patients respond to case management interventions.
- Case management models will move from an illness model to a wellness model. There will be a major focus on teaching patients disease prevention strategies.
- Protocols will be established that assist clients to move through the life cycle with an emphasis on health and the prevention of disease.
- Patients will be active participants in case managed systems and assume more responsibilities for their own health maintenance. They will have an increased awareness of care alternatives.

- Case management will focus more on the family as a unit, working together to maintain health through supportive relationships.
- A wider array of health services will be made available to patients through more comprehensive and elaborate case management systems.
- Patients will choose their providers in the future based on quality outcomes. Case management systems will drive these outcomes.
- Case management systems will incorporate models of patient focused care with the patient at the center of all health care activities.

REIMBURSEMENT SYSTEMS

Case management models and reimbursement systems will be intimately linked. Payers will support the delivery of care via case management systems. Capitation and capitated systems of reimbursement will play a major role in these emerging trends:

- Case management systems will be designed to be more efficient in the use of resources for the delivery of care.
- Capitation will drive more explicit budgeting of health care dollars and will control excessive costs within case management systems.
- Case management systems will be the vehicles that result in the delivery of quality care in capitated reimbursement environments.
- There will be greater attempts to integrate health care financing and the delivery of health care services to populations.
- Case management will focus on developing more proactive ways to improve efficiency in acute care hospitalization to prevent third-party payer denials and thus reduce costs.
- Models of case management systems for home care will flourish, thus reducing further the need for expensive hospitalizations.
- There will be financial incentives for organizations that can develop innovative case management systems demonstrating significant reductions in health care costs.
- Financial experts will assume important roles in the development and evaluation of cost-effective case management systems.
- Nurse case managers will coordinate the delivery of care in fiscally sound ways.

EVOLVING GOALS

As our health care system moves toward further transformation, new goals for case management will be defined. These defined goals will be instrumental in reshaping care delivery through case management. These goals will also serve as critical indicators for evaluating newer models of case management. Some of the future goals of case management are to:

- publish outcomes assessments of case management. This will assist the public in making better informed choices about its care.
- focus on long-term patient outcomes rather than short-term assessments
- develop quality provider networks of case management systems
- link case management systems for the purpose of providing full continuity of services across the life span
- develop needed specialized case managers in expanded roles, such as geriatrics and pediatrics
- develop case management systems that focus on developmental disabilities
- develop improved quality measurement tools that will more adequately assess case management outcomes
- develop elaborate information systems that support care delivery through case management and provide for more detailed assessment, compilation and analysis of outcomes, and tracking of clinical pathways that include the cost of interventions and resources
- develop electronic patient records and data bases that allow a smoother transition for patients moving from one case managed system to another
- unify and standardize generic protocols for use in case management systems
- promote the continual evaluation of case management models through the evaluation of data about the system accumulated over time
- move from a case management model of illness to a case management model of wellness
- develop a unified definition and understanding of case management
- integrate all health care disciplines into the case management model of care delivery
- prepare the community, through education, to receive health care services via case management systems

EVOLVING ROLES

As case management systems evolve and are transformed, so too case manager roles will change. Such changes will be necessary to drive new models of case management in the future. Some of the role changes that are likely to occur include:

- All professional health care roles will be integrated into a more unified model of care.
- Nurse case managers will be prepared at the graduate level and will function as professional case managers leading the delivery of health care.
- Physicians will play more active roles in the delivery of care through case management.
- Theories and concepts of case management will become a common component of undergraduate programs in nursing.
- Nurse researchers will focus heavily on assessing the short- and long-term outcomes of case management systems.
- Health care executives will study case management systems and assist in developing more efficient and effective models of care.
- Discharge planners and professional social workers will be in collaborative practices with professional nurse case managers to coordinate more fully the delivery of health care.
- There will be a surge of nurse entrepreneurs who will market their case management services to organizations and payers.
- Third-party payers will employ professional case managers to work collaboratively within integrated networks and systems.
- Professional nurse case managers will become more active in government legislation and consult on government activities related to the delivery of health care.

CONCLUSION

This presentation examines and predicts emerging trends related to case management. The information provided is not exhaustive, rather it is a beginning, designed to explore the likelihood of future transformations in health care delivery. Although many of the defined trends may or may not occur, what is important is that nurses have always managed care and always will. Case management is the vehicle that nurses and other health care professionals will use to move health care delivery well into the next century.

Appendix A
Discussion Topics for Each Chapter

1—Case Management: Delivering Care in the Age of Managed Care

1. What are the seven major trends shaping managed care?
2. What is the American Nurses Association's definition of case management?
3. What are the major goals for any case management model?
4. What is a clinical practice guideline, a CareMap®, and a critical path?
5. What two major trends are increasingly driving the redesign of case management systems?

2—The Early Years: The Evolution of Nursing Case Management

1. What did the Pratt 4 study reveal?
2. Why were nurses the most likely candidates to introduce critical paths and case management?
3. What are the chief deficits of critical paths?
4. What does a complete CareMap® system include?
5. What are the three stages of market evolution?

3—New Challenges and Opportunities in Integrated Health Care Systems

1. What is the relationship between managed care and integrated health care systems?

2. How can integrated systems be defined from the following perspectives: organizational, social systems, and strategic management?
3. What are the forms of integration that create the system needed to enhance the health of a community?
4. What are the attributes of successful integrated health care systems?
5. How is clinical integration measured?

4—Developing a Successful Hospital Case Management System

1. What two features of managed care are encouraging the growth of hospital case management?
2. What is required for effective hospital case management?
3. How can we change to improve outcomes?
4. What are the common features of effective guideline development programs?
5. What are the five process steps for creating an effective hospital case management program?

5—Developing and Implementing Critical Paths in Case Management

1. How can critical paths be used?
2. What are the different types of variances?
3. What are the steps in developing critical paths?
4. What strategies can be used to promote compliance in using critical paths?
5. In what ways is the critical path for the patient different from the health care team critical pathway?

6—Documentation To Achieve Patient Outcomes through Critical Pathways

1. What is the difference between case management and outcomes management?
2. What are the five stages in the outcomes management model?
3. What is a variance?
4. What are the three types of variances?
5. How can the collection of data assist in managing patient outcomes?

7—Outcomes Assessment through Protocols

1. What is the impetus for protocol development?
2. What is the impact of benchmarking on protocol development?
3. What is the importance of variance analysis as it relates to assessment of outcomes for the individual, clinician, or health system?
4. How do outcomes have an effect on/dictate the direction/future of health care institutions?
5. Why is a multidisciplinary approach to protocol development important?

8—Improving Quality through Nursing Case Management

1. What are the seven attributes Donabedian recommends in defining the quality of health care?
2. How are quality and cost interrelated?
3. What measures of quality encompass both the patient and provider perceptions of quality?
4. What is nursing case management's impact on patient care as identified in the literature?
5. What internal constituency groups must be recognized during the planning and implementation of case management?

9—Evaluating the Effectiveness of Case Management Plans

1. What are the two types of variance data?
2. What is a positive variance?
3. What are clinical quality indicators?
4. What are discharge patient outcomes?
5. What is the definition of outcomes measurement?

10—Variance Analysis

1. How can variance analysis data be used to improve processes of care, attain financial goals, and assist in achieving patient outcomes?
2. What are key elements of infrastructure necessary to support variance analysis?
3. What technologies are available for collecting and processing variance data?

4. What are the approaches for collecting variance data?
5. Which groups in your organization would use outcome variables, and why?

11—Improving Accreditation Results through Case Management

1. What is the basic tenet of accreditation?
2. What are patient-focused function standards?
3. In what way does case management support the achievement of standards for organizational performance?
4. How does the case management process enhance efforts to achieve standards compliance in preventive health services?
5. What are the five major comparisons of case management to the Joint Commission performance improvement model?

12—Strategies for Operationalizing Case Management

1. What are the essential components of a case management proposal?
2. What two strategies can be used to reduce costs for a patient undergoing surgery?
3. What are the necessary steps in the implementation process of case management?
4. What strategies can be used to educate patients and staff about case management?
5. What are some outcomes measures of case management?

13—Training and Education Needs of Case Managers

1. What are the 10 tasks in which the nurse case manager is required to be astute?
2. What are the skills required of the nurse case manager?
3. What are some of the goals for establishing a nurse case manager training and education program?
4. What are the most important topics that should be included in the training and education program of nurse case managers?
5. How can nurse administrators demonstrate competency of nurse case managers?

14—Roles of the Professional Registered Nurse in Case Management and Program Direction

1. What are the differences and similarities of the patient advocate role as a direct care giver and as a case manager?
2. How can Mark's dimensions of nursing practice models be related to the roles of a case manager?
3. How would the case management director's role of care coordination at the program level influence the quality of care individual patients receive?
4. How can care paths be useful tools in a quality management program?
5. What leadership behaviors can you use to make a case management program successful when there is resistance to the program by physicians and staff?

15—Alternate Case Management Models

1. What is the major advantage of the private case management model to the consumer?
2. What four populations can benefit from social/community-based case management?
3. How do clients typically enter the primary case management network?
4. What ways can a nurse case manager control costs in the vendor/gatekeeper model?
5. What is needed to demonstrate the success of any of the models of case management?

16—Relationship Building in Developing the Continuum of Care Concepts

1. What two concepts lead to 83 percent of the health care dollar savings as researched by the Health Care Advisory Board?
2. What are the benefits of having a care provider from home health as a member of the team developing critical pathways?
3. What are the four relationships identified in this chapter, and what is one outcome to be achieved with each of the relationships?
4. Why do you think the total joint replacement patients' length of stay was able to be decreased?
5. What is the role of case managers, and what outcomes should they help achieve?

17—Physician/Nurse Collaboration in Case Management

1. What are the components essential for collaboration to occur between physicians and nurses?
2. How might a clinical model of physician/nurse collaboration be initiated?
3. Why is physician/nurse collaboration essential in the managed care environment?
4. What is the value of clinical variance screens used by nurse case managers?
5. What questions would you ask if you were interviewing for a job as a nurse case manager?

18—Managed Care and the World of Capitated Payment

1. What are the four major reimbursement structures of the health care market?
2. What is capitation?
3. What are the five stages in the evolution of managed care networks?
4. What is managed competition?
5. What is the key to successful integration?

19—Working with Managed Care Networks: Strategies for Success

1. What two clinical issues are related to interacting with managed care representatives in relation to home care patients?
2. What administrative issues do home health care staff experience when interacting with the staff of managed care companies?
3. What four areas do the National Committee on Quality Assurance evaluate for each managed care plan?
4. What communication strategies may be used to ensure successful relationships with managed care companies?
5. What are some of the advantages for home health care agencies contracting with managed care companies?

20—Cost Savings and Financial Analysis of Case Management Models

1. Why is it necessary to establish standards for case management?
2. When assigning DRGs, what information needs to be contained in the medical record?

3. What are the reimbursement trends that an organization needs to identify?
4. What two statistics for critical pathways are used for evaluation?
5. What is a variance analysis?

21—Data Management through Information Systems

1. In 1995, what were the most pressing information system needs identified?
2. What is a CHIN?
3. To negotiate managed care contracts effectively, an organization's information system must have what capabilities?
4. Why do nurse case managers need computer fluency?
5. What are the major steps in planning and implementing an information system?

22—Case Management As a Service Economy Job Design: Toward a Theoretical Model

1. What criteria are commonly cited as the distinguishing characteristics of service organizations?
2. What is job characteristics theory?
3. In addition to primary nursing, collaborative practice initiatives include what other elements?
4. What are the components of a successful case manager's role?
5. What is meant by role overload?

23—Legal Liabilities in Case Management

1. What are standards of nursing practice, and how do they relate to a lawsuit in negligence?
2. What are the elements of negligence?
3. What are the case manager's duties concerning patient confidentiality?
4. What is the role of the case manager in benefit decision making and the risk of legal liability?
5. What is the relationship between professional responsibility and legal liability?

24—Ethical Issues in Case Management

1. What is the relationship between autonomy and patient advocacy?
2. What two mandates within the case manager's role are likely to be in ethical conflict?
3. How can autonomy be compromised in the health care setting?
4. What assistance can an ethics committee provide a case manager?
5. What are the ethical dimensions of the less frequently addressed ethical issues of gender, race, and class?

Index

A

Abandonment, legal issues, 437–438
Accountability, 400
Accreditation
  case management, 224–238
  Joint Commission on Accreditation of
    Healthcare Organizations, 224
  National Committee for Quality
    Assurance, 224
Achievement, 411, 416–417
Admission/daily orders, stroke, 331–332
Advance directives, 451
Advanced practice nurse, case
  management, 13
Advocacy, 444–446
  justice, functioning at interface,
    448–450
Affiliation, 412, 416, 417
AIDS, ethical issues, 451–452
Algorithm, stroke, 330
Analysis of variance, statistical terms, 202
Anesthesia care unit, critical path,
  113–115
Assisted suicide, 451
Asthma, quality indicators, 187
Authority, 400
Autonomy, 400, 406
  ethical issues, 445–446, 447

B

Benefit decision making, case
  management, compared, 432–436
Budget, case management, 243

C

Capitation, 42
  case management strategies, 42
  managed care, 2, 336–346
    market evolution stages, 339–342
    model, 345–346
    success factors, 342–343
    system evolution, 336–339
  mapping strategies, 42
  trends, 42–43
Care giver variance, critical path, 107, 109
CareMap, 138
  congestive heart failure, 17, 18, 19–22
  development, 27
  outcome, 18, 19–22
  protocol, 7, 8
  system, 37
  tools, 36
Carondelet Saint Mary's Hospital, 23
Case management, 196–200. *See also*
  Specific type

accreditation, 224–238
acute care nursing case management system, 296
advanced practice nurse, 13
alternate models, 295–303
benefit decision making, compared, 432–436
brokerage of services, 11
budget, 243
classic model, 38–41
clinical resources management, 343–345
concept development, 239–240
continuity, 5
continuous quality improvement, 176
continuum of care, 12
coordination of services model, 295–303
cost, 362–378
    control, 5
    critical path development, 367–369
    critical path result evaluation, 369–372
    critical path selection, 366–367
    data collection, 364–366, 376–377
    finance department data, 365
    medical records, 364–365
    patient care project team, 367
    reimbursement maximization, 376–377
    sponsor, 364
    standards, 363
    steering committee, 364
    utilization review data, 365–366
    variance analysis, 372–375
critical path, development, 244–247, 367–369
defined, 175, 196–199
    American Nurses Association, 4
    National Case Management Task Force, 4
dispositional differences, 410–412
education program, 247–248
    elements, 249
    outline, 249
elements, 4–6

evaluation, 184–191
evolution, 23–44, 175
family focused, 6–7
family satisfaction, 248
financial analysis, 362–378
    critical path development, 367–369
    critical path result evaluation, 369–372
    critical path selection, 366–367
    data collection, 364–366, 376–377
    finance department data, 365
    medical records, 364–365
    patient care project team, 367
    reimbursement maximization, 376–377
    sponsor, 364
    standards, 363
    steering committee, 364
    utilization review data, 365–366
    variance analysis, 372–375
future trends, 13, 461–465
goals, 5–6, 175
groundwork laying, 239–244
implementation process, 244–248
job design, reintegrating labor, 401–402
Joint Commission on Accreditation of Healthcare Organizations, 229–232
    compared, 230, 231
length of stay, 5
logistics, 240
managed care, 348–350
    compared, 348–350
    relationship, 2–3
method for evaluating outcomes, 240–242
multidisciplinary, 9–11
multiservice, 11
National Committee for Quality Assurance, 233–237
nurse driven, 6
nursing as industry catalyst, 24–27
nursing job enrichment, 402–403
operationalization strategies, 239–253
outcome driven, 9, 20

outcomes, 248–250
outcomes management, 100–103
   compared, 100–103
   outcomes measurement, 190
   outcomes monitoring, 190
   tool development, 189–190
patient satisfaction, 248
physician, 244, 246
physician/nurse collaboration, 315–328
   clinical collaboration model,
      316–317
   clinical variance graph, 320–322
   clinical variance screen, 320–322
   peer review committee letter,
      322–323
   physician/nurse liaison committee,
      318
   restorative care path development,
      323–327
   transition from managed care to
      case management, 319
plan excerpt, 27, 28
prevention, 13
primary care case management,
      297, 301
private case management, 296–298
professional advances, 39
program assessment, 197–198
program description, 230, 232
proposal, 240–243
protocol, 7
quality of care, 5, 175–181, 248–250
   constructs, 176
   evidence in literature, 177–178
   leadership, 179–181
rationale, 240
registered nurse, roles, 272–294
research, 199, 403–406
research based, 12
resource utilization, 5
results dissemination, 242–243
service economy job design, research
      opportunities, 417–418
situational constructs, 406–410
social/community-based case
      management, 297, 298–301

specialized, 11–12
steering committee, 244
support for, 243
system characteristics, 6–12
system classification, 295–296
theory base loss as application
      expands, 35
turnover rate, 248
variance analysis, 185–187
vendor/gatekeeper model, 297,
      301–302
wellness, 13
Case management association, case
      manager, 292–293
Case management director, registered
      nurse
   ethical practice, 291
   financial management, 286–287
   leadership, 290–291
   outcomes management, 288
   program level care coordination,
      285–286
   project management, 289–290
   as resource, 290
   roles, 284–291
Case management team, role clarity, 74
Case manager. *See also* Specific type
   appointment, 243
   case management association,
      292–293
   certification, 292–293
   common tasks, 257
   description, 245–246
   education, 254–270
   enactment of role, 251
   as enriched job, 401–406
   evaluation, 266–270
   graduate program, 292
   issues, 250–251
   performance appraisal tool, 267–269
   performance evaluation, 266–270
   registered nurse
      care coordination, 276–277
      care evaluation, 277–278
      case finding/screening, 274
      clinical roles, 274–278

education, 291–292
as educator, 282–284
implementation, 276
negotiator, 279–280
outcomes/quality manager, 280–281
patient advocate/facilitator,
278–279
patient assessment, 275
planning, 275–276
political activist, 284
resource manager, 276–277,
281–282
roles, 273–284
relationship building, 309–310
roles and responsibilities, 243–244
selection, 250–251
service economy job design, 388–418
skills, 256
training, 254–270, 291–292
curriculum goals and objectives,
256–257
curriculum knowledge base,
255–256
curriculum length, 255
curriculum outline, 257–265
preceptorship program, 265–266
transition to, 251
utilization management, 281–282
Center for Case Management, 43
Centralized accountability, hospital case
management, 72–73
Centralized authority, hospital case
management, 72–73
Certification, case manager, 292–293
Certified Professional in Healthcare
Quality, 292–293
Clinic without walls, integrated delivery
system, 55
Clinical collaboration, model, 316–318
Clinical guidelines. See Protocol
Clinical outcomes, 187, 188
Clinical path, 8
outcome-based, 35–38
Clinical quality indicator, 187
Clinical resources management, case
management, 343–345

Clinical variance, 142
Collaboration
concept analysis, 316
defined, 315
elements, 316, 317
outcomes management, 109–110
Commission for Case Manager
Certification, 293
Communication
hospital case management, 75–78
integrated delivery system, nurse
executive issues, 64
Community Mental Health Act, 295–303
Community variance, 185, 186
Competition, 47
Comprehensive medical service
organization, integrated delivery
system, 62
Concurrent utilization review, legal
issues, 434
Confidentiality
documentation, 429–431
deniable information, 430
nonprivileged information, 430
privileged information, 430
legal issues, 429–431
Congestive heart failure, CareMap®, 17,
18, 19–22
Consumer
information system, 382
relationship building, 308–309
Continuity of care
case management, 5
defined, 272
future trend, 461–462
Continuous quality improvement, 225
case management, 176
integrated delivery system, 58
Continuum of care
case management, 12
healthcare provider, 310–314
integrated delivery system, 52–53,
52–54
relationship building, 305–314
Contracting, legal issues, 440
Control, 406–407

influence with other professional
  coworkers, 407
physician/physician collaboration, 407
Coordination of care, defined, 272
Cost
  case management, 362–378
    control, 5
    critical path development, 367–369
    critical path result evaluation,
      369–372
    critical path selection, 366–367
    data collection, 364–366, 376–377
    finance department data, 365
    medical records, 364–365
    patient care project team, 367
    reimbursement maximization,
      376–377
    sponsor, 364
    standards, 363
    steering committee, 364
    utilization review data, 365–366
    variance analysis, 372–375
  quality of care, relationship, 174–175
Cost-effectiveness, integrated delivery
  system, 47, 48
Coworker relationships, nurse
  satisfaction, 413–416
Critical path, 138, 362
  anesthesia care unit, 113–115
  care giver variance, 107, 109
  case management, development,
    244–247
  components, 84
  definition, 80–82
  delayed discharge, factors, 81
  development, 27, 82–85
    purchasing compared, 83–84
    steps, 89
  deviation, 87–88
  documentation, 81–82
  early discharge, factors, 81
  education program, 85–86
  evaluation, 88
  format, 84
  functions, 105–106
  implementation, 85–86

information management, 206–220
  card scanner, 212–215, 216
  data collection, 206
  data collection methods, 208–215
  data collection resources, 206–208
  integrated computer systems, 209
  intermediate semiautomated
    methods, 209–215
  laptop computer, 210–211
  manual data collection, 208–209
  Newton hand-held computer,
    211–212
  transformation of data into
    information, 218–220
intervention, 17
limitations, 27–28
multidisciplinary committee, 82–83
outcomes management, 104–109
  variance, 106–109
patient education, 84
patient variance, 107, 108–109
pilot test, 86
program assessment, 197–198
protocol, 7, 8
purchasing, 83–84
samples, 91–99
software program, 84
staff compliance, 86–87
staff education, 84
system variance, 107
time line, 84
tools, 36
uses, 80–82
variance, defined, 106–109
variance record, 29
variance report, 113–115

D

Data management, information system,
  379–387
  benefits, 383–384
  increased need for information
    access, 379–380
  nursing management impact,
    384–385

Decentralization, managed care, 3
Decision-making, ethical issues, 456–457
Delayed discharge, critical path, factors, 81
Deniable information, 430
Diagnosis-related group, protocol, 8
Diagnosis-specific restorative care path, 323–327
Discharge patient outcome, 188
Documentation, 100–110
    confidentiality, 429–431
        deniable information, 430
        nonprivileged information, 430
        privileged information, 430
    critical path, 81–82
    visiting nurse, 165–169

E

Early discharge
    critical path, factors, 81
    vaginal delivery
        multidisciplinary plan of care, 154–155, 161–162
        protocol, 149–153, 157–159
Economically integrated primary care, integrated delivery system, 55
Education, case manager, 254–270
Educational program
    case management, 247–248
        elements, 249
        outline, 249
    critical path, 85–86
End-of-life issues, ethical issues, 451
Equity model, integrated delivery system, 62
Ethical issues, 443–458
    AIDS, 451–452
    autonomy, 445–446, 447
    cultural perspectives, 452–453
    decision-making, 456–457
    end-of-life issues, 451
    gender, 455
    HIV, 451–452
    justice, 446–448

    multicultural issues, 452–453
    race, 455–456
Ethics committee, 454
Evaluation
    case management, 184–191
    case manager, 266–270
    variance analysis, 185–187

F

Family satisfaction, case management, 248
Fee-for-service, 42
Financial analysis, case management, 362–378
    critical path development, 367–369
    critical path result evaluation, 369–372
    critical path selection, 366–367
    data collection, 364–366, 376–377
    finance department data, 365
    medical records, 364–365
    patient care project team, 367
    reimbursement maximization, 376–377
    sponsor, 364
    standards, 363
    steering committee, 364
    utilization review data, 365–366
    variance analysis, 372–375
Financing, integrated delivery system, nurse executive issues, 64
Flow sheet, post anesthesia care unit, 119–121
Foundation model, integrated delivery system, 62
Friendly Hills Health Care Network, 345–346

G

Gender, ethical issues, 455
Governance, integrated delivery system, nurse executive issues, 64
Graduate program, case manager, 292

Group practice, integrated delivery system, 55
Group practice without walls, integrated delivery system, 62

H

Health care delivery, strategic changes, 195–200
Health care provider
continuum of care, 310–314
relationship building, 309–310
variance, 185, 186, 202–203
HIV, ethical issues, 451–452
HMO, 2
Home care
managed care, 348–360
managed care *vs.* case management, 348–350
performance improvement, 355–360
quality assessment, 355–360
service authorization progress note, 354, 355
managed care company
contracting advantages, 350
contracting disadvantages, 350–351
National Committee for Quality Assurance, 355–360
quality of care, 355–360
relationship building, 352–354
Home care case manager, 348, 349
goals, 349
role, 351–352
Home care clinical case manager, payer case manager, compared, 351–352
Hospital administrator, protocol, 139
Hospital case management
centralized accountability, 72–73
centralized authority, 72–73
communication, 75–78
effective program creation, 75–78
historical aspects, 68–79
organizational mandate, 70

organizational structure, 72–74
organizational vision, 70–71
performance data, 71–72
physician, cultural and financial alignment, 74–75
product line organization, 73–74
requirements, 69–75
system development, 68–78
Hospital-owned practice, integrated delivery system, 55
Hughes v. Blue Cross of Northern California, 435

I

Incentive system, integrated delivery system, 58–59
Incompetence, reporting, 439–440
Individualism, 447–448
Influence, 411–412, 416–417
Information linkage, integrated delivery system, 58
Information management
critical path, 206–220
card scanner, 212–215, 216
data collection, 206
data collection methods, 208–215
data collection resources, 206–208
data transformation into information, 218–220
integrated computer systems, 209
intermediate semiautomated methods, 209–215
laptop computer, 210–211
manual data collection, 208–209
Newton hand-held computer, 211–212
variance analysis, 206–220
card scanner, 212–215, 216
data collection, 206
data collection methods, 208–215
data collection resources, 206–208
data transformation into information, 218–220
integrated computer systems, 209

intermediate semiautomated
   methods, 209–215
laptop computer, 210–211
manual data collection, 208–209
Newton hand-held computer,
   211–212
Information system
   consumer, 382
   data management, 379–387
      benefits, 383–384
      increased need for information
         access, 379–380
      nursing management impact,
         384–385
   implementing, 385–386
   managed care, 2
   needs, 380–382
   patient satisfaction, 382
   planning, 385–386
   system readiness, 380–382
Insurance company, managed care, 3
Integrated delivery system, 3
   attributes, 55–59
   boundaries, 56
   clinic without walls, 55
   communication, nurse executive
      issues, 64
   comprehensive medical service
      organization, 62
   continuous quality improvement, 58
   continuum of care, 52–53, 52–54
   cost-effectiveness, 47, 48
   defined, 49–50
   dimensions, 50–54
   driving forces, 47–49
   economically integrated primary
      care, 55
   equity model, 62
   financing, nurse executive issues, 64
   forerunner hospital system, 59–60
   foundation model, 62
   fully integrated, 54
   generic model, 61
   governance, nurse executive
      issues, 64

group practice, 55
group practice without walls, 62
hospital-led model, 61
hospital-owned practice, 55
hybrid hospital/physician-led
   model, 61
incentive system, 58–59
information linkage, 58
insurance-company-led model, 61
integration, 50–52
management, nurse executive
   issues, 64
management service bureau, 62
model systems, 60, 61, 62
new management culture, 56
nurse executive challenges, 63–65
organization, nurse executive
   issues, 64
organizational outcomes, 61–63
organizational perspective definition,
   49–50
patient care coordination, 52
patient management system, 57
physician, 56
physician-hospital organization, 62
physician-led model, 61
population-based needs assessment, 57
provider alliance, 55
provider-hospital organization, 55
regional network, 55
social systems perspective, 50
sponsorship, nurse executive issues,
   64
staff model, 62
strategic management perspective, 50
surrogate terms, 54–55
technology management system,
   57–58
vertically integrated system, 54–55
Integration of care
   defined, 272
   managed care, model, 345–346
Intermediate patient outcome, 187–188
Intervention, critical path, 17

J

Job characteristics
  model, 395–397
    job enrichment, 393–397
    nursing job enrichment, 397–401
    assessment of characteristics,
      397–399
    effects, 397–399
    evaluation, 399–401
Job design
  case management, reintegrating
    labor, 401–402
  service economy, 389–393
Job design theory, 393–406
  nursing, 392
Job enrichment, 393–397
Joint Commission on Accreditation of
  Healthcare Organizations, 226–232
  accreditation, 224
  agenda for change, 226
  case management, 229–232
    compared, 230, 231
  mission, 226
  organizational functions, 229–230
  organizational performance
    improvement model, 229, 230
    case management compared,
      230, 231
  patient-focused functions, 227–229
  standards, 227–230
Justice
  advocacy, functioning at interface,
    448–450
  ethical issues, 446–448

L

Leadership
  case manager, 290–291
  quality of care, 179–181
Legal issues, 424–441
  abandonment, 437–438
  concurrent utilization review, 434
  confidentiality, 429–431
  contracting, 440
  malpractice, 431–432
  negligence, 431–432
  negligent referral, 436–437
  patient discharge, 437–438
  professional responsibility, 426–427
  prospective utilization review, 434
  retrospective review, 433
  standards, 427–429
  utilization review, 433
  vicarious liability, 438
Length of stay, case management, 5

M

Malpractice
  legal issues, 431–432
  reporting, 439–440
Managed care
  capitation, 2, 336–346
    market evolution stages, 339–342
    model, 345–346
    success factors, 342–343
    system evolution, 336–339
  carve-out, 3
  case management, 348–350
    compared, 348–350
    relationship, 2–3
  characteristics, 68–69
  data required, 385, 386
  decentralization, 3
  home care, 348–360
    managed care *vs.* case
      management, 348–350
    performance improvement,
      355–360
    quality assessment, 355–360
    service authorization progress note,
      354, 355
  information system, 2
  insurance company, 3
  integration, model, 345–346
  Medicaid, 3

Medicare, 3
  outcomes, model, 345–346
  physician control, 2–3
  relationship building, 319
  as strategic initiative, 195–200
  trends, 2–3
Managed care company, home care
  contracting advantages, 350
  contracting disadvantages, 350–351
Management, integrated delivery
  system, nurse executive issues, 64
Management service bureau, integrated
  delivery system, 62
Medicaid, managed care, 3
Medicare, managed care, 3
Mentoring, case manager, 265
Misconduct, reporting, 439–440
Multicultural issues, ethical issues,
  452–453
Multidisciplinary committee, critical
  path, 82–83
Multidisciplinary team, relationship
  building, 309–310

N

National Commission for Certifying
  Agencies, 292
National Committee for Quality
  Assurance
  case management, 233–237
    accreditation, 224
  history, 233
  home care, 355–360
  preventive health services, 235–237
  quality of care
    quality improvement, 233–234
    quality management, 233–234
  utilization management, 237
National Organization for Competency
  Assurance, 292
Need for achievement, 411, 416–417
Need for affiliation, 412, 416, 417
Need for influence, 411–412, 416–417

Need theories of motivation, 392, 411–
  412, 416–417
Negative variance, 186
Negligence, legal issues, 431–432
Negligent referral, legal issues, 436–437
New England Medical Center Hospitals,
  23–26, 30–35
Newborn care, 125–129
Newborn nursery, nurses' admission
  assessment, 160
Nonprivileged information, 430
Nurse. See Specific type
Nurse manager, outcomes
  management, 110
Nurse satisfaction, 413–417
  coworker relationships, 413–416
  dispositional need strength
    differences, 416–417
  role ambiguity, 415
  role conflict, 415
  role overload, 415
  role stressor, 415
Nurses' admission assessment, newborn
  nursery, 160
Nursing
  changing job structure, 391–392
  job design theory, 392
Nursing job enrichment
  case management, 402–403
  job characteristics, 397–401
    assessment of characteristics,
      397–399
    effects, 397–399
    evaluation, 399–401
Nursing practice, 392
Nursing record, post anesthesia care
  unit, 119–121

O

Operational variance, 185, 186, 202
Organization, integrated delivery
  system, nurse executive issues, 64
Organizational structure, hospital case
  management, 72–74

Organizational vision, hospital case
  management, 70–71
Outcomes
  CareMap®, 18, 19–22
  case management, 248–250
  characteristics, 145
  defined, 143
  expected outcomes of care, 187–188
  indicator, 187, 188
  managed care, model, 345–346
  measurement, 190
  resource management, 145
  utilization, 145
  variance, 188
Outcomes assessment
  protocol, 136–146, 149–169
  variance analysis, 142–145
Outcomes management, 188–191
  benefits, 103–104
  case management, 100–103
    compared, 100–103
    outcomes measurement, 190
    outcomes monitoring, 190
    tool development, 189–190
  collaboration, 109–110
  critical path, 104–109
    variance, 106–109
  defined, 101
  model, 102
  nurse manager, 110
  outcomes manager, 110
  patient outcome defined, 104
  physician, 109
  staff nurse, 109–110
Outcomes management/critical path,
  variance report, 122–124
Outcomes manager, outcomes
  management, 110

P

Parent teaching/infant care checklist,
  163–164
Paternalism, 446

Patient advocacy, 444–446
Patient care coordination, integrated
  delivery system, 52
Patient care coordinator, 307–308
  position description, 307–308
Patient discharge, legal issues, 437–438
Patient education, critical path, 84
Patient management system, integrated
  delivery system, 57
Patient satisfaction
  case management, 248
  information system, 382
Patient variance, 141–142, 186,
  200–201, 203
  critical path, 107, 108–109
Patients' rights movement, 445
Payer case manager, 348, 349
  goals, 349
  home care clinical case manager,
    compared, 351–352
  role, 351–352
Performance appraisal tool, case
  manager, 267–269
Performance data, hospital case
  management, 71–72
Performance evaluation, case manager,
  266–270
Physician
  case management, 244, 246
  hospital case management, cultural
    and financial alignment, 74–75
  integrated delivery system, 56
  outcomes management, 109
  protocol, 139
  quality of care, 180
Physician-hospital organization,
  integrated delivery system, 62
Physician/nurse collaboration, case
  management, 315–328
  clinical collaboration model, 316–317
  clinical variance graph, 320–322
  clinical variance screen, 320–322
  peer review committee letter,
    322–323
  physician/nurse liaison committee, 318

restorative care path development, 323–327
transition from managed care to case management, 319
Physician/nurse liaison committee, 318
Physician-patient relationship, interference with, 439
Physician/physician collaboration, control, 407
Positive variance, 186–187
Post anesthesia care unit
flow sheet, 119–121
nursing record, 119–121
Post-partum self care teaching, 156
Practice parameter. *See* Protocol
Practitioner variance, 185, 186
Pratt 4 Project, 24
Preceptorship program, 265–266
Prevention, case management, 13
Preventive health services, National Committee for Quality Assurance, 235–237
Price competition, 47
Primary care case management, 297, 301
Primary nursing, 39
Private case management, 296–298
Privileged information, 430
Product line organization, hospital case management, 73–74
Professional practice, developmental stages, 25
Professional responsibility, legal issues, 426–427
Prospective payment, 42
Prospective utilization review, legal issues, 434
Protocol
benefits, 7–8
CareMap, 7, 8
case management, 7
critical path, 7, 8
defined, 138
development, 8–9, 138–141, 139
multidiscplinary participation, 139
diagnosis-related group, 8
early discharge/vaginal delivery, 149–153, 157–159
goals, 139
hospital administrator, 139
implementation, 138–141
multidiscplinary participation, 139
nomenclature, 7, 8
outcomes assessment, 136–146, 149–169
overview, 137–138
physician, 139
stroke, 329–335
Provider alliance, integrated delivery system, 55
Provider-hospital organization, integrated delivery system, 55

Q

Quality of care
care giver *vs.* patient perceptions, 173–174
case management, 5, 175–181, 248–250
constructs, 176
evidence in literature, 177–178
leadership, 179–181
cost, relationship, 174–175
defined, 171–172
growing interest, 170–171
home care, 355–360
managing key constituencies, 180
National Committee for Quality Assurance
quality improvement, 233–234
quality management, 233–234
patient perceptions, 173–174
patient-focused definition, 173
physician, 180

R

Race, ethical issues, 455–456
Regional network, integrated delivery system, 55

Registered nurse
   case management director
      ethical practice, 291
      financial management, 286–287
      leadership, 290–291
      outcomes management, 288
      program level care coordination,
         285–286
      project management, 289–290
      as resource, 290
      roles, 284–291
   case management roles, 272–294
   case manager
      care coordination, 276–277
      care evaluation, 277–278
      case finding/screening, 274
      clinical roles, 274–278
      education of, 291–292
      as educator, 282–284
      implementation, 276
      negotiator, 279–280
      outcomes/quality manager, 280–281
      patient advocate/facilitator, 278–279
      patient assessment, 275
      planning, 275–276
      political activist, 284
      resource manager, 276–277
      roles, 273–284
      utilization/resource manager,
         281–282
Reimbursement, future trends, 463
Relationship building
   case manager, 309–310
   consumer, 308–309
   continuum of care, 305–314
   health care provider, 309–310
   home care, 352–354
   managed care, 319
   multidisciplinary team, 309–310
   payer relationships, 319
Resource management, outcomes, 145
Resource utilization, case management, 5
Restorative care path, 323–327
   stroke, 333–335
Retrospective review, legal issues, 433

Role ambiguity, 410
   nurse satisfaction, 415
Role conflict, 409–410
   nurse satisfaction, 415
Role overload, 409–410
   nurse satisfaction, 415
Role stressor, 408–410
   nurse satisfaction, 415
Role theory, 392

S

Service economy job design
   case management, research
      opportunities, 417–418
   case manager, 388–418
Social ethics, 447–448
Social integration, 408
Social/community-based case
   management, 297, 298–301
Software program, critical path, 84
Sponsorship, integrated delivery system,
   nurse executive issues, 64
Staff compliance, critical path, 86–87
Staff education, critical path, 84
Staff model, integrated delivery system, 62
Staff nurse, outcomes management,
   109–110
Standards, 363
   legal issues, 427–429
Steering committee, case management,
   244
Stroke
   admission/daily orders, 331–332
   algorithm, 330
   assessment profile, 117–118
   intermediate outcomes worksheet,
      130–135
   protocol, 329–335
   restorative care path, 333–335
System variance, 142, 185, 186
   critical path, 107

T

Technology management system,
   integrated delivery system, 57–58

Time line, 27, 28
  critical path, 84
Tort of interference with physician-
  patient relationship, 439
Total quality management, 225
Training, case manager, 254–270,
  291–292
  curriculum goals and objectives,
    256–257
  curriculum knowledge base, 255–256
  curriculum length, 255
  curriculum outline, 257–265
  perceptorship program, 265–266
Turnover rate, case management, 248

U

Unmet clinical outcomes, 203
Utilization, outcomes, 145
Utilization management, National
  Committee for Quality Assurance, 237
Utilization review, legal issues, 433

V

Variance
  classification of causes, 202–204
  components, 141–142
  critical path, defined, 106–109
  defined, 185, 201–202
  negative, 186
  outcomes, 188
  positive, 186
  statistical terms, 202
Variance analysis, 141–142, 194, 200–
  220, 372–375
  case management, 185–187

data quantity, 204–206
data relevance, 204–206
evaluation, 185–187
information management, 206–220
  card scanner, 212–215, 216
  data collection, 206
  data collection methods, 208–215
  data collection resources, 206–208
  data transformation into
    information, 218–220
  integrated computer systems, 209
  intermediate semiautomated
    methods, 209–215
  laptop computer, 210–211
  manual data collection, 208–209
  Newton hand-held computer,
    211–212
  models, 373–375
  outcomes assessment, 142–145
  results, 215–218
  source of patient outcomes, 200–201
Variance on admission, 185
Variance report
  critical path, 113–115
  outcomes management/critical path,
    122–124
Vertically integrated system, 54–55
Vicarious liability, legal issues, 438
Visiting nurse, documentation, 165–169

W

Wellness, case management, 13
Wickline v. California, 434
*Wilson v. Blue Cross of Southern
  California,* 435
Work redesign, 392
  behavioral approach, 394–395